The Medical Formulary of Al-Samarqandī

The Medical Formulary of Al-Samarqandī

and the Relation of Early Arabic Simples to Those Found in the Indigenous Medicine of the Near East and India

MARTIN LEVEY
Rockefeller Institute
and
NOURY AL-KHALEDY
Middle East Studies Center
Portland State College

Philadelphia
University of Pennsylvania Press

Published in Great Britain, India, and Pakistan
by the Oxford University Press
London, Bombay, and Karachi

Library of Congress Catalogue Card Number: 66-14525

7504

Printed in the United States of America

In Memory of
John Farquhar Fulton
and
Max Meyerhof
For Their Contributions to the History of Medicine

Preface

Very little research has been carried out in the study of early mediaeval Eastern Arabic pharmacology. This book, together with some earlier work of one of us, is part of a continuing effort to remedy this lack.

We have not attempted to draw too many final conclusions in this work. These will have to await the study and publication of further related texts which should prove of assistance in the understanding of this almost virginal field. Therefore, because of this, we have chosen to concentrate on the gathering of facts detailed in the section, "Notes and Comments." In this latter part of the book, attention has been drawn to the present day usage of old Arabic drugs, the employment of the drugs in the much earlier al-Kindī *Medical Formulary*, and to the etymological discussion of Arabic plant names not studied in previous works on the subject.

It has been difficult to offer a study which must, at best, contain many uncertainties. We have, therefore, for the sake of our own work and for the benefit of our colleagues in the scholarly community, not hesitated to note questionable identifications of plants and other incomplete areas of knowledge when discussing the al-Samarqandī text.

As much as possible, one of us has gone over the work of the most important of our scholarly predecessors of the past thirty years both by review of their studies and by examination of thousands of unlisted manuscripts in the many branches of medicine in the Arabic belt stretching from Morocco to India. He has also taken much time in his travels to chat with drug sellers in the bazaars with regard to present day indigenous medicine particularly outside the large cities. He also had the unhappy misfortune of spending a month in a Cairo hospital on the occasion of a recent illness.

On various other occasions we have visited North African and Asian hospitals which practice the particular kinds of medicine indigenous to the areas.

We should like to thank the Turkish Government and its library officials for the generous use of their manuscripts, their ready aid to scholars, and for permission to publish the photocopy from the Aya Sofya collection. We are also deeply obligated to Arabic manuscript libraries in Leiden, Patna, Oxford (Bodleian), Rabat, Fez, Tunis, Cairo, Teheran, Hyderabad, Madras, Calcutta, and others for their assistance in diverse ways.

Dr. W. B. McDaniel, 2d, of the Library of the College of Physicians of Philadelphia, was very kind to furnish the authors technical information on ancient medical apparatus. Mary McG. Levey carried out the difficult task of checking for technical and other errors as well as suggesting many important ideas. We are grateful for this. M. L. is indebted to the Public Health Service (RG-07391) for the assistance which made it possible for him to carry out this research.

MARTIN LEVEY
NOURY AL-KHALEDY

Contents

The Medical Formulary of Al-Samarqandī

Introduction

"To know and to sleep is better than to pray and be ignorant." —Ancient Arabic proverb

The period from the ninth to the twelfth century and perhaps the thirteenth century may be considered as the Golden Age of Arabic science. One of the earliest sciences to be developed by the Muslims was pharmacology and it was also one of the last to be supplanted by modern science. Its dominant position in western Europe lasted until the beginning of the nineteenth century. Today, Arabic drugs are used in much of India and the Near East as well as in backward areas in the West.

That Muslim[1] pharmacology could last over one thousand years until the advent of modern chemistry is an amazing point in itself. This gives rise to the question of why Arabic medicine, pharmacology, and other Muslim sciences are of such great interest to present day historians of science.

One reason for it is that the Muslim world during its Golden Age and later aided and supported these studies at a time when western Europe was experiencing an almost hopeless decadence. It was the Muslims who contributed so much to the rebirth of European culture. In regard to pharmacology and chemistry,[2] the Arabs were responsible for their development both theoretically and practically. Not only were the Muslims transmitters of early Greek atomic theory, for example, but they also contributed many original ideas on the nature of the atom, its association with other atoms, matter in relation to the atom, and numerous elaborated theories on what occurs in the mixing and solution process. Expanded views on pharmacology are also to be found in al-Samarqandī's work. A great material aid in the growth of Muslim pharmacology was that the Arabs established hospitals for the first time which were much like those known today. Licensing procedures of medical practitioners by legal authorities were developed. Relevant teaching illustrations were used in medical works. Finally, the practice of medicine was raised from a menial to a learned profession. All these factors had a profound influence on the exponential growth of the new Muslim chemistry and pharmacology.

There are many fascinating aspects of the history of the far reaching branches of Arabic medicine. One of these is the path of transmission of pharmacology from the ancients to the Muslims; following this is the middle period from the ninth to the thirteenth century; and finally there is the passing on of knowledge to Western Europe. One of the reasons for study of al-Samarqandī's text (early thirteenth century) is to determine what took place in this middle or golden period beginning with al-Kindī (ninth century).[3] Both of these physician authors reflect the knowledge of medical practice prevalent in Baghdad in their respective periods.

A question which frequently arises is how dependent the Arabs were upon Greek medicine, and correlatively whether or not the Muslims displayed originality in their work or whether they were merely transmitters of knowledge. These questions received a partial answer in a previous work on al-Kindī. However, these questions as phrased are prejudicial. What has been omitted is any reference to an appraisal of the importance of Indian pharmacology and ancient Babylonian materia medica in so far as they affect the development of Arabic studies in this field.

The original correlative question, it would seem, is a very significant one in the history of Arabic pharmacology. Investigation of this problem has been pursued along three general lines. The first direction was to determine the methods of study in the form of the kinds of literary models used by the Muslims in this area and to determine their relation to those used earlier in other cultures. Secondly, the etymology of hundreds of terms from the Arabic materia medica [3a] has been determined and analysed to obtain the relative number originating in the Indian and Persian, Mesopotamian, North African, and Greek pharmacopoeias. Thirdly, the theoretical ideas of al-Samarqandī's text were studied in relation to pre-ninth-century pharmacology to determine, if possible, original steps made by the Muslims beyond the well established humoral concepts of antiquity.

Al-Samarqandi and His Works

In the early thirteenth century, the long symbiosis of the Arabs, who loved knowledge and their religion, and the Persians, who possessed a rare scientific acumen, was broken asunder by the incursions of northern armies. The immediate result of this sad event was the sweeping victory of the barbarian hordes over much of the Asiatic Near East going as far as Baghdad. In one of these early invasions, the entire city of Herāt, said to have a population of one and a half million, was put to the sword.

The devastation was far reaching in that the great centers of culture were sacked, libraries were destroyed, and scientists and writers were wiped out. As a result of this holocaust, Persia remained almost a complete cultural vacuum until toward the end of the century when the invaders began to foster the growth of astronomy and medicine.

Al-Samarqandī, whose full name was abū Ḥāmaid M. b. ᶜA. ᶜO. Najīb al-Dīn al-Samarqandī,[4] met his death in the pillage of Herāt, Persia, by the Tartars in 1222 A. D. He was an eminent physician who flourished in the time of Fakhr al-Dīn al-Rāzī (d. 1210), the great philosopher.

Of his various medical works, all written in Arabic, the most important is "Etiology and Symptoms [of Diseases]," of which many manuscripts are known. This best known work of al-Samarqandī is called in Arabic *Al-asbāb wa' l-ᶜalāmāt*. It is known also in the commentary of Nafīs ibn ᶜIwad al-Kirmānī (d. 1449) who wrote *Sharḥ al-asbāb wa'l-ᶜalāmāt*.[5] As late as 1700/01, M. Arzani wrote a larger work based on this commentary. He called it *Ṭibb-i-akbarī*.[6] According to ibn abī Uṣaibiᶜa,[7] al-Samarqandī also wrote a book on the treatment of diseases by diet, and two medical formularies, a large and a small one. A treatise[8] on the principles of compounding of drugs is also ascribed to al-Samarqandī in the early bibliographical literature; it is called *Uṣūl tarkīb* [*al-adwiya*]. Other works still extant on the subject of medicine are listed below:

Al-adwiya al-mufrada, "Simple Drugs."

Aghdhiyat al-marḍā, "Diet for the Ill."

Al-aghdhiya wa' l-ashriba wamā yattaṣil bihā, "Food and Drink and What Is Basic in Them."

*Fī mudāwāt waja*ᶜ *al-mafāṣil,* "On the Cure of Pains of the Joints."

Fī al-ṭibb, "On Medicine."

*Fī kaifīyat tarkīb ṭabaqāt al-*ᶜ*ain,* "On the Kind of Composition of the Layers of the Eyes."

Tractatus de medicamentis repertu facilibus.

Aqrābādhīn, "Medical Formulary."

Fī ᶜ*ilāj man suqiya al-sumūm au nahashahu al-hawāmm waghairhā,* "On the Treatment for One Who Has Been Given Poison, or Bitten by Vermin, and Similar Cases."

*Ghāyat al-gharaḍ fī mu*ᶜ*ālajat al-amrāḍ,* "The Last Word on the Goal of Treating the Ill."

*Fī ittikhadh mā' al-jubn wamanāfi*ᶜ*ihī wakaifīyat isti*ᶜ*mālih,* "On Administration of Water of Cheese, Its Benefits, and the Kinds of Its Uses." [9]

*Fī al-adwiya al-musta*ᶜ*mala* ᶜ*inda al-ṣayādila,* "On Drugs Prepared by Pharmacists."

The extant works of al-Samarqandī thus are devoted largely to simple and compound drugs and their preparation. The *Aqrābādhīn,*[10] the subject of this book, is also called *Kitāb al-qarābādhīn* ᶜ*ala tartīb al-*ᶜ*ilal,* "Book of the Medical Formulary on Compounding for Diseases." The translation was done mainly from the Aya Sofya MS 3555 with aid from the Leiden MS 1353. The former manuscript, which is far superior to the Leiden, Patna, and Bodleian copies,[11] the only others extant, has forty-one folios with seventeen lines to the page in a Naskhī hand.

In addition to a lengthy introduction, the text is divided into nineteen chapters: 1. syrups and robs, 2. stomachic confections and electuaries, 3. pills and aperients, 4. decoctions and infusions, 5. clysters, suppositories, and pessaries, 6. emetics, 7. lohochs, 8. lozenges. 9. powders and stomachic powders, 10. dressings, coatings, and cataplasms, 11. balms, 12. collyria, 13. poultices and aromatic powders, 14. dentifrices, 15. gargles and confections, 16. snuff remedies, 17. sternutatives, fragrances, and inhalants, 18. bath aromatics, and 19. hair medicines.

Literary Models of Muslim Pharmacological Texts

In regard to the question already posed as to whether the Muslims were original or merely transmitters of Greek knowledge, one aspect of the answer has already been considered in a statistical study of the origins of Muslim simples.[12] Another facet of study should take account of the types or models of pharmacological literature existing before the hijra. In the ancient and mediaeval periods and up to the early part of the nineteenth century, new qualitative levels of understanding in medicine brought on varied rhetorical forms for the requisite literary explanation. Arabic pharmacology was not an exception to this.

In ancient Mesopotamia, medical knowledge was partly in rhetorical form; chemical, astronomical, medical, and other scientific data were also organized into long lexical lists. Usually, these lists contained related names side by side. The following, an excerpt from a long medical list which is representative, gives the corresponding Sumerian and Akkadian terms in their respective columns.

DISEASE LIST (incomplete)

Sumerian	Translation	Akkadian	Translation
DUB	comes out	*šu-ú-lu*	comes up
DUB	comes out	*um-ṣa-tum*	sore
GUG.SU.GUG	increasingly light	*pi-in-du-ú*	pustule
SU.UM	flesh	*ḫa-šá-lu*	to rub
SU.TAB	a sickness	*um-ṣa-tu*	paralysed hand
$UM.DU_{11}.GA$	excrescence	*ka-tar-ru*	dry rot

It was primarily the Sumerians, Akkadians, and Hittites who organized these lists. These were the earliest attempts to organize facts on science and other subjects. For example, in the *ḪARRA-ḫubullu* lexical series, written in cuneiform, tablets three to seven give the names of trees, parts of trees, products of trees, and objects made of wood; tablets eight and nine give names of reeds and objects made of reed; tablets ten to twelve give names of vessels, ovens, clay objects, hides, chemicals, objects of bronze, copper, silver, and gold; tablet sixteen contains names of stones; and tablet seventeen has names of plants. In the medical area in other series, there are lists of anatomical terms, names of diseases, pharmaceuticals, and types of symptoms.[13]

The text of Dioscorides on materia medica in the time of the Greeks treats each drug separately giving its origin, description, and the pharmacological uses of the effective morphological parts of the plants. It is divided into five major books: aromatics, oils, resins, and trees; animal products and sharp herbs; roots, juices, and herbs; drugs useful for poisons; and vines, wines, minerals, and stones. Galen wrote books on the strength of purgative drugs, on simple drugs, on compounded drugs, on nutritive drugs, drugs which purge and improve, and three books relating to theriacs.[14] The medical encyclopedia of Paul of Aegina (*fl. ca.* 640) contains much pharmacology in the seventh book on simple and compound remedies. The simples are arranged alphabetically together with their properties and uses. Paulos took his material on this subject mainly from Galen who, in turn, owed much to Dioscorides. The compound remedies fall into such groupings as purgatives, salves, emmenagogues, antidotes, pastilles, powders, mouth salves, sweet drinks, collyria, plasters, oils, and aromata.[15]

The Muslims, on the other hand, elaborated on the Greek classification and originated new major types of pharmacological literary models. The Muslim approaches to pharmacology became not only more numerous but more flexible. Since the pharmacological literature flowered into works which considered the subject from a great variety of new directions, there resulted new understanding and new lines to investigate.

Arabic pharmacological texts may be divided mainly into those bearing directly on the subject and others which are closely related. In the case of the latter, which reveal much of the Arabic materia medica, there are many works on travel, the *ḥisba,* which is the common law regulating particularly medicine and pharmacy, medical biography and bibliography, botany, zoology, the lapidaries, and others.

Since the Muslims were excellent organizers of knowledge, their purely pharmacological texts were carefully directed along many directions. As a result, these books generally fall into more or less well delineated groups. Some of these major types of Arabic pharmacological literature may be categorized as follows:

1. Medical formularies
2. Books on poisons
3. Synonymic lists of simples usually in alphabetical order

4. Tabellar, synoptic treatises
5. Alphabetical lists of materia medica including therapeutic considerations and opinions of various writers on the subject
6. Substitute drugs
7. Methods for testing purity of drugs
8. Works on drugs for particular diseases concerned with the heart, eyes, sexual organs, and others.

In the case of the medical formularies, there are varied types. One of these is the abbreviated text, "Compounded Drugs Used in Most Ailments." It is called *Mukhtaṣar fī al-adwiya al-murakkaba al-mustaᶜmala fī akthar al-amrāḍ* by Sahlān ibn Kaysān (d. 990). Included in this book are chapters on myrobalan confections, electuaries, pills, aperients, pastilles, powders, syrups, lohochs and robs, gargles, collyria, suppositories, pessaries, cataplasms, oils and lotions, oral medicines and dentifrices, and ointments.[16]

A better known example of the medical formulary, and one from which much of the preceding one was taken, is *Al-dustūr al-bīmāristānī fi'l adwiya al-murakkaba of Abu'l Faḍl Dā'ūd b. a. al-Bayān al-Isrā'īlī* (b. 1161). Bayān practised in the famous al-Nāṣirī Hospital in Cairo. This treatise is divided much like the previous one of Sahlān.

Al-Kindī (ninth century) also wrote a text of this type called *Aqrābādhīn.*[17] It is a compilation of prescriptions falling into the same general categories as those of Bayān and ibn Kaysān. Al-Samarqandī's present text is similar to this.[18]

Texts on poisons are very old and were known to the Greeks and Indians. An early one in Arabic is the *Kitāb al-sumūm* of ibn Waḥshīya (fl. before 912). The author was born of an Aramaean family in Iraq. He was much interested in agriculture, alchemy, and in the occult sciences generally. His book on poisons is largely a translation from the Syriac authors Yārbūqā and Sūhāb Saṭ whose works came originally from Indian and perhaps old Babylonian sources. Ibn Waḥshīya gives many names of poisons known today as mythical. Antidotes to ward off the supernatural poisons are described.[19]

There are many alphabetical lists of materia medica in the Arabic literature. These generally include the preparation, description, therapeutic usage of drugs, and the opinions of other writers on the remedies. Although most of these are based on the organization and on much of the contents of Dioscorides' famous book, nevertheless, the Arabic works are much fuller, both in the number of drugs discussed and in the extent of the particular discussions.

Ibn al-Baitār (thirteenth century) [20] is probably the best known writer in Arabic who followed the Greek pharmacological tradition. It is known, however, that much of his compilatory work is based upon the earlier treatise of al-Ghāfiqī (twelfth century).[21] This text is a compilation also from earlier authors as Dioscorides, Galen, abū Ḥanīfa (d. 895), al-Rāzī (d. 923/4), ibn Sīnā (980-1037), al-Majūsī (d. 994), ᶜĪsā b. ᶜAlī (ninth century), al-Bīrūnī (973-1048), al-Idrīsī (1100-1166), Maimonides (1135-1204), ibn Jazla (d. 1100), ibn Riḍwān (*ca.* 980-1060), and others.

A typical entry in the abbreviated version is that of *utrujj*.[22] The authors quoted are abū Ḥanīfa, Dioscorides, ibn Sīnā, Galen, ibn Māsawaih, and Isḥāq b. Sulaimān al-Isrā'īlī of Qairawān. This text gives a Greek synonym, botanical and therapeutic facts, and also some physical properties of each of the plant's morphological parts.

Being excellent synthesizers of knowledge (which was then growing by leaps and bounds) the Muslims were fond of building tables for their data to give a ready reference form. An excellent example of this is the work of ibn Biklārish (fl. 1106) called *Kitāb al-Mustaʿīnī,*[23] In the five columns on two facing pages, the following is given for each drug: name, Galenic nature and grade, synonyms in Persian, Syriac, Greek, Latin, and Spanish, substitute drug and preparation, therapeutic value, and therapeutic uses of the drug.

This last type of pharmacological literary model, the synoptic tabellar text, was original with the Muslims and served an effective purpose in view of the quickly rising quantitative level of the Muslim materia medica.

Although some of the Arabic types are related to the Greek models in varying degrees, a successful effort was constantly being made by the Muslims to expand and improve over the previous models so that the huge body of pharmaceutical knowledge would be more readily available to the physician in need.

Geographic Origins of al-Samarqandī's Materia Medica

A. INDIAN INFLUENCE

In view of the fact that the Muslims were the dominant power in most of the early mediaeval world and were also great seafarers and travelers having contact with Eastern Asia and East Africa, it is of interest to examine how this affected their materia medica.

In the Golden Age, the Arabs expanded their trade and commerce to the point where they acted as intermediaries between the Far East and the West as far as Spain, Morocco, and Italy. Arab ships went from Baghdad, the home of the ᶜAbbāsid Empire, to ports in China, India and up the Indus River, to Ceylon, and to East Africa. They also sailed the Mediterranean, the Black and Caspian Seas, as well as up and down the Nile.[24]

The learned V. Minorsky, in his translation of a Persian geography of 982 A. D., states that there were many Muslims in Canton in Muhammad's time. This anonymous treatise gives excellent descriptions of the caravan routes of the early Arabs and Persians to India and China.[25]

How much did the Arabs depend on the pharmacology of other peoples with whom they were acquainted in trade? Did the difficulty of obtaining simples from distant places affect their usage by the Arabs? As to the Muslim knowledge of the ancients, there is evidence that the Sumerians and Akkadians had transmitted their learning in medicine to the Arabs through various intermediaries. Since ancient Mesopotamian pharmacology is still imperfectly known, it will be more rewarding to commence by looking into the early Greek period to determine some of the latter's sources of drugs.

In the Hippocratic period, the materia medica used came not only from Greece and its colonies but also from foreign countries. For example, some of the vegetable and mineral simples came from Egypt, which had already been known in Homeric times as a land of great physicians. In the Hippocratic corpus are to be found many simples with the adjective "Egyptian," as for example Egyptian alum, Egyptian bean, Egyptian cumin, and Egyptian salt. Some believe that they are found in these works because Hippocrates is presumed to have traveled in Egypt. However, trade among some of the highly civilized Greek islands and Egypt throve throughout the first millennium B.C. and earlier. Egypt enjoyed a fine reputation as a great center of culture at that time.

Many simples of the Hippocratic corpus were derived

from India. Some scholars have been of the opinion that Pythagoras and others had been in India and had brought back to Greece the Indian medical lore.[26] Theophrastus [27] remarks in his work on plants that the aromata for salves came by ship from India. Some of the botanicals used by the Greeks and which originated in India were cardamom, certain species of nard such as *Valeriana Jatamansi* Roxb., camel hay, *Cymbopogon Schoenanthus* Spreng., Indian sesame which is *Sesamum indicum L.*, and various species of cinnamon.

Much of the early Greek materia medica came from Persia, such as sal ammoniac and coriander. From Arabia came myrrh and frankincense, and from locations north of Greece came other remedies, aside from the vast majority of simples which were native to Greece, its colonies, and its neighboring shores on the Mediterranean.

The Muslims inherited the Hippocratic pharmacology together with the further works of, among others, Theophrastus, Dioscorides, Galen, and Paul of Aegina. Thus, in inheriting the Greek medicine, the Arabs came to know simples from many distant parts of the then known world. After this, they added to their oral store of Babylonian medicine the early medical knowledge of the writings of the Indians and Egyptians.

Laufer [27] has pointed out the intensive commercial and cultural intercourse in drugs between India and Persia. As a result, when studying these in the light of their origin, it is helpful frequently to place those drugs coming from Persia and India under one heading. The reason for this may be seen, for example, in the Indian drugs or products which occur in abū Manṣūr's (fl. *ca.* 961-976) *Kitāb al-abnīya ʿan ḥaqāiq al-adwiya* "Book of the Foundations of the True [Foundations] of Remedies." This was originally a Persian treatise on the materia medica of the time, containing in all close to 600 simples. Abū Manṣūr's information, from Persian, Syriac, Greek, and Indian sources, came largely from his own personal experience and extensive travels in Persia and India.

In discussions on the origin of Persian materia medica in regard to India, the Babylonian contribution has been almost entirely neglected or obscured. As a result, Lauter [28] has ascribed an Indian origin to Arabic and Persian drugs which are properly Babylonian such as, for example, soda, Ar. *ushnān,* and mungo bean, Ar. *māsh, mangu* in Akk. Indian remedies in abū Manṣūr include rice, Ar. *aruz,* Pers. *bitrinj (Oryza sativa);* citron, Ar. *utrujj,* Pers. *turunj (Citrus medica)* from Sans. *mātuluṅga;* myrobalan, Ar. *ihlilaj,* Pers. *halīla, (Terminalia chebula),* Sans. *harītakī;* belleric myrobalan Ar. *balīlij,* Pers. *balīla* (*Terminalia bellerica*), Sans. *vibhītaka;* emblic myrobalan, Ar. *amlaj,* Pers. *amīla (Emblica officinalis),* Sans. *amala,* Chin. *an-mi-lo;* croton, Ar. *dand* from Sans. *dantī (Croton polyandrus);* Himalayan cedar, Pers. *dīvdār (Pinus* or *Cedrus Deodàra*) from Sans. *devadăru;* ginger, Ar. *shangalīl,* Middle Pers. *shangavir,* Ar.-Pers. *zanjabīl* (*Zingibir officinale*) from Sans. *çṛṅgavera;* scammony, Ar. *saqmūniyā* (*Convolvulus scammonia*)*;* sugar, Ak. *sukkar* from Prakrit and Pāli *sakkharā,* Sans. *çarkara;* coconut, Ar. *narjīl (Cocos nucifera)* from Sans. *nārikelo;* also indigo, lesser cadamom, mandrake, sandalwood, pepper, cloves, and a score of others. Laufer [29] gives a total of 52 out of 466 botanicals as Indian, or 11 per cent. This percentage is low since Laufer, it seems, mentions only those plants as being of Indian origin which are native to India and rarely found in Persia. Not taken into account are those botanicals growing in both Persia and India and found in the older Indian medical literature.

When the fossil evidence obtained from botanonymic

evidence is considered, then it appears that the combined Persian-Indian origin of abū Manṣūr plant simples approaches much closer to the statistical results obtained in a similar study of the geographic distribution of the origins of al-Samaraqandī's materia medica. In the latter, the Persian-Indian simples account for 54 per cent of the materia medica; the Babylonian, 20 per cent; the Greek, 17 per cent; the pre-Islamic Arabic, 6 per cent; Egyptian, 2 per cent; and the Chinese, less than 1 per cent.

A typical etymological account used in the above determination of a botanical term may be seen in the outline for *wajj*.

Ar. *wajj, Acorus Calamus* L., sweet-flag.

Sum. *GI.DÙG*	Sans. *vucha* or *vacā*	
Akk. *qanū ṭābu*	↓	
Gr. ἄκορον ἀσπλήνιον	Guzerat	*vaz*
↓	Deccan	*bache*
Modern Ar. *aikar, ighir, ikkur*	Malabar	*vazabu*
↓	Concan	*vaicam*
Turk. *egur*	Hindi	*gora vach*
	↓	
Hieroglyphic Egyptian *kš*	Pers. *vāj*	
↓	↓	
Coptic *kas*	Ar. *wajj*	

The sweet-flag is from China, Japan, and India.

At this point, it is of some interest to compare the sources of Arabic names of the materia medica in al-Kindī's *Aqrābādhīn* with those in the work of the same name in al-Samarqandī. In time and place, there is a great difference between these two men. Al-Kindī, who worked in the ninth century and whose parents came from Arabia, wrote his work in Baghdad, a crossroad of the ancient caravan routes and an intellectual center.[29a] Al-Samarqandī, who was in Baghdad for a time, lived and worked hundreds of years later in Herāt, an important city of ancient Persia having many cultural ties with India and the East. It would be logical, therefore, to assume, a priori, a difference between the materia medica of the Persian and that of the Baghdad physician.

The statistical results bear this out. In al-Kindī's *Aqrābādhin,* 31 per cent of the materia medica comes from Persian-Indian sources, 33 per cent from Mesopotamia, 25 per cent from Greek origins, 5 per cent from Arabic, and 3 per cent from ancient Egyptian origins.

It appears then from examination of these figures that it probably was not a particular author on pharmacology, such as Dioscorides or any other, who exerted the greatest influence on the choice of simples. A more important factor seems to have been the geographic availability of the botanicals, minerals, and zoologicals. Since the evidence is not yet complete in regard to the botanonymic and botanical studies of the materia medica of other regions like Egypt, North Africa, and Spain, the above conclusion must, of necessity, remain tentative.[30] One fact is certain, however; this is that Arabic writers on pharmacology, such as al-Kindī and al-Samarqandī, increasingly owed much as time passed to Indian medicine for its contribution of materia medica.

With the establishment of the Muslim hegemony in the Near East, trade with the Middle and Far East prospered so that Indian and also some Chinese simples found a permanent role in Muslim chemistry and pharmacology.

B. BABYLONIAN INFLUENCE ON ARABIC PHARMACOLOGY

An important factor much neglected by historians is the oral transmission of ideas and technical know-how in ancient and mediaeval times. A very difficult period having little scientific manuscript material in Semitic languages is from 300 B.C. to the beginning of Islam in Mesopotamia and Egypt. As a result of this, the Semitic continuity in the knowledge of technical terminology and technological methods must have been passed down orally, to a considerable extent, from father to son. The pre-Islamic oral literature, in its terminological richness, is partial evidence of this.

The Akkadian knowledge must have found its way, at least in part, into the succeeding Semitic Aramaic, Hebrew, and Syriac cultures and literatures. Linguistically, it was much simpler for the early Arabs to have translated these languages or to obtain oral material through them rather than through the Indo-European group of languages such as Persian and Greek. However, Persian physicians and scientists gathered much material from the Indo-European Sanskrit and related tongues in India.

In the case of the transmission of pharmacology to the Arabs, the two largest groups of origin would be expected to be the Indian (through the Persian) and the Semitic sources going back to the Akkadian in ancient Mesopotamia. The evidence of many Indian loanwords and plants in Muslim pharmacology has already been demonstrated. To a lesser extent, depending somewhat on the geographic area, the Muslims derived much of their materia medica from the Semitic Babylonian sources.

Some examples of simples in al-Samarqandī that were originally Babylonian are lead, Ar. *abār,* Akk. *abaru,* Sum. *A.BAR;* myrtle Ar. *āss,* Akk. *āsu;* onion, Ar. *baṣal,* Akk. *biṣru,* Heb. *bĕṣĕl;* lupine, Ar. *turmus,* Sum. *TAR.MUŠ,* Syr. *turmᵉsā;* thyme (*Thymus vulgaris* L.), *ḥāshā',* Akk. *ḫašū;* mustard, Ar. *khardal,* Akk. *ḫaldappānu;* lettuce, Ar. *khass* or *khas,* Akk. *ḫassu,* Sum. *ḪI.IS.ŠAR,* Heb. *khasā;* peach, Ar. *khaukh,* Akk. *ḫaḫḫu,* Syr. *ḫaḫḫā;* and others according to the evidence in the notes to the translation.

In these examples, based on botanonymic studies, i.e. the etymological explanation of botanical terms, the results are fairly obvious. For others, the relevant data must come from other directions such as the geographic indigenousness of the botanicals in ancient times, the number of species and varieties in various geographic areas, archeological remains of plants and their representations, ancient agriculture, modern uses and occurrence in the Near East, Asia, and North Africa, and the names, both in the professions and in the bazaars, presently in use in India, Persia, Iraq, Egypt, China, and North Africa. The materia medica and botany of ancient Babylonia are well worth studying in this connection. The method of botanonymic study has been described elsewhere.[31]

Al-Samarqandī's Pharmacotherapy

A. THEORETICAL ASPECTS

A direction to explore which may help to clarify the relationship of al-Samarqandī's ideas to those of the Greeks concerns the development of a chemical-pharmacological theory among the Muslims.

The basic theory of matter which the Greeks held was that there are four elements: air, fire, earth, and water. These, according to Aristotle, composed the substance of man; the "accidents"[32] of man are the four humors, cold, hot, dry, and moist.

In the Hippocratic corpus, the writings ultimately rely upon empirical evidence (when this was possible) rather than theory in the actual dispensing of drugs to the patient. It was the theoretical which issued from the practical experience, and not vice versa. Furthermore, remedies were chosen to bring the patient back to health in the most direct way possible. Thus, compounded remedies were preferred by the Hippocratic physicians.

In addition, the earliest Greeks believed that many illnesses could be cured by the *vis mediatrix natural,* that man finds his own way to health very often through the unconscious intervention of natural reactions in the body. One of the purposes of drugs in Hippocratic works was, then, to aid nature to carry out this healing reaction.[33]

With time, the humoral theory became entrenched in Greek medical thought as may be seen in Galen and Dioscorides. It was this idea that was inherited by the Muslims. But the latter went a step further; to explain the next development, it is first necessary to discuss atomicity very briefly.

The development of atomic theory by the Arabs is closely allied with the particulate theory of medicine. In the tenth and eleventh centuries, generation (the coming into being) and corruption (the passing away) were of great interest to philosophers. Earlier there had been the monists and pluralists. The former believed that generation and corruption were processes of the same substances; the latter contended that generation was the combination, and corruption the dissociation of elementary bodies making up a whole.

Ibn Rushd, or in Latin Averroës (1126-1198), was a great admirer of Aristotle as had been ibn Sīnā (Avicenna, b. 980 in Bukhara). Furthermore Averroës was Aristotle's most famous interpreter in the great Islamic period. In relating how composite bodies originate from the elements, he wrote: [34]

> Since we maintain that hot and cold may be absolute and may also be subject to increase and decrease, we say that

which is generated out of them is not absolutely hot or absolutely cold, but rather do we say that it is hot and cold simuletaneously just as we say of intermediates, i.e. hot relative to the absolutely cold at the extreme and cold relative to the absolutely hot at the extreme. . . . It takes place by way of mixture.

Mixture was then an important subject. Averroës writes: [35]

Mixture occurs when each one of two contraries acts upon the other with nearly equal force in such a way that the miscibles acquire a single property intermediate between these two contraries. The substratum for this property will necessarily be the combined magnitude of the miscibles, as is the case when each one of the miscibles ,as it is altered by the other, acquires a given property to an equal extent so that when each attains the intermediate property which is naturally a single property of a single substratum, the substratum of both is their combined magnitudes.

All these ideas are transferable and applicable to the humoral theory. It is no coincidence that Averroës was a strong exponent of this idea [36] as were so many of his fellow Muslims. At the same time, he opposed any extension of his ideas to the concept of atomicity.

In order to appreciate more fully what Averroës, al-Samarqandī, and many more Arabic physicians stated in regard to theories of pharmacology and medicine, it should be remembered that they carried out their work with a new background of thinking somewhat removed from that of the Greeks. It cannot be denied that much of the Greek influence persisted, but, through the intensive development of atomicity in Arabic philosophy, chemistry, and, in turn, pharmacology, many of the old Greek terms took on new meaning.

The particulate idea, as expounded by the *mutakallimun,* expositors of the *kalām* ("conversation" or controversy in the first century and a half to answer objectors to the Islamic thought), is described by Maimonides.[36a]

Some of the important bases of this concept, as given by Maimonides (who, by the way, rejected it), influenced the Arabic idea of the humoral theory. Briefly, some of the points of the atomic theory are:

1. Every corporeal substance is made up of very small parts called atoms. The atoms have no quantitative properties or relationships but may at different times possess qualitative values.
2. To the atom may be appended certain properties called "accidents," such as rest, motion, life, death, ignorance, knowledge, combination, separation, cold, and so on.
3. Atoms themselves must have the attached "accidents," and only atoms have "accidents."
4. Matter is inseparable from "accidents."
5. There are only material atoms and their accompanying "accidents." The nature of the "spirit" was a great difficulty for Arabian theologians and scientists.[36b]

Not all Arabian theorists believed exactly in the atomic idea as expressed above. There were many variations as well as objections throughout the entire Arabic period. It is not too difficult to see, however, that the Arabian physicians, many of whom were also philosophers of note, looked beyond hot and cold, and moist and dry. As a result, the rigidity of the application of humoral therapy was ameliorated by a flexibility frequently alluded to by Muslim medical men. Al-Samarqandī comes out openly with his reasons for following a more elastic approach:

For one who wishes to obtain benefit from a [compounded remedy] and for one who uses it, it must be exposed to the rules of compounding and he must be free in dealing with it accordingly until he attains the right thing. Then he tries it.

Some "accidents" are mentioned in a passage in al-Samarqandī:[36c]

Whoever notices the differences [in amounts] these prescriptions and their frequency in the *aqrābādhīn,* sees the variations among them, and that each kind is taken for a specific ailment, will realize then that the differences occur because of the variations in the state of the illness. The latter would be in the acuteness, weakness, sharpness, and chronicity; and the variations in the quantity of heat and cold, the state of thickness, gentleness, whether it be compounded or simple, and excessive. It is also according to the different conditions of the patient in strength and weakness, the periods of his sickness to excess, the beginning, decline, and end, and the "accidents" which happen to the patient during illness.

To describe the reluctance of some physicians to allow for growth and development of knowledge, al-Samarqandī quotes the poet al-Mutanabbī:[36d] "Their works remain after the masters because of cowardice. Perdition may touch them but they are still followed."

To return to al-Samarqandī, it is significant that he does not rely entirely on the humoral theory, and, in the practical art of compounding, does not consider the theory of decisive importance. In general, however, al-Samarqandī is aware of many "accidents," and attempts to consider all of them in the preparation of a remedy. In a sense, the pharmacotherapeutic ideas of al-Samarqandī are somewhat akin to those in the Hippocratic corpus; but al-Samarqandī has come forth with the further step of not only considering the humors but also taking account of many "accidents" in a much broader theorization of the basic pragmatic value of drugs.

Similarly, al-Samarqandī agrees with a basic idea also manifested throughout the Hippocratic corpus, that of the importance of nature in healing.

> The physician should not treat everything of a minor character or small change occurring in the body with a drug. Rather, he should treat it by changing the method of management and by adjusting the necessary basic conditions. He must not stir up anything nor impair the body in its natural functions. It is more difficult to quiet the stirring than to stir the quiet. Whenever we can, we should treat by nutritive drugs, and, if compelled, by pure drugs not going beyond the simples as much as possible.[37]

In contrast with al-Kindī, al-Samarqandī describes in detail the theoretical pharmacology of his day. It must be remembered, however, that the ideas expressed by al-Samarqandī do not find their proper and logical expression in his pharmacological practise. To more clearly understand al-Samarqandī's ideas of pharmacology in its truly empirical content, it is important to examine the manner of and his actual reasons for the compounding of drugs.

B. METHODS OF COMPOUNDING DRUGS

According to al-Samarqandī, "there are reasons which compel one to compound [drugs] in the absence of a simple which attains the desired goal. It is partly because of the aspect of the nature of sickness and diseases, partly because of the state of the organs, and partly because of of the drug."

Fourteen practical reasons are given for the use of compounded drugs:

1. The first concerns the extent of the ill humor if

there is no drug opposite to it in its strength. It is then compounded from one which is stronger in the quantity of its [humor] with one which is less so. From these a blend is put together to resist that ill humor.

2. The next is concerned with the strength and acuteness of the illness when there is no single drug which is effective. It is then compounded so that the constituents may have a synergistic action.

3. There are differences in the state of a disease and associated circumstances and its treatment; a drug is unknown which performs at the same time opposite actions like absorbing and bringing up in chest ailments or the abetting and hindering of tumors. Compounding is then necessary.

4. To counteract many poisons and different ailments, a compounded drug is necessary so that it may possess a strength superior to the strengths of all simples.

5. The distance of an ailing organ from the stomach is important in that a useful drug must be compounded with one which will help it to reach the ill organ quickly.

6. The strength and importance of the ill organ must be taken into account. Usually a drug to dissolve a tumor and one to ease the symptoms are compounded together in a remedy.

7. The distastefulness of a drug must be remedied with one which can improve it.

8. The excessive strength of a drug may be taken care of, for example, by mixing it with turpeth.

9. A drug may be added to prevent harm by the original drug as in the use of correctives with purgatives.

10. Sometimes a single drug like gum in the collyrium of verdigris is inadequate.

11. The evil property of a drug may be destroyed by another as by mixing castoreum with opium.

12. An added drug may have the power of keeping the original strength of an important drug for a long time.

13. There is a difference in drugs in their doses and usages. A mixture of both may be desired.

14. In order to use a single drug effectively, sometimes it is necessary to mix it with another, as, for example, an unguent with verdigris for wounds.[38]

In the calculation of the weights of the drugs to be used, there are seven simple determining factors to be considered:

1. Strength of the drug's natures.
2. Its effectiveness.
3. Its benefits.
4. Its usefulness, alone or with other drugs.
5. Distance from the stomach of the ailing organ.
6. Drugs in the compounded remedy which weaken its strength.
7. Ill effects of the drug on other organs.

It is perhaps worthwhile to quote al-Samarqandī on the subject of experience with prescribing and compounding:

> The method of analogy is safe and is used dependably in all medical practice. The fact that it is difficult should not lead to its not being employed. Earlier workers compounded according to the analogical method. After experience, they found that it gave the best of what they had expected from it so that they wrote it down and immortalized it in books. This was done so that it should be an example for us in using compound remedies according to the kind of need and the satisfaction of self interest; the exception is in the compounded ones for which the rules are known and also the purpose. . . . I have proved by example some of what the hands of experience have been bequeathed in turn, and elucidated it from the force to the action.[39]

Chemistry in al-Samarqandi's Aqrabadhin

For the student of thirteenth century Arabic chemistry, this text is exceedingly rich in the names of botanical, zoological, and mineralogical chemicals and their mixtures. Further, the pharmacological theory of the introduction is in accord with the chemical theory of writers on the structure of matter and how it reacts.

Although al-Samarqandī mentions the humoral idea from time to time, the predominantly stressed consideration in his pharmacotherapy is the therapeutic property of a particular drug when it acts upon a bodily organ. This action was considered by the mediaeval Muslims as a specific characteristic of a substance, and, in turn, of the particles or atoms of which it is composed. These properties were called the "accidents" of the atoms.

Essentially, there are two major theories or ideas of the working of chemistry and of pharmacology; the first is based on empirical data, and the second is humoral which is but rarely employed before the fact but used post-factum as a scholastic kind of interpretation.

This method of the operation of Muslim chemistry and the pharmacological sciences has escaped to a large extent the observations of many students of these areas. One source of confusion in the past has been that part of the humoral theory is often confused with the hot, cold, dry, and moist conditions found in actuality as, for example, excessive perspiration, fever, and so on. Even though these are almost always mere symptoms, they are still medically treated in modern as in ancient times to reverse them without the need of a humoral or any other theory. In other words, no theory is considered necessary but it is simply an empirical normalizing operation. The same held true for many chemical processes, both in and out of al-Samarqandī.

An excellent example is in another text of the thirteenth century by an Iraqi, abū al-Qāsim n. ibn Ahmad al-ᶜIrāqī.[40] In a discussion of the prime matter upon which the elixir is based, he writes:

> . . . mercury mixes with copper and tinctures it, but lacks permanency and power of completion. So that which we seek is not to be found among the elementary minerals; hence the substance must be a compound possessing the powers mentioned, and we examined the metallic chemicals suitable for this purpose. We found no substance from which it was proper to compound the elixir except gold, for gold is fusible, stable, and perfecting, since the agent should be better than all else in its power of completion . . . nor does it contain excess of heat to heat the silver and fix it, and to give the fire power to accelerate the reaction with it.
>
> And so it is necessary that we should feed it with moisture of its own kind united with dryness of its own kind, so that when the hotness is increased in it, the food combines with the gold, and the gold changes the food into its own essence; and the gold is the cause of its permanence in the fire and the food is the cause of its tinctorial power and purple color. It becomes hot, dry, red, and easily fusible. When it is projected upon silver, it tinctures it. . . .

Abū al-Qāsim then goes on with a comparison of the powers of plants and animals with metal. In fact, throughout much of the book, this analogy is maintained and expanded upon.

In the description above, it is obvious that the author knows many facts about the chemicals with which he is concerned. At the same time, all references to the humors are completely uncorrelated with and irrelevant to the primary chemical reactions described. It is thus an "idea after the fact" and not worthy of being called a theory since it cannot be used *a priori* for unknown chemical reactions. This procedure is carried out in al-Samarqandī's pharmacology with the reservation already mentioned of the pragmatic aspects of hot, cold, dry, and moist.

How closely Arabic ideas in chemistry and medicine are linked may be seen in another section of the same book.

> It appears that these six metallic forms [i.e. gold, silver, copper, iron, lead, and tin] are all of one species, distinguished from one another only by different 'accidents'; their extreme limit is reached when they become gold. Now that which is free from any 'accident' is gold, while what possesses these becomes either silver or the two leads, if it has the quality of coldness, or copper, or iron, if it has the quality of hotness. And these six species are similar merely to health and fever in man. When the fever is treated so that it departs and the man returns to freedom from disease, he regains the most perfect state of health.[41]

From this, it is seen that hotness and coldness are "accidents" which are the chemical and physical properties of a body, and so in turn are determined which of the six metals it is to be.

Further, in this text and also implied in al-Samarqandī's are the close relationships among chemistry, pharmacology, and pharmacotherapy.

In chemistry, as in the compounding of materia medica, analogical reasoning was often considered sufficient. Al-Samarqandī describes its use in pharmacology as having been originated by earlier workers in the field. Credit is thus given to al-Samarqandī's predecessors for the experience they handed down.

With the Arabs, the most common division of chemicals was based upon their origins in the vegetable, animal, or mineral kingdoms. By far, most of the chemicals and simples used came from botanicals. These are fully described in the notes to the translation. Materials of animal origin include the white and yolk of egg, castoreum, the excrement of bats and mice, milk, sour milk, and mother's milk, broth meat, honey and oxymels, fish, butter, the fat of the camel's hump, duck, chicken, bees-wax, shell, ambergris, cheese water, and the gall of cows and birds.

The mineral materials, mostly of Persian origin, include burned lead, burned copper, stibnite, ceruse, soda, borax, haematite, scales of iron and copper, tutty, scoria of iron, gold, and silver, Darānī salt, dough salt, *nafṭī* salt, Indian salt, malachite, red vitriol, arsenic, red arsenic, Armenian bole, pitch, verdigris, vermilion, mercury, "sea crab" (an Indian stone), alum, Isfahan clay, potters' clay, sealing clay, sulfur, lapis lazuli, litharge, marcasite, quicklime, and ammonium chloride.

From the three kingdoms, al-Samarqandī employed over 600 chemical materials whose properties were well known to him. This implies an enormous store of chemical knowledge when it is considered that each of these had to be prepared to the purest state possible and that purity tests had to be devised for many of these to thwart the frequent substitutions common in the pharmaceutical and other trades of the time.[42]

Muslim Materia Medica in Contemporary Medicine

At the time of the Golden Period of the Arabs, Muslim medicine was recognized as the most forward and progressive. Although formal medical practice at this time was more widespread than it had ever been previously, it was confined mainly to the large cities of the Near East and North Africa. Much of the evidence for this is attested in works relating to the Crusades.[43]

In spite of the advances of modern medicine and its

spread throughout much of the civilized world, it is still, nevertheless, unknown to more than half of the global population. To many more in the Near East, it is intermixed with native medicinal practises both subjective and objective in nature.

The *Aqrābādhīn* of al-Samarqandī makes use of many simples which are found in use today in the native medicine of India, Persia, and the Arab countries of Asia and North Africa. These drugs are not only employed by individuals as home remedies handed down from generation to generation. Rather, they are used on a much larger scale in the well organized present-day Ayurvedic system in India by Hindus, and also by the school of practitioners, mainly Muslims, who use Avicenna's *Canon* as their Bible of Medicine. The latter group is well developed in India and has a number of large warehouses at strategic locations. These store the raw material of the botanical, zoological, and mineralogical simples found in Muslim works. Large medical schools, as in the case of allopathic medicine, are devoted to the teaching of the Ayurvedic system and others to Avicenna's method.[44] The latter is the major ingredient of Yunani medicine. "Yunani" refers to the "Greek" medicine from which it is assumed in India that Avicenna's method originated.[45]

In order to better understand the two major native Indian systems, one of the possible directions of investigation is to assess the influence of ancient Arabic pharmacology particularly in present day Arabic and Indian pharmacology. Study of the Ayurvedic system and its influences, unfortunately, cannot be undertaken in the present work. However, many hundreds of mediaeval Muslim simples have found their way into modern native Indian and other medicines. Some of these are described below.

Lavender (*Lavandula Stoechas* L.), native to the Mediterranean region, was known to the Arabs through the description of Dioscorides who used it for the thorax and in antidotes. In Muslim times, it was employed therapeutically for the chest. In India today, the juice expressed from the leaves is used for cyanche. It is also used as a carminative and resolvent. In modern Egypt, it is an antispasmodic and stimulant.[46]

Wormwood (*Artemisia Absinthium* L.) was known to the Akkadian people for swellings, bruises, in clysters, for fumigation, and as a stomachic. In India today, it is used as a stomachic, as a deobstruant and antispasmodic. It is also a stomachic in Persia and China.

Fleawort (*Plantago Psyllium* L.) grows in India, Burma, Sudan, and in the Himalayas. In India, it is used for rattlesnake bites whereas in Egypt fleawort is employed as a drug for the kidney, urinary difficulties, and for internal haemorrhoids. The Persians consider it effective for gonorrhoea and as a diuretic. The Chinese, at present, approve of it as a diuretic and antirheumatic.

Another example, hemp (*Cannabis sativa L.*), is an interesting simple. Today, it is indigenous in Persia, Western and Central Asia, and almost all over India. In Yunani medicine, it is known as a retentive, anaesthetic, and astringent. In the Ayurvedic system, is is an aphrodisiac with narcotic properties. It is also an anaesthetic in China as well as a diuretic, emmenagogue, and anthelmintic. Hemp is used in Egypt today to excite one to delirium.

In more advanced circles, Muslim pharmacology persisted strongly in the West throughout the eighteenth century as may be seen in the London Dispensatory and similar works, and then into the early part of the nineteenth century. It is still known and used in Western

Europe and the United States particularly in rural areas in medicines based on home remedies.

Very frequently, a simple shows evidence that it has one important therapeutic use common to the various contemporary civilizations in which it is found. For example, wormwood is known mainly as a stomachic, gum ammoniac as a resolvent under certain conditions, lavender for chest conditions, fleawort for diuretic purposes, maiden hair for tracheal mucus, and hemp as an anaesthetic.

This common denominator which threads through the present native medical practices of Egypt, India, Persia, and Morocco (also Greece, Babylonia, and ancient Egypt if these are to be considered), it appears, may be its significant therapeutic property. On the other hand, in addition to this use common to various cultures, the drugs are noted in the literature as having other widely varying effects. This may, in part, be attributed to the widespread knowledge of the drug and its partial or chance effectiveness in other directions; thus people are led to ascribe various valuable attributes to it as they did with sociological phenomena like the philosopher's stone, the universal remedy, etc. Comparative study, therefore, of the uses of ancient materia medica in widely different cultures, present and past, assists in the determination of its best known, and perhaps most useful and effective therapeutic virtues.

Because of their relative cheapness, many simples of indigenous medical systems have a place in the pharmacopoeias of China, India, and other poor countries of the Near East. It is the duty of Eastern and Western pharmacologists to study this rich source of knowledge not only as an aid to the people using these simples but also for the unearthing of new products as part of a rational system of medicine.[47]

Although the ancient use of these drugs was not based on a scientific system as we know it today, it was, nevertheless, founded on empiricism. Many examples of modern, commonly known drugs which have been derived from a knowledge of their ancient usages may come to mind. One interesting example from the Chinese pharmacopoeia which, by the way, had an influence upon Muslim pharmacology, is that of the powdered heads of toad-fish as a remedy for heart trouble. It has been found that there are glands in the head of that fish which contain adrenalin. Another example is the nutritive value of liver. It is said that the American Indians first ate the liver of an animal and that the white hunter, when sharing an animal, always preferred the flesh.

Out of the large number of simples used by the Kavirages and Hakims in the past and present, there may be drugs which still deserve their old reputations.[48] In the case of the Muslim simples, fortunately, a fairly large body of manuscript material particularly on botanicals and other drugs is still extant. Many of these never reached the printed pages of early Western pharmacopoeias. It is, therefore, of some importance, that these be identified and thoroughly studied in the laboratories. Much of the information in the "Notes and Comments" after the tranlation, is given for this purpose.

Drugs in the Aqrabadhins of al-Kindi and al-Samarqandi

About four centuries intervened between al-Kindī and al-Samarqandī. It is known that al-Kindī practised in the great Baghdad hospital of his day. Furthermore, although al-Samarqandī was a native of northeast Persia, now a locality within the borders of modern Afghanistan, he also was acquainted with medical practise in Baghdad because in his introduction to the *Aqrābādhīn* he writes, "I have seen physicians of the hospital in the city of Baghdad. . . ." [49] He goes on to quote these medical men as objecting to the use of complex electuaries and mentions that they agreed with Mithridates, saying, "We did not find them of value because of the corruption of the compounding and the use of substitutes for drugs which were difficult to locate."

It is a fact, however, that both of the physicians mentioned availed themselves of complex remedies which were well known in their respective periods. These included some from Greek sources. But, in al-Samarqandī, there are many more of these name-designated compounded remedies than in al-Kindī; they were, in the main, complex drug preparations of Indian and Persian origin.

As to the drugs themselves, according to the statistical studies of their origins, al-Samarqandī derived many more from Persia, India, and China than did al-Kindī. As may be reasonably supposed, the Greek influence in the hospital during the time when al-Kindī practised was greater than at the time of al-Samarqandī. The net result is that the number of Greek simples remained more or less stationary and the number of drugs coming from the East was greatly increased. Thus, the percentage of drugs of Greek origin was markedly decreased in al-Samarqandī's work.

It may also be noted from examination of the etymology and the indigenousness of a number of drugs that their origin was Spanish or Moroccan. However, in order to state as a fact that the major knowledge of pharmacology among the Arabs proceeded from East to West, it is necessary to substantiate it by study of Western Arabic pharmacology. Much of the previous work in this area, particularly in the scientific determination of Arabic plant names and their botanonymy, must be rechecked and new manuscript material consulted.[50]

The organization in the medical formulary of al-Samarqandī is much more detailed than in the similar work of his famous predecessor, al-Kindī. The titles in al-Samarqandī's text of the nineteen chapters are sufficient to bear this out. The more exacting arrangement in the later work makes it simpler to be used as a handbook for practising physicians. The accretion of pharmacological knowledge in the four centuries became so great that the medical formulary model of drug text had to be supplemented by other forms of description.

A gnawing question usually asked of mediaeval Arabic culture, here applied to pharmacology, is if al-Samarqandī, for example, displayed movement away from Greek or Indian pharmacological theory and practice. Although discussed earlier in this book, it may be answered within this particular frame of reference by stating that al-Samarqandī definitely showed dissatisfaction with full acceptance of earlier drug theory. To have done so head-on would not have been psychologically proper in al-Samarqandī's culture. Without objecting too much to the ideas of others, the author stated his own reasons for compounding drugs and their weights used. This was done very clearly and forcefully.

The search for a better and more acceptable pharmacological theory in the Arabic period brought about a complex groping along a tortuous path similar in many ways to that found in the development of chemistry, astronomy, and other sciences.

Translation and Analecta

An attempt has been made in the translation to contain the vocabulary and ideas within the cultural confines of the early thirteenth century in Persia. The passive is used as consistently as reasonably possible although this has not always proved to be expedient. The primary emphasis in the translation is placed on the scientific aspects rather than on its value from the literary point of view. The latter is not for the scholar of ancient science to determine.

In transliterating Arabic words, the system of the United States Library of Congress as generally employed. In the case of diphthongs, au and aw are alike, and also ai and ay. In the case of names, the transliterations often follow the most common usage in this field. For other languages, the common transliterations have usually been used. For Indian languages, the diacritical marks have generally been omitted for simplification. In Sumerian and Akkadian, the determinatives *šar, iṣ* and *riq* denoting plant, tree, and resin respectively have been omitted since the context will indicate which should apply.

Abreviations of languages used are Af. for Afghan, Akk. for Akkadian, Ar. for Arabic, Aram. for Aramaic, Armen, for Armenian, Assam for Assamese, Ben. for Bengali, Ber. for Berber, Bokh. for Bokhara, Bom. for Bombay, Burm. for Burmese, Can. for Canarese, Chin. for Chinese, Cop. for Coptic, Duk. for Dukni, Gr. for Greek, Guj. for Gujarati, Heb. for Hebrew, hiero. Egypt. for hieroglyphic Egyptian (mostly Middle Kingdom), Hind. for Hindustani, Hit. for Hittite, Kon. for Konkani. Lat. for Latin, Mand. for Mandean. Os. for Osmanli, Pah. for Pahlevi, Pers. for Persian, Port. for Portuguese, Punj. for Punjabi, Sans. for Sanskrit, Sind. for Sindhi, S. for Sinhalese, Sp. for Spanish, Sum. for Sumerian, Syr. for Syriac, Tam. for Tamil, Tel. for Telugu, Turk. for Turkish, and Ug. for Ugaritic.

The foreign words are usually accompanied by their language designation. Where this is omitted, the word is Arabic. Words in capitals are Sumerian.

In the designation of references, the numbers refer either to pages or paragraphs. Which one it is will readily be evident to the reader since that one is used which makes it easier to check the information.

According to Hinz, in Iran when al-Samarqandī practised, the *mithqāl* or dirham weighed 4.3 grams. The following relationships based on the above value of the dirham are to be considered only approximate until more definite evidence of Iranian metrology is available.[51]

1 grain is 1/60 to 1/48 of a dirham or .072 to .090 grams
1 *qīrāṭ* is 1/20 of a dirham or .215 grams
1 *istār* is 4 1/2 *mithqāls* or 19.3 grams
1 ounce is 1/12 *raṭl* or 34.63 grams
1 *manna* is 260 dirhams or 1118 grams

In the glosses to the text, other values are given. The text glosses date from the time the manuscript was copied or earlier since both handwritings are the same. The year noted in the colophon is 857 H. or 1453 A.D. The date of the gloss is then 1453 or earlier. Based on the value given of the dirham, the following relationships follow from the glosses:

1 *ṭassuj* is 1/24 of a dirham or .179 grams
1 grain is .0895 grams
1 *dāniq* is .716 grams
1 *istār* is 6 1/2 dirhams or 28 grams
1 *qīrāṭ* is four grains or .3580 grams

Notes to the Introduction

For abbreviations, *vide* Bibliography

1. The words Muslim and Arabic, for want of a better expression, refer to the entire cultural system which included Persians, Arabs,

Jews, Spaniards, North Africans, and other ethnic groups which participated in this great movement.

2. Evidence for the close relations between Muslim chemistry and pharmacology is discussed at length in M. Levey, *Mediaeval Arabic Bookmaking and its Relation to Early Chemistry and Pharmacology*, published as vol. 52, part 4 of the *Transactions of the American Philosophical Society*, Philadelphia, 1962.

3. For this early period, *cf.* M. Levey, *The Aqrābādhīn or "Medical Formulary" of al-Kindī with a study of its Materia Medica*, University of Wisconsin Press, 1965.

3a. Cf. M. Levey, *Transactions and Studies of the College of Physicians* 4 ser., *30*, 157–161 (1963).

4. GAL I, 491; GAL S I, 895; IAU–B II, 47 gives his name as Najīb al-dīn abū M. b. ᶜA. B. ᶜO. al-Samarqandī:

5. Leclerc II, 128–129; Ḥājjī Khalīfa no. 846.

6. Wüstenfeld, H. F., *Geschichte der arabischen Aerzte und Naturforscher*, Goettingen, 1840, p. 119.

7. ibn abī Usaibiᶜa, *Kitāb ᶜuyūn al-anbā' fī tabaqāt al-atibbā'*, Beirut, 1956, part II, pp. 47–48.

8. Leclerc II, 127–128.

9. GAL I, 491; GAL S I, 895–896.

10. This is a loanword from the Greek which means a list or registry. *Cf.* extended discussion on the *aqrābādhīn* and its history in al-Kindī, Introduction.

11. *Cf.* GAL I, 491–492 for library numbers. All of these have been examined.

12. al-Kindī, Introduction.

13. *Cf.* Levey CCTM, Introduction.

14. Anawati, G. M., *Drogues et Médicaments* (Ar. text), Cairo, 1959, pp. 117–118.

15. *Cf.* also A. Fonahn, *Janus* 14, 347–353 (1909).

16. Berendes, I., *Paulos' von Aegina*, Leiden, 1914, p. 606 ff.

17. For the text by Sahlān ibn Kaysān (d. 990 H.), *cf.* Paul Sbath and C. D. Averinos, *Deux Traités Médicaux*, Cairo, 1953.

18. In al-Kindī.

19. To be published by M. Levey from MS Velieddin 2542 and others.

20. *Cf.* Leclerc.

21. Half of this text is preserved in Bibliotheca Osleriana, McGill University. Part of this text is said to be in a depository in Tripoli (E. Rossi, *Oriente Moderno 33*, 67–68 (1953). An abbreviated version by Bar Hebraeus (thirteenth century) was partially translated by M. Meyerhof and G. Sobhy, *The Abridged Version of "The Book of Simple Drugs,"* Cairo, 1932–1940.

22. Citron, *Citrus medica* Risso var. *Limonum*. Cf. Meyerhof and Sobhy, *op. cit.*, pp. 78–79.

23. Leiden MS 1339, Rabat MS 481, and Salar Jung MS used by the author. *Cf.* H.-P.-J. Renaud, *Bull. soc. franc. hist. med.* ***21***, 345 (1927); *Hespéris* ***10***, 135–150 (1930–1931).

24. *Cf. The Encyclopedia of Islam*, Leiden, 1963, 2nd edition, ***11***, 582–587 by S. Maqbul Ahmad for geographical references. *Vide* also Heyd; A. Dietrich, *Zum Drogenhandel im islamischen Aegypten*, Heidelberg, 1954; I. Galdston, *Bull. N.Y. Acad. Med* ***13***, 512–538 (1937); P. Kahle, *Opera Minora*, Leiden, 1956, p. 326 ff. on Chinese poreclain in Islamic countries.

25. *Ḥudūd al-ᶜālam*, London, 1937, translated by V. Minorsky. This work is anonymous.

26. von Schroeder, L., *Pythagoras und die Inder*, Leipzig, 1884.

27. Laufer, p. 580 ff.

28. *Ibid.*

29. Laufer, pp. 581–585.

29a. Hamarneh, S., *Middle East Forum* ***39***, 35–38 (1963).

30. For a fuller discussion, *cf.* al-Kindī.

31. *Ibid.*

32. "Accidents" are the properties or characteristics of matter more definitely and fully discussed in the later Arabic atomic theory. *Cf.* Levey, M., *Chymia* ***7***, 40–56 (1961).

33. von Grot, R., "Hippokratischen Schriftensammlung enthaltenen pharmakologischen Kenntnisse," *Historische Studien aus dem Pharmakologischen Institute der Kaiserlichen Universität Dorpat* ***1***, 72 ff. (1889).

34. Kurland, S., *Averroes on Aristotle's "De Generatione et corruptione: Middle Commentary and Epitome"* Cambridge, 1958, p. 94.

35. *Ibid.*, pp. 65–66.

36. Levey, M., *Chymia* ***7***, 50 ff. (1961).

36a. Munk, S., ed. *Guide des égarés*. Paris, 1856–1866.

36b. Levey, M. *op. cit.*, 41–42.

36c. Al-Samarqandī MS 3555 of Aya Sofya, fol. 25a.

36d. *Idem.* fol. 15a.

37. Introduction to present manuscript, fol. 3b–4a.

38. *Ibid.*, fol. 4b–5a.

39. *Ibid.*, fol. 6a.

40. Holmyard, E. J., ed., *Kitāb al-ᶜilm al-muktasab fī ziraᶜat al-dhahab*, Paris, 1923, p. 20.

41. *Ibid.*, p. 13.

42. Levy, R., ed., *Ibn al-Ukhawwa's maᶜālim al-qurba fī aḥkām al-ḥisba*, London, 1938, p. 150 ff.

43. *Cf.* for example P. H. Hitti, *An Arab-Syrian Gentleman and Warrior . . . Memoirs of Usāmah ibn Munqidh (Kitāb al-iᶜtibār),* New York, 1929, pp. 213 ff. *et passim.*

44. Frequently, no clear dividing line between Ayurvedic and Yunani medicine in India may be discerned. During the Pathan and Mogul dynasties, Muslim medicine had intimate contact with the old Hindu medicine for many centuries so that they intermingled and they used the materia medica of the other. As a result, though both systems declined, a rich materia medica was left behind (R. N. Chopra *Indigenous Drugs of India,* Calcutta, 1933. p. 6). With the coming of the Europeans, the Portuguese, French, and English, the decline was accelerated. This decline was arrested when India became independent; since then, medical schools based upon Ayurvedic, and also upon Yunani medicine have been supported by the government in the same manner as the more modern schools.

45. This nomenclature recalls to mind the similar occurrence of the term for us of Arabic numerals but known to the Arabs as Hindu numerals.

46. *Cf.* "Notes and Comments" for complete descriptions of the drugs here mentioned.

47. Nadkarni, I, p. xxi.

48. Chopra, p. 15 ff.

49. al-Samarqandī, fol. 3b.

50. It is necessary to recheck, for example, IB, ibn al-ᶜAwwām, Bik., al-Zahrāwī, al-Ghāfiqī, Maim., and others.

51. Hinz, W., *Islamische Masse und Gewichte* in *Handbuch der Orientalistik,* Erganzungsband I, Leiden, 1955.

Translation of Aqrabadhin of M. b. 'Ali b. 'Umar al-Samarqandi

A Book Concerning the Fundamentals of the Preparation of Drugs in Medicine, and Smaller Works on Medicine which are Precious to the Utmost.[1]

In the name of Allah, the Compassionate, the Merciful.[2]

Praise be to Allah, Lord of all the worlds. Prayers and peace to the best of creations, Muḥammad and his family. As to the *imām,* scholar, and master of the sages Najīb al-dīn, the heir of the past and the teacher of the coming generation, may Allah sanctify his dear soul. It is the obligation of every intelligent person to seek close relationship with the exalted God and to beg him for all that he can secure of nearness and the appropriate ways after having obeyed the commands and [abstained from] that which is forbidden. This is what brings good to all people and especially repels harm. It is also to discuss the science of medicine, to be concerned with the ill, to be interested in their cure, and to seek their health with whatever search it involves. This is to set the Muslims on the correct path and to win the reward of Allah. It is to demonstrate the God of all the worlds by uncovering the miracles of nature, the soul, and that which is tangential, to understand and receive this knowledge, power, generosity, and grace on all.

Since I am concerned with the subject of the practise of medicine, I like to gather [material] from books on medicine for those in this profession who practise it. [I gather] preparations of drugs, making them brief both in time and conditions, explaining the benefit to be derived, and making it simple for those who desire to make use of them. I have seen physicians of the hospital in the city of Baghdad,[3] may the exalted Allah guard it, confine themselves to a number of duplicates of compounded [drugs] which may be found in a limited number of small treatises and to reject the more complex electuaries. This is because of the lack of the drugs since some are in small demand. They agreed with Mithridates[4] saying, "We did not find them of value because of the corruption of the compounding and the use of substitutes for drugs which were difficult to locate."

The physician should not treat everything of a minor character or every small change occurring in the body with a drug. Rather, he should treat it by changing the method of management and by adjusting the necessary basic conditions. He must not stir up anything nor impair the body in its natural functions.[5] It is more difficult to quiet the stirring than to stir the quiet. Whenever we can, we should treat by nutritive drugs, and, if compelled, by pure drugs, not going beyond the simples as far as possible. It is easier on nature and more effective in illness as Galen has stated in regard to the compound drugs that those [simples] known to be very useful for a certain disease will not be effective in a compound drug since they will be in insufficient amount in a dose to be useful. They never reach that quantity sufficient to saturate the ailment which they [are intended to] cure.

In this [present time], there is evident a disappearance of the guide posts of the sciences, and unsalability of the products of the arts to the extent that the greater part of the noble drugs is lost and only their names are left. Whatever may be found is adulterated or old and weak since it has stayed for a long period. The strength of most drugs does not remain after two or three [months (?)]. Therefore, the mixed, large [6] compounded ones are preferably ignored in these days. One is then restricted to the smaller of the compounded ones which are preferable when necessary so that one may procure beneficial results. It is not true what people say in this respect. It is more untrue than the [actual] medical formulary [7] of the physicians.

The drugs are compounded for the particular circumstance and at the moment with attention to the rules of composition according to the need of an ailment and the sufficiency of the humors [in the patient]. It is better than copying from editions of the medical formularies [8] which are overstuffed, officious, erroneous, and not put together correctly, omitting some parts and reading incorrectly. Some people regard it like God's Book which should not be changed or altered and that neither the genii nor mankind can produce one like it. They are the ones whom Galen blamed and ridiculed. He said that many whose copies were lost died of grief, and the others remained perplexed, until they died, without any guidance. He gave assurance for those who perfected the knowledge of the strengths of drugs and the rules of their compounding that compounding could be carried out whenever it was desired and whenever better remedies were desired and more effectively in that [medium] which was wished.

There are reasons which compel one to compound [drugs] in the absence of a simple which would attain the desired goal. It is partly because of the aspect of the nature of sickness and disease, partly because of the state of the organs, and partly because of the drug. For the use of compounded drugs there are fourteen reasons. One of them is due to the extent of the ill humor if there is no drug opposite to it in its strength. It is then compounded from one which is stronger in the quantity of its [humor] with one which is less so. From these a blend is put together to resist that ill-humor. The second is concerned with the strength and acuteness of the illness when there is no single drug which can resist it. It is then compounded so that the constituents may assist one another in resistance. Thirdly, there are the differences in the state of the disease and associated circumstances, and its treatment; a drug is unknown which [by itself] performs opposite actions like absorbing[9] and bringing up[10] in chest ailments, and the freeing[11] and hindering of tumors so that one must be compounded. Fourth is a basic one, a means to counteract many poisons and different ailments. This is the noblest of compounded ones because it protects one from constriction with a strength superior to the strength of any simple. The effectiveness is due to the presence of its simples. The fifth has to do with the remoteness of the ailing organ from the stomach. It is compounded with a drug which is useful for it and [with one which] makes it reach [the organ] quickly as saffron with camphor [12] and Chinese cinnamon [13] with haematite.[14] The sixth concerns the strength and importance of the organ and its size and functions. A drug is mixed to dissolve tumors and to ease [at the same time] the properties which lessen [a drug's] effectiveness to act as a restraining remedy. The seventh relates to the unsavoriness of the drug and its disagreeableness until it is improved to the point of acceptability by nature. The eighth has to do with the increase of potency of a drug as in mixing ginger with turpeth.[15] The ninth protects some organs against the harmfulness of a drug as by correctives with purgatives, and the tenth is the inadequacy of a drug like gum arabic in the collyrium of verdigris.[16] The eleventh concerns the destruction of the evil [property] of a drug as mixing castoreum [17] with opium. The twelfth is for keeping the strength of the compounded drug for a long time as in mixing opium [18] with the major electuaries. The thirteenth is concerned with the difference of drugs in their sizes and usages in the desired direction as mixing a *qīrūṭī* [19] unguent with the essentials [20] in poultices. The fourteenth is the need of a single useful remedy for the illness as in mixing the unguent with verdigris to form an effective drug for wounds when there are no drugs good for wounds. There are, then, valid reasons for compounding. One is forced to it when a single remedy is needed to produce all that is desired.

As to the reasons for the differences in weight, there are seven simple ones, and other combinatory reasons of these simple ones. As to the seven simple ones, the first is the strength and weakness in its [the drug's] natures. Second is the abundance or lack of its usefulness. Third is the importance or lowliness of its benefits. Fourth is its partnership in usefulness or its being alone. The fifth is concerned with the location of the ailing organ in regard to its proximity to or distance from the stomach. Sixth is the existence or non-existence of drugs in the compounded one which weakens its strength. Seventh is the existence of harmfulness in it for some organs, or for the inadequacy of drugs of their sufficiency.

However, the differences in weight vary according to the strengths and weaknesses. The strength of the power of the drug in [over] heating and [over] cooling requires its decrease in a compounded one; the weakness of its power necessitates an increase so that its abundance will assure the strength desired of it. In regard to a greater or lesser usefulness, a greater effectiveness requires an increase, and the lesser, i.e. the drug having one single use, indicates a decrease. As to the importance of its usefulness, the amount requires an increase, and if lowly, a decrease.[21] As to its being in partnership with others or being alone, the latter demands an increase, and the former, the opposite. When [the organ is] far from the stomach, then an increase is required so that the weakness, because of the length of the distance, be obviated; for its nearness, the opposite. When drugs are present in a compounded remedy, then some drugs annul the strength of others, so that the useful drug must be increased, and vice versa. Should a drug be harmful to an organ, it is decreased; if not, then its opposite does not require anything.

These are the reasons for increasing and decreasing [the amounts] and the rules which are to be followed according to whether it is alone [or compounded]. In the latter, it depends on the binding conditions and the compounding of certain drugs. If the binding conditions improve by a single drug in greater quantities, then its quantity is increased; if the opposite, then it is decreased accordingly. If [the optimum condition] is obtained for an equal quantity of simple drugs, then its measures are purposely made in equal amounts. This is from the rules and regulations which are dependable in the preparation of drugs and wherever drugs come to be well known in their characteristics, goodness, evil, strength, and action.

The best, new, superior one is chosen and compounded from the least [number] of simples according to the rules of compounding and according to each ailment and its severity. It is thus more effective and more apt to lead to success in it [i.e. treatment] rather than when one applies it to another patient because of similarities in the symptoms of disease. This [latter] is what old women do and those who have no understanding of this art, its principles, and consequences. One may try this by tested analogy. I swear by my religion that making a decision is difficult but experimentation is dangerous.

The analogical method is safe and is used dependably in all medical practice. The fact that it is difficult should not lead to its not being employed. Earlier workers compounded according to the method of analogy. After experience, they found that it gave the best of what they had expected from it so that they wrote it down and made it permanent in books. This was done so that it should be an example for us in using compounded remedies according to the kind of need and for the satisfaction of the individual interest; the exception is in the compounded ones for which the rules are known and also the purpose. So, it happens that we have the opportunity as they did, and thus existing thoughts will coincide with existing thoughts as the hoof tread falls on the hoof tread. I have proved by example some of what the hands of experience have bequeathed in turn and elucidated it from the force to the action. From this example, benefit may be derived when it strikes the spot and is used in its proper place. The rest is considered accordingly.

There are nineteen chapters.

1. Syrups and robs
2. Stomachic confections[22] and electuaries
3. Pills and aperients
4. Decoctions and infusions
5. Clysters, enemas, suppositories, and pessaries
6. Emetics
7. Lohochs
8. Lozenges
9. Powders and stomachic powders
10. Dressings, coatings, cataplasms
11. Balms
12. Collyria
13. Poultices, aromatic powders
14. Dentifrices
15. Gargles and confections
16. Preserves
17. Sternutatives, odorants, fumigants
18. Aromatics for baths
19. Hair medicines

Chapter I
Syrups and Robs

The special drink is extremely simple; it is clear water which is the most useful drink for those afflicted with sharp fever[23] for it possesses a strong gentleness, is quickly penetrative, and has a lightness in nature.[24] The Prophet, may the grace and peace of God befall him, said that fever is the exhalation of hell and to cool it with water. This is because all drinks aside from it contain nutrition which requires nature to work on it. Its presence then will be a retardant during its strong activity in combating sickness and enduring its heavy matter so that there is no benefit as there is from water. In some cases, it may be necessary to compound it with others as ice to increase its cooling [power] or vinegar for the same reason. It may also be required for its penetration to the extremities of the body and to reach the utmost of cooling, or sugar may be necessary to strengthen its moistness and extension to the main parts of the organs through the acquired sweetness. Or both together may be necessary in a malabathrum oxymel.[25]

Oxymel is a syrup which is beneficial in acute fevers since it calms the heat, prevents putrefaction, stops the confusion [of humors], and opens obstructions. The ratio of its parts differs from one to the other because of the difference in vinegar and sugar, depending on the heat of the fever, its humor, and the attributes of the nature of the drinker. In this regard, the kind made from vinegar sharply sour with a double quantity of very white sugar, cooked finely, is good to drink for fevers which are extremely acute and hot. It is good for those who can endure it and do not dislike it. The viscous kind made from strong wine vinegar with three times it of red sugar is for compound fevers from yellow bile and phlegm. The vinegar may also be reduced from that to the ratio of one fifth or less. It is necessary that the sugar be washed a little at first, then thrown into the pot; on it the vinegar is poured. It is placed over a slow burning fire until the sugar dissolves. Then water in the same amount, more or less, is poured on it according to the requirement. It is boiled, and then its froth is removed. Honey [26] is not good for acute fevers; it is effective for the compound ones whose humors are cold. The ratio of the vinegar to the honey depends on the thickness of their humors,[27] viscosity, thinness, and strength of putrefaction. The vinegar cools and quiets; honey is a warming and easing agent.

Vinegar of onion [28] may be taken in very cold illnesses; this vinegar is hot, sharp, active and good. The seedy oxymel is a compound with seeds to increase its cabability to open obstructions.[29] In acute fevers, cold seeds are used but in the fevers whose humor is cold and in the case of other illnesses, then hot seeds are indicated. In the compounded one, with hot and cold together, one is concerned with the ratios as regard to those of the humors and to the organs. For example, if it is to be taken for acute fevers, choleric humors, and for venal obstructions, then it is made up of seed of the endive [30] and the rind of its root, the seed of the cucumbers, and the water melon seed so that it is from seeds which are cold and cause diuresis; it is especially effective against blockage of the veins and for allowing the bile to flow.

It is made from seed of the two cucumbers [31] and the melon in greater quantity since it is weak and its pathways are distant; there is less of the rinds of the root of endive because of the existence of its association in the stomach with the decreasing effectiveness from its seed. More of the seed of the endive than the rinds of its root increases its usefulness and effectiveness, and because, as usual, it is depended upon for the clearing of obstructions of the veins in acute fevers. There is less of the seed of the two kinds of cucumbers and melon because they are strong.

Preparation

Two kinds of cucumber	5 dirhams
Melon	5 dirhams
Rinds of the root of the endive	2 dirhams
Endive	3 dirhams

In fevers whose humor is cold, take celery [32] seed, anise,[33] and endive seed which is used because it is of compounded attributes and of common effectiveness, seed and root of fennel,[34] celery root, agrimony,[35] and rhubarb.[36] It is made from three dirhams each of the seeds, and five dirhams [each] of the roots because of the strength of the seeds and the weakness of the roots, and three dirhams of the dodder because of the value of its effectiveness, and two dirhams of agrimony for its strength and its strong bitterness, and of rhubarb less than that because of the excess of its co-partners in its action accompanied by an excess of constipation for it is like a protective agent for the liver.

A *raṭl* of sugar [37] should be in each of the two recipes [above].

In compound fevers, the warm seeds are gathered with the cold in accord with the superiority of one of the two mixtures over the other. In the case where there is no fever, for example, hardness of the spleen, this is what is essential: the seed of the chaste tree, rind of the root of the caper,[38] and endive seed in equal amounts as a secondary mixture. It is taken in large amounts because of the value of its effectiveness. With it is taken fennel seed, the rind of fennel root, and anise in moderate quantity for its strength and its great usefulness in diuresis. Put in it seeds of the two cucumbers, the melon, and the purslane [39] when it is necessary to moderate it because of its antagonism to the melancholic humor. Make its quantity greater since it is weak.

However, if it is taken for hardness of the liver, add to it rhubarb, *lukk*,[40] and lemon-grass.[41]

When seed of the chaste tree [42] is taken to promote menstruation, one adds to it dittany,[43] lichen, and seed of rue. Dodder [43a] may also be added.

In black bile illnesses, the method of preparing the drugs should be that they be pounded coarsely, soaked in vinegar and water for one night, and cooked the next morning in three times the quantity of water in which they were soaked until a third [of the mixture] remains. It is filtered, then returned to the pot and cooked with sugar. The froth is removed and vinegar is prepared in ratio to the sugar and the ratio of all the drugs[44] so that neither strong taste nor smell overtake it so that it would be hated and disliked by most of the natures. It is best to pour the juice of the seeds and the filtrate on the sugar in sufficient amount so that the sugar is dissolved. It [the sugar] is added and dissolved until the taste is adjusted. Then stop and do not add any more.

As for the robs,[45] each one [when used] alone is stronger, but when put with sugar, it becomes gentler. The robs may be put together in compounds with each other to assist in cooling[46] and in constipation. The compound is called "robs." It is from apples, quince,[47] verjuice,[48] pomegranate,[49] Chinese pear,[50] lemon,[51] sorrel, barberry,[52] ribes,[53] grains of myrtle,[54] sumach,[55] white mulberry[56] [57] that is close to being unripe, and the azarole,[58] which is called *nārsinjid.*[59] Tabasheer[60] is added to it and also cooked gum when it is badly needed for cooling and constipation.

The juices of these fruits are gathered when robs are needed and enough crystalline sugar is thrown in to make it sweet-sour. It is cooked until viscous. The juice of some of the fruits is used instead of the water in the oxymel. It is either to do away with some of the harm of the vinegar, to increase its cooling power, or to strengthen some of the organs. Some are quince, apple, and pomegranate; oxymel is related to them.

That of quince, which is one of them, may be mixed[61] with strengthening drugs for the stomach like Indian aloeswood,[62] Chinese cinnamon, rose, mastix,[63] and so on.

In the case when cardiac drugs are needed, there are greater cardamon,[63a] clove,[64] saffron,[65] and so on. If there is no hindrance by the heat of the humor, then its mixture is such that it is not an oxymel or syrup for healthy people that must be counteracted.

Of the syrups, the syrup of the minted pomegranate is to calm disturbance and vomiting in jaundice. Take juice of sour pomegranate; mix with it, over a fire, an amount of sugar which will not be enough to annul its sourness completely. On it, pour enough mint juice so as to produce a bitterness in it. Add also a small amount of cooked rind of Barānīyye[66] pistachio[67] and enough leaf or rind of citron[68] to impart an odor. It is cooked until it is viscous, then removed [from the fire]. The patients suck it. The mint may be cooked in the juice of the sour pomegranate until it is viscous, then removed [from the fire].

Syrup of poppy.[69] Take thirty white pulpy poppies, the moist is the best, and remove the seeds. These are pulverized finely, gathered with the rinds, soaked in rose water a night, and then boiled carefully until it is evaporated to a third. It is filtered and squeezed well. On it is thrown one *raṭl* of white sugar. It is made viscous. With it there is soaked once one ounce of the filtrate and once with water of the barley compound[70] together with the filtrate according to the heat of the humor and the thickness or thinness of the rheums.

Syrup of rose, violet, nenuphar,[71] borage,[72] mountain-balm,[73] wormwood, and so on. The way to prepare it is to cook it in enough water to absorb its strength, taste, and color. Then it is filtered. On it is thrown white sugar to sweeten it a little, with the taste and coloring remaining. It is made viscous over a good fire which will not allow it to boil. If it boils, the top of the pot is wiped with a wet cloth after it has settled so that nothing in it will burn.[74] If mixed into the solution of another which is boiling, it will spoil. It may be mixed with the syrup of borage, mountain balm, juices of fruits to increase its pleasantness and effectiveness and to decrease its sweetness when necessary.

Then there is the syrup of hyssop [75] to ripen the thick phlegm in the channels of breath [76] in asthma.

Rind of root of celery	5 dirhams
Rind of root of fennel	5 dirhams
Rind of root of marshmallow [77]	5 dirhams
Rind of root of caper	5 dirhams
Celery seed	3 dirhams
Fennel seed	3 dirhams
Hyssop	4 dirhams
Sticky fig	10 dirhams
Raisins without pips [78]	10 dirhams

After peeling the roots, the rinds are made wet for one night. They are cooked in three *raṭls* of water until one *raṭl* remains. It is filtered. The dose is five *istārs* with fifteen dirhams of galingale.[79] When it is necessary to increase the strength, root of the blue lily, root of the lily,[80] and maiden hair [81] are added. Some of the hot drugs are decreased when the humor is hot and violet is substituted together with seed of marshmallow, quince seed, jujube, sebesten,[82] and poppy. This is when it is necessary to rub the chest and prevent cold.

Water of cheese purgates the burned humors. The milk [used] is two *raṭls* of boiled milk [83] of a goat. On it after two boilings, is poured five *istārs* of sour oxymel. It is removed and filtered through a finely woven cloth. The dose is ten *istārs* with the oxymel. It is taken for purgations of yellow bile and black bile according to the need.

Syrup of sandalwood[84] [85] for heat of the heart. The Macassar sandalwood is taken in an amount of thirty dirhams, then filed, soaked in a half *raṭl* [of water] one day and one night, cooked the next day in three *raṭls* of water until one *raṭl* remains, and then filtered. To it is added a half *raṭl* of juice of sour pomegranate, a half *raṭl* of juice of tamarind,[86] and three *raṭls* of crystalline sugar. It is made viscous over the fire and left until it is cool. On it is thrown two dirhams each of tabasheer and sandalwood, both pulverized, with one half dirham of pulverized camphor and three dirhams of saffron.

Syrup of jujube to quiet the overheating of the blood and ailments of the blood as excess of its humor. One *raṭl* of pure Jurjani jujube,[87] fifteen dirhams of dry coriander,[88] one hundred dirhams of peeled lentils,[89] and a bunch[90] of endive roots[91] are all soaked in vinegar for three days and then boiled once vigorously and filtered. Oxymel[92] is made from it. Every day ten dirhams of it is soaked in a glass containing a dilution of barberry whose preparation is as follows.

One *raṭl* of Jurjani jujube without seeds, one *raṭl* of fresh barberry without seeds, one *raṭl* of cuscuta, one handful of endive seed, and one handful of genuine rhubarb, altogether three dirhams, are gathered in a vessel. On it is poured enough water to cover it and to exceed it by two fingers in width. It is put in the summer sun for three days or in the winter for four days. Allah is omniscient.

Chapter II
Electuaries and Confections

Honey contains favorable properties and has good action.[93] It prevents whatever is mixed with it from changing and deterioration. When honey is used, one may expect it to be an assist in curing. It is delightful and appealing to nature for its properties besides being nutritious, pleasant, and removing the distastefulness and disagreeableness of medicines, it clarifies and ripens the thick remainders, purifying them. Also, in regard to its properties, it mixes with the particles of what is compounded with it, extracts its strength, and mixes them together. It ferments it in order that a second mixture will be derived thus preparing it to have in it a strength which emanates from its favorable properties and actions which are not to be found in single drugs. That is why it is chosen for all drugs and their confections.

Those electuaries whose rules of compounding are well known and whose drugs are available and tested by our contemporaries are the myrobalan confections.[94] The word *iṭrifl*[95] is arabized from the Indian language in which it applies to Kabul, belleric, and emblic myrobalans.[96] The three of them strengthen the nervous organs, aid the organs of nutrition[97] in regard to waste excesses.[98] They are gathered and compounded because they all agree in usefulness and help each other. They are made up in equal weights since their strength and usefulness are the same.

Yellow Basran[99] myrobalan may be added to it and also black Indian, as much as their weights,[100] since they are so close to them in nature in usefulness in strengthening and cleansing. It is also so since it is then more perfect and stronger in activity.

It is pulverized and immersed in ghee or almond oil to destroy the strength of its dryness. This is because dryness[101] is harmful for the digestive forces. When it surpasses the limit of the strengthening of the organs of nutrition then the continuing use of myrobalan confection causes leanness. Butter is preferable since it is the strongest of all oils which agree with the humors of man if it is used immediately. If its use is delayed, then almond oil is preferable since the butter would be rancid and its smell is altered[102] quickly. The belleric myrobalan which has been soaked in milk so that its dryness disappears is called *shirāmulaj*.[103] It is preferred over non-myrobalan confections. The honey should be double the amount of the drugs in myrobalan confections when their effectiveness and perfection are desired. It may be made as much as three-fold so that it may be warmer and gentler and less unpleasant. It may be put in other confections, those in which fermentation is desired.

Raw honey is warmer, sharper, and closer to being a medicament. The cooked whose froth is removed is less sharp. Water should be poured on it and cooked so that it may return to its original viscosity. If its decoction is desired, the myrobalan confection may be made of the three myrobalans [104] when the purpose of cleansing is more important than that of strengthening. It may be confined to the three [105] together with turpeth and false bdellium [106] in equal parts for hemorrhoids accompanied by dryness of the faeces. The turpeth may be changed if there is no drying in the nature or if it is with constipating drugs which coagulate the blood such as yellow amber,[107] pomegranate flower,[108] tamarisk gallnut,[109] burned shell, especially prepared royal cumin,[110] [111] coral,[112] and so on according to the weights [113] less than it. If hemorrhoids are present, the bowls loose, and blood flowing, Kabul myrobalan, belleric myrobalan, and emblic myrobalan are fried in fat which has strength to stop looseness and constipation. The fat will keep it so for a long time. Ghee is the best of the fats for that.

Honey is removed from it [114] to the extent that it possesses sharpness, opening ability, and power in loosening the bowels. It is gathered with blue bdellium, dissolved in juice of the leek which is specially for hemorrhoids and the coagulation of blood. It is made into pills so that its dissolution may be easier and ease its flowing to the lower parts. It is called "pill of the rear." [115]

Added to the myrobalan confection may also be those drugs which are good for the stomach when it is disturbed and for the gathering of moist humors in it. These are mastix, ginger,[116] pepper,[117] long pepper [118] and Indian aloeswood. The quantity in number and weight is relative to the quantities of the humors. The weight is made according to the seven rules mentioned and the ratio of all of it to the drugs of the myrobalan confection is as the ratio of the coldness of the stomach to its moistness.

For disturbance of the humors, heat, and yellow bile,

senna[119] and red rose are added to it. It is soaked to saturation with almond oil and mixed with tamarind syrup, siracost,[120] and rose syrup.

For mange, it is squeezed on the three myrobalans, and senna and mandrake fruit[121] are put in it. It is gathered with dried currants[122] for its moistness and because it has less heat. When it is needed to keep hot moistness from the head, put dry coriander in it. When it is necessary to evacuate the black bile, it is compounded with agaric,[123] common polypody,[124] turpeth, wormwood,[125] and lavender.[126] These five are increased with an opposite five. Their weights are made equal since their usefulness is equal and their strengths are close, and in half of the weights of the myrobalan confection drugs because of the sharpness of the latter's strength in comparison with it.

Turpeth may be added, as much as five or six dirhams of the whole, for phlegmatic black bile. When it is desired to strengthen [the bowels for] looseness, it is called "confection of success."

Galen pulverizes the drugs of the myrobalan confection and the electuaries not too finely[127] to roughen the lining of the stomach and to lengthen its duration in it.

The first three[128] may be increased to four with tamarisk gall[129] to strengthen the binding action. It may be made five with scoria of iron[130] soaked in ripe vinegar many times for that. The amount of scoria of iron is double the quantity of one of the four because of its great usefulness, important purpose, for its effectiveness in calming the stomach, for continuous diarrhea[131] and hemorrhoids.

Warm binding drugs are added to these five but the heat is to moderate the five cold drugs, to warm the stomach and to clear the confusion.

As to constipation, it requires rinds of frankincense,[132]

sweet Cyperus,[133] nard,[134] lemon-grass, royal cumin together with vinegar in a ratio less than it in the association of one to another as we wish it. Sugar and rose may be added to it for increased constipation so that it becomes more moderate. It is called the "electuary of the scoria" and "*penjanush*" [135] arabized from Persian for the five equivalent to the fundaments.

As to the heart strengtheners, they are used with the original and what follows it in making the ill tempered gentle, in spreading, and collecting the softness and strengthening it, and with its quantity in protecting one from most of the aspects of the spirit. It should be compounded according to the need for it. If there is weakness without ill temper, then the cold is compounded with the hot to moderate the original. The essences are gathered and when it is activated its special property is intensified. There is no substance binding it. It is pulverized to an extreme, washed, and then used.

The use of purgatives for black bile in heart strengtheners is not commendable because it excites the black bile. It is unable to expel it and so is harmful, unfortunately. It also competes with others. It may be compounded with heart medicines and medicines which are not for the heart like seed of the two cucumbers, purslane, pumpkin,[136] lettuce,[137] and so on when it is needed to break the dryness of cardiaca and to strengthen cooling and drugs which cool if very cold like saffron and ambergris.[138] It may be taken in purgative medicines. It ameliorates electuaries which are administered for ailments when there is need and when time allows its compounding.

Electuary of purging cassia [139] for hot colic, bilious elements, and phlegm in the intestines.

Isfahan violet	40 dirhams
Turpeth	40 dirhams
Indian salt [140]	7½ dirhams
Fennel seed	5 dirhams
Anise	5 dirhams
Mastix	5 dirhams
Licorice rob [141]	2 *istārs*
Scammony	15 dirhams
Pods of purging cassia	100 dirhams

It is weighed after being sieved and then gathered with the pulp of the purging cassia and one hundred dirhams of sugar candy. The dose is from five to ten dirhams so that in a complete dose there will be a dirham of root of turpeth, a dirham and 2 *dāniqs* of violet and a *ṭassūj* [142] of scammony. This is the complete drink of it for a serious case. In rapid purgation, the amount of salt is reduced and the latter ingredients are diminished in weight in the other electuaries because of their strength and heat.

One of them, the electuary of colchicum [143] is for pains of the joints if it arises from yellow bile and phlegm. It is compounded from purgatives especially for the joints, for diuretics, and pain relievers. It is also to prevent the flow of the thick humor and the narrowing of its ducts. These humors are the problem in treating these ailments.

White colchicum	6 dirhams
Orchis (?) [144]	2 dirhams
Juice of *mīzamiraj* [145]	2 dirhams
Caper root rind	2 dirhams
Cumin [146]	2 dirhams
Indian leadwort [147]	2 dirhams

Yellow myrobalan rind	7 dirhams
Celery seed	1½ dirhams
Fennel seed	1½ dirhams
White pepper	1½ dirhams
Thyme [148]	1½ dirhams
Indian salt	1½ dirhams
Henna leaves [149]	1½ dirhams
Jelly-fish	1½ dirhams
Red rose	3 dirhams
Sesame [150]	3 dirhams
White turpeth	5 dirhams [151]
Ginger	3 dirhams
Scammony [152]	3 dirhams
Honey	150 dirhams
Almond oil [153]	1 *istār*

The dose is one *istār* with hot water, or five depending on the time [in between].

This electuary [154] is weakly purgative along with a balanced strength since every type of drug has its opposite in nature, weakening it and preventing it from full activity. Since the activities of the three [155] make a strong base in treating these diseases, it appears from the combined action of the three, even if weak, that there is a strong effect against disease.

The antidote of the four is useful against poisons. This is for poisons of animals which kill by stinging especially the scorpion and for phlegmatic diseases.

Greek gentian [156]	1 part
Sweet bay grain [157]	1 part
Meccan myrrh	1 part
Long Aristolochia [158]	1 part

All are pulverized, and then kneaded in honey whose froth has been removed. The dose is a *mithqāl.*

Royal cumin electuary for the crumbling of calculi and the cleansing of the urinary organs. Royal cumin is pulverized finely and kneaded in honey. The dose is a *mithqāl.*

Electuary for cleansing of the lungs. Equal parts of blue lily and licorice root are both rubbed, pounded, and sieved, if ripe, and when purity is desired. One may be more than the other according to the desirability of the properties of one or the other. It is kneaded in honey. The dose is a *mithqāl,* more or less, depending on the difference in weights and the condition of the patient in his strength or weakness, and the ripeness of his humors according to their saturation or deficiency.

Electuary for the purification of the intestines from phlegm. Pith of the seed of carthamus [159] and fig are both pounded or their juices [used]. Both are used equally in the mixture. The dose is one ounce.

Electuary for phlegmic coughing. Flax seed [160] is baked well to remove excess moisture, make it viscous, and warm it. It is kneaded with honey.

The confections [161] are like the electuaries except that the latter are sweet and bitter, and spherical or non-spherical. The confections are not the best. The word *jawarishin* comes from the Persian which means "composed" and the best is *jawārishnāt.*

The best is the aloeswood confection. It strengthens the stomach and warms it quite well. It is mixed with a *raṭl* of sugar and two dirhams of pulverized Indian aloeswood. It is placed over a fire. To it are added saffron, clove, cardamom, and so on, one after the other. The sum total is according to the need for it. It may be mixed with lemon rob in a quantity to make it pleasant. Lemon juice may be used instead. It is yellow and pretty.

The fragrances that are used in confections are aloeswood, ginger, [white and black] pepper, clove, lesser cardamom,[162] saffron, cardamom, galingale, Chinese cinnamon, rose, mastix, mace,[163] cubeb,[164] musk,[165] ambergris, cinnamon,[166] malabathrum,[167] lichen,[168] inferior cinnamon,[169] nard, lemon-grass, nutmeg, ironwood tree,[170] thyme, and basil.[171] These are gathered according to the reckoning of necessity for them in the warming of the stomach. It is good for it. It removes the moistness[172] and [aids] the digestion of the excess. Binders may be added to it such as myrtle grain, wild pomegranate flower, tabasheer, and so on. It is gathered with the pulp of quince softened by cooking in syrup or in vinegar, and made viscous with crystalline sugar. Or it is gathered with rob of quince and crystalline sugar. It is spread out on a flat plate and cut up to improve its appearance.

One may add to it, instead of the binders, scammony and turpeth according to the [desired] ratio. They are soaked in the syrup of the compounded [material]; for each of the two of them a syrup [is made]. It is gathered like that and is called purgative quince confection. It is salutary for serious colic.[173] It makes colic disappear and quiets the blood. One may gather that fragrance with honey; it is kneaded like the rest of the electuaries. It is related to every one of those [latter] fragrances and to the successful major confections for the lungs.

Cumin confection. Take cumin, rue,[174] ginger, pepper, and *bauraq*[175] in the ratio required of them according to the condition. When the humors are weak, increase the *bauraq* and add to it wormwood and white [and black] pepper. It is kneaded with honey from which the froth has been removed.[176] The drugs are well pounded. If the condition remains so that the humors are colic and weak, then decrease the *bauraq;* take away the wormwood and instead put in royal cumin if urinary incontinence is present. The drugs are well pounded and kneaded with honey bereft of froth. In it is put black pepper because this is beneficial for urinary incontinence and for diarrhea.[177]

In this method, one thing that is necessary is that the cumin be soaked in vinegar and fried after that. Vinegar is like a corrective and a strengthener.[178] It makes it mild. The confections may be made from the warm binding fragrances which are put with them as myrtle berries to overcome them. It is kneaded with the honey of Tabrazd,[179] known as the "big Khūzī," named after the first [man] who adopted it; it is good for diarrhea of the stomach which has cold humor.

The "small Khūzī" is what is prepared from the fried seed of raisin, myrtle berries, Nabataean carob,[180] [181] pomegranate blossom, tamarisk gallnut, powder of frankincense, and royal cumin prepared by kneading it with honey of Tabrazd or quince rob. It is good for diarrhea with a warm humor if the greatest part of the ingredients is made up of raisin seeds then myrtle berries since they suit the instruments of nutrition.[182] It contains more nutrition and usefulness than other drugs. The powder of frankincense and royal cumin are in the smallest quantities. It may be necessary to increase them so that they will follow the next category in weight when the warmth of the humor is less.

Electuaries may be prepared from stinking, distasteful

drugs for different ailments as colic, pains of the joints, diminution of semen,[183] and others. They are called confections[184] since they soothe the hearts of those who take them. It cannot but have the same effect on some people. It relieves them. If the electuary is to be taken, it should be put in a clay vessel, not full. Some space should be left in which it may rise and expand if it boils and bubbles in fermentation. The top should not be tightened so that no opening is left for the vapors to escape. The clay vessel is placed in barley[185] to keep the heat and to reflect it. It will ferment very well. After the fermentation, when the volume has resumed its original one, it is removed from the barley and the top is tightened. The most preferred containers for electuaries are those which are not affected by them. They are chinaware and what is like them in characteristics[186] and resembles them practically. These are glassware[187] and the ware of metals as gold and silver since they do not rust as other metals do but keep their strengths.[188]

If the electuaries are to stay a long time, their softness, flexibility, taste, and odor are to be safe from opposing conditions, then Allah is omniscient.

Chapter III
Pills and Aperients

On Purgative Pills and Hieras [189] Which Are Purgative Drugs Compounded with Their Correctives to Reduce Ill Effects, to Help in the Easing [of the Condition], and Preparing Medicines That Are Gentle and Flowing.

Iyārij means "noble," and it is meant as a purgative corrective. It is explained as a derived medicine. The reason that purgative medicines are specified as derived is that, although all existing things are from the Blessed and the Exalted, the strength of purgatives is not from the world of creation and nature but from the world of instruction. That is, I mean the use of aperients is more ancient than [the use] of pills.

The ancients used it but were not exposed to the ill effects because of the abundance of correctives and the benefit that is derived from honey in fermentation and mixing. Later, pills were used.

The aperients are easy to store and improve with

time, opposite to pills which are good until they begin to dry up.

The regulations given for using the pills is to gather the purgative[190] drugs in a complete dose. It is assembled with its correctives. The number of purgatives is counted[191] and it is all divided according to this number. If it has two, it becomes two parts [i.e. halves]; three, three parts; four, four parts; five, five parts. Each part is a complete dose. However, we do not have need for all the purgative medicines which are compounded in the pills nor for the same intensity of action all the time. Our needs are sometimes more or less. We must produce a remedy which is complete but if [the drugs] are compounded and then divided by the number of them, then a single dose [should be] active but [may] fall short of our purpose. When the dose is weak, it is unsuccessful. The rest dries, weakens, and disappears. Because of this, we rejected this procedure and abandoned it. We give priority to the prescription which contains a basic remedy. That is the one upon which we rely for our purpose.

We formulate the weights in the dosage according to the exigencies of the situation and the strength required. It is followed by other purgatives for which there may be need, more or less, according to their weights. The minimum dose is three dirhams; the maximum is four. We write the corrective of each one beside it as one fourth of it or one third. If we want to weaken its strength, we mix all of it with bdellium and gum tragacanth[192] if it is included.

It is made into large pills if we want it for the brain and the stomach so that its going down will be delayed; it is made small if we want it for the lower parts and organs so that it will not stay long in the stomach. Thus we have a satisfactory dosage which satisfies our goal and purgates according to our need. I shall write some prescriptions [193] as an example. This is a rule to be followed in whatever is compounded.

There is a pill to cleanse the body of different humors.

Turpeth	1	*mithqāl*
Yellow myrobalan rind	½	dirham
Wormwood	1½	*dāniq*
Agaric	½	dirham
Antiochan scammony [194]	1½	*dāniq*
Indian salt	1½	*dāniq*
Colocynth pulp [195]	1½	*dāniq*
Ginger	1½	*dāniq*
Mastix	1	*dāniq*
Anise	1	*dāniq*
Bdellium	2	*dāniqs*
Gum tragacanth	¼	*dāniq*
Red rose	1	*dāniq*

Another which eases the black bile and phlegm and cleanses the brain.

Turpeth	1	*mithqāl*
Fīqrā aperient [196]	1	dirham
Lavender	2	*dāniqs*
Agaric	½	dirham
Antiochan scammony	1½	*dāniq*
Ginger	1	*dāniq*
Red rose	1	*dāniq*
Bdellium	2	*dāniqs*

The *fīqrā* aperient [acts] as a corrective for the scammony in that it contains the fragrances. When they are together, the corrective is sufficient.

Another which eases yellow bile and is good for the chest.

Grain [197] of violet	2	dirhams
Violet	2	dirhams
Turpeth	1	*mithqāl*
Antiochan scammony	1½	*dāniqs*
Licorice rob	½	dirham

If the turpeth is white, strong,[198] and gummy, it is rubbed very well, pounded and sieved. The first sieving is used. A corrective is not necessary in this pill since the moistness of the violet and its viscidity do to it what almond oil would do. Also the scammony when pulverized with quince juice or with sweet almond oil corrects it especially if it is used in cold pills.

Another which is for pains of the joints

Turpeth	1	dirhàm
Colchicum	1	dirham
Orchis	2	*dāniqs*
Shīramaraj juice [199]	2	*dāniqs*
Indian salt	1½	*dāniqs*
Antiochan scammony	1	*dāniq*
Lesser cardamom [200]	1	*dāniq*
Red rose	1	*dāniq*
Mastix	1	*dāniq*
Bdellium	2	*dāniqs*

Another that is stronger than this.

Turpeth	1	*mithqāl*
Colchicum	½	dirham

Colocynth pulp	1½	*dāniqs*
Indigo grain [201]	1½	*dāniqs*
Aperient	1	dirham
Indian salt	1½	dirham
Ginger	1½	*dāniqs*
Antiochan scammony	1½	*dāniqs*
Rose	1	dirham
Mastix	1	dirham
Anise	1	dirham
Bdellium	2	*dāniqs*

The gum tragacanth and scammony may be omitted from the pills in the case of weakness and for those for whom it may be dangerous. The pills will be effective without harm or the occurrence of strong thirst.

In most pills, turpeth is included as almost an entire dose because of its minimum danger. It eases phlegm, yellow bile, and the thick and thin moistnesses when ginger and others like it are used as assistants.

Pills for asthma [202] which expel dampness from the chest.

Turpeth	1	dirham
Agaric	1	dirham
Aperient	1	dirham
Iris [root] [203]	½	dirham
Scammony	1	*dāniq*
Bdellium	2	*dāniqs*
Violet	½	dirham

Pill of agaric for those who are weak. A *mithqāl* of white, soft, sieved agaric kneaded with honey is made into pills. It is taken before going to sleep.

Pills for acute dropsy. A *mithqāl* of agaric and two *dāniqs* of agrimony are made into pills with honey.

Pill for easing phlegm gently, the turpeth remedy. Two *mithqāls* of turpeth and half a dirham of ginger are made into pills with honey.

Pill for gently easing yellow bile and phlegm. Two dirhams of violet and a *mithqāl* of turpeth are made into pills with rose syrup.

Pill which reduces heaviness. Inhaling it aids digestion and stimulates desire. It is the pill of fragrances.

Mastix	10 dirhams
Cinnamon	10 dirhams
Ginger	10 dirhams
Clove	10 dirhams
Pepper	10 dirhams
Long pepper	10 dirhams
Ironwood [204]	10 dirhams
Scammony	10 dirhams
Sugar	10 dirhams

It is made into pills as large as chick peas from one to two *dāniqs*.[205] One takes one of them and it remains in place, or two and they remain in place [for smelling].

A pill which makes the breath of the mouth agreeable. It is put in the mouth in the morning and evening and its juice swallowed.

Sukk [206]
Clove
Cinnamon

Ginger
Nutmeg
Sweet Cyperus
Nard
Citron rinds
ᶜUdnī[207]

Equal parts are gathered in apricot rob,[208] and made into pills [the size] of chick peas.

Pills of kings for those who dislike purges. It causes vomiting.

Turpeth	1⅔ dirham
Agaric	⅔ dirham
Yellow myrobalan	1½ *dāniq*
Black myrobalan	1½ *dāniq*
Bindweed	½ dirham
Mastix	¼ dirham
Borage[209]	⅙ dirham
Saffron	⅙ dirham
Mint[210]	⅙ dirham
Red rose	⅙ dirham

All are kneaded in rose water[211] and then made into pills.

Important aperients attributed to ancient physicians such as Hermes,[212] Rufus,[213] Galen, and others because they are ancient have gone through the hands of copyists very often and have become varied in mixture. Because of this, they were discarded. Most of the compounded ones which are left are wrong. There are many who are interested in these mixtures and are in favor of their reproduction. They are like miracles of a long time ago which have completely disappeared and their traces effaced with nothing left except the name.

Al-Mutanabbī[214] has a poem:

> "Their works remain after the masters because of cowardice. Perdition may touch them but they are still followed."

For one who wishes to obtain benefit from it [i.e. the compound] and for one who uses it, it must be exposed to the rules of compounding and he must be free in dealing with it accordingly until he attains the right thing. Then he tries it. After that, hoping that Allah made him fit for it and helped him to attain the truth in it and to renew that gifted intelligence[215] to His people—the exalted Allah is the first and last leader and guide.

I have taken *lūghāzujā*[216] aperient according to the written copy and existing medicines. I found a strange matter in what was used in that he used to place them side by side with the three humors, each being distinct from the other. The rule of administering the big aperient is that a dose of it is taken kneaded with a dirham of dough salt and dissolved in a concoction. This is its description: four dirhams of bindweed, ten dirhams of raisins bereft of seeds, seven dirhams of black myrobalan, three dirhams of lavender cooked in a *raṭl* and a half of water until half a *raṭl* is left. Then it is filtered and the aperient is dissolved in it. It is then administered orally. During [an attack of] diarrhea, he [i.e. the patient] should be given honey juice and sugar water. After the diarrhea [has subsided], he is given marshmallow seed and mallow[217] with rosewater and almond oil.

The *fīqrā* aperient, meaning "bitter" is [used] with its correctives since aloe in itself is slow in relief. In its correctives are many whose easing effects become slower. It takes a day or two when administered alone and when not strengthened with other purgatives which give quick relief. Though aloe [218] is mainly to ease yellow bile, it will also ease phlegm. If it is compounded with aromatics and very warm drugs, it eases the phlegm further. Therefore, it is useful for ailments of contagious phlegm and of the brain. These medicines are nine in number: seed of balm of Gilead and its stem, nard, cinnamon, wild ginger, mastix, Chinese cinnamon, saffron and then twice as much aloe as the rest. Latecomers have been free with these. They have added some drugs and substituted some for others depending on their purpose. This is proper if it is administered alone and if put in purgative pills and what is added to it is what the ailment and the patient's condition require, then it has been enriched.

The best liberty taken is when saffron is replaced by red rose to make sure in certain cases that headache and nausea not be caused. If bdellium is added in the weight of one of the correctives of the aloe, harming of the lower part is avoided. Aloe is washed with the juice of endive and dried for those with warm ailments. That which remains of it is made into particles which become weak quickly.[219]

The one kneaded with honey is a stronger and warmer purgative. Its strength remains from six months to four years. It is made into cakes [220] with bdellium and so is safer from danger. The single complete dose is three dirhams.[221]

Chapter IV
Decoctions and Infusions

The decoctions are either soothers or purgatives for the humors, but the soothers are the bases of the warm drugs. They are either roots like those of celery, fennel, iris, caper, marshmallow, licorice, sweet flag,[222] pyrethrum, ginger, costus,[223] leadwort,[224] rhubarb, madder,[225] greater Aristolochia, orchis; or seeds like those of fennel, celery,[226] endive, bishop's weed, rue, wild carrot,[226a] black cumin,[227] caraway,[228] parsley,[229] anise, bastard cumin, dodder,[230] flaxseed, origan of Egypt,[231] fenugreek and cumin; or herbs like thyme,[232] hyssop, thyme, marum,[233] lemon-grass, centaury,[234] maiden hair,[235] nard, origan of Egypt, mountain-mint,[236] borage, and basil (?);[237] or fruits like fig, raisin, date, jujube,[238] sebesten, and others similar to them like honey, sweetmeat, and sugar.

The decoctions are compounded of these to bring the humors to maturity according to their types and kinds, and according to the degree of their coldness, their thickness, and the combination of them.

As to the purgatives of the decoctions, the rule of their

compounding is similar to the rule of compounding pills and aperients depending on the differences between the dose quantities and those of the decoctions. They [the aperients] are more gentle than the former, and softer and lighter on the natures. They are less warm and dangerous, faster in purging, and more proper for delicate matter since the strength of purging medicines is extracted from their matter by water. Thus, their dense bodies are exchanged for a gentle compound [239] which flows in it, in the vessels of the chyme. It attracts it,[240] together with its properties and helps in its purging; purging cleanses. Purging is easy and certain in a short period. After the purging, nothing is left in the body which might be a cause of leaving its symptoms such as depression, nausea, loss of desire, and thirst. Nor does purging return as when parts of the pills from the bodies of the medicines become lodged in the rough surface [241] of the stomach and grooves of the intestines.

Taking it is easier for those who live in ease and for those who cannot swallow unbroken pills and those simple decoctions in which *sārdarūj* [242, 243] is not thrown in. It is good when the humors are little [disturbed] and gentle. It is good when the stomach and brain are full of the windy and vaporous humors; as a whole, it is effective for an easy and light purging.

There are also decoctions which are strengthened by some purging medicines which are pulverized and thrown on it after it has been cooked and filtered at the time of drinking it. It is sought to purge some of the thick humors and for strengthening. The purging drugs are known and retained for those who wish to benefit from them in this formulary with their quantities and the degree of their qualifications and the properties of all in purging all kinds of humors, the specialization of each one of them in the organs, the quantity of each going into a dose in the decoctions, with the knowledge of their correctives.

The decoctions are compounded according to the need for them. For example, if it is desired to prepare a decoction to purge black bile from the entire body, except in case of fevers, it is compounded from Kabul myrobalan, black Indian [myrobalan], dodder, common polypody,[244] and levender. Their weights are adjusted perfectly as I described. Then, the correctives are added to it and whatever assists the purging of the mild [drugs].

One must strive that it be pleasant for the heart and strengthening for the spirit so that the black bile[245] will be freed especially in its movements and its disturbances from its positions. One adds to it mountain-balm, borage, rose, lesser cardamom, and mint. Also that is added which opens ducts and clears blockages such as anise, agrimony,[246] cuscuta, celery seed, fennel, and those which ripen like figs, raisins, licorice root, and whatever concerns the principal organs and which maintain their strength as rhubarb, seed of endive for the liver, and aromatic, fragrant drugs like those previously mentioned for the heart and brain.

That which is solid is pounded. All of it is moistened except the dodder and then left for a night. The next morning, three *raṭls* of water are poured on it and then cooked until it becomes one *raṭl*. It is then filtered while it is boiling. The dodder is mashed well by hand after it has been soaked in very hot water for a night. It is filtered with a piece of cloth and then all of it is gathered and left until clarified. The clear part is decanted. An ounce of cassia pods is dissolved in part of it, then decanted or sieved. In another part, three ounces of *shirbakht*[247] (?) or manna[248] cleaned of thorns and earth[249] is put. It is all put together and drunk in the morning early if the weather is hot, or later in the day if the weather is cold so that the purging may take place at the best and moderate time of the day. Nausea is prevented, if it occurs however, by sucking quince and apple and smelling them. Also one smells rosewater and vinegar which are sprinkled over sun baked clay. Also tarragon [250] and mint are chewed. Both upper arms are tied by a bandage. All this is to calm the soul and to strengthen the natural spirit and gather it, and prevent it from moving upward. The chewing of the quince and sucking its juice after the decocting is good if its action is slow, and also after the pills, if their descent is slow, after their dissolution to strengthen the opening of the stomach,[251] and to squeeze it over it until it pushes the medicine to the lower part of the stomach. The drinking of hot water after taking the decoctions is something which gives it strength by washing it. This is contrary to pills. It makes them fine [in size] and carries them down where they begin their activity. This is the simple decoction.

If it is desired to strengthen it to purge thick black bile also, the following is to be added at the time of drinking: one dirham of sieved agaric which has not been pounded, a *dāniq* and a half of *nafṭi* salt,[252] two thirds of a dirham of emetic earth, a *dāniq* of scammony, and a *dāniq* of mastix. The best is that which is kneaded with a part of the decoction and then dissolved in it. This addition may be administered as pills and is taken two or three hours before the decoction is taken.

If the black bile is caused by burning of the bile, yellow myrobalan is added to the decoction as well as senna, fumitory,[253] and wormwood. If it is caused by burning of the phlegm, emetic earth is added to it as well as belleric myrobalan and emblic myrobalan, and in the *sardārūj*, ginger and aperient. Similarly, if the illness is composed of two or more humors, the decoction is compounded accordingly. If the trouble is rooted in a certain organ, then whatever is good for that organ is added to the decoction, and belongs for it after the common medicine useful for the entire body [is put in].

As an example, if it is taken for pain of the joints, colchicum is put in it, and orchis and cocculus.[254] A superaddition is pulp of colocynth and grain of indigo. If it is taken to clear up the chest, put in it maiden hair, marshmallow seed and its root, hyssop, jujube, sebesten, root of licorice, and raisins. Put myrobalans in it instead of violet, and so on. Also if it is taken for fevers, the myrobalans are thrown into it [for them] as well as to correct and dry the passages after purging. The latter causes narrowness and blockages.

The keynote in treating fevers is the opening of blockages which cause putrefaction of humors. In fevers, there is added whatever purges by loosening by means of violet and fruits like plums,[255] tamarisk, apricot, jujube, and sebesten, and whatever opens blockages as the root of endive and its seed, rhubarb, agrimony, and cuscuta. If it is administered to clear the brain, it is to be drunk with rose syrup. In addition, an aperient is put in. For the stomach there is wormwood; for the spleen, roots of caper; for the liver, the leaf of black nightshade; [256] and so on.

Wormwood is for the intestines to cleanse them of worms, mucus, vitreous moistures, or for the skin to rid it of pimples, or for the kidneys and bladder to rid them of gravel and stones. It may be added to whatever is specific for an organ or for a [general] condition. Each time, something is more, and another is less, it is added or decreased accordingly.

The infusions are gentler than the simple decoctions. It is so in comparison to the simple decoctions as the simple decoctions are to the strengthened decoctions with the *sardārūj*. This is because boiling and cooking make the medicines stronger by drawing out their strength and mixing some of their particles with water to dissolve the fine parts especially of those medicines whose properties are soft and loose. Cooking draws out their strength by dissolving [plants] like dodder and many herbs. If the fineness of their matter and the softness of the composition come to the point where steeping will take up their strength like endive and other similar ones, then strong heat and long cooking are indicated to dissolve their strengths [completely].

The infusion is lighter than the decoction, and also colder. It does not acquire from the heat of the fire what the decoction does. That is why it is more suitable for fevers and hot natures and for well-to-do people who dislike medicines which have bad tastes and odors.

The major requirements for infusions in fevers is to soften the abdomen, lower the temperature, and in other than fever cases to force out [certain] matter gently, little by little.

Of those infusions used for fevers, there are fruit infusions like those of tamarind, plum, medlar,[257, 258] apricot, *Cassia Fistula* L., jujube, sebesten soaked in rosewater, and juice of sour pomegranate oiled and soaked with a like amount of siracost [259] or *taranjubīn* or sugar or rose syrup or violet syrup [260] to the extent of the necessity of sweetness, the sweet and sour state, and sourness. This is the gentlest of all infusions and the best.

The scrapings of *Cassia Fistula* L. may be soaked in the juice of squeezed endive, leaves of black nightshade, and juice of fennel for ailments of the liver.[261]

It is soaked in the juice of fumitory, juice of cuscuta, juice of ivy,[262] and juice of endive for eruptions in hot humors. On it is thrown scammony, violet, and yellow myrobalan to give it strength when necessary.

The infusions are made from drugs that are found in decoctions which are proper in composition according to necessity. If taken, they are soaked in water in a measure equal to the water above it by two or three fingers. During the day, it is put in the sun in a bottle with a stoppered top, at night in straw and felt. It is given to be drunk after three days, after it has been squeezed by hand and filtered through a piece of cloth, strengthened or not strengthened.[263] Aloe is soaked in the extract.

Infusions may be useful to purify the stomach and the brain. For most patients, it is harder to drink the aloe infusion than to bear the illness. If there is no other way, it should be made into pills with each pill coated with treacle.[263a]. It is soaked an hour before infusion.

One may soak mashed turpeth. It is then put in the sun for days until the water takes up its strength. Whatever dissolves in it is mixed with some of its curd, gum, and some of its small particles. Then that water is thickened in the sun so that it becomes very gentle and light in nature and far from being dangerous. The same is done with yellow myrobalan.

Chapter V
Clysters, Suppositories, and Pessaries

The preparation of purging clysters resembles that of the decoctions since they are compounded of purgatives and soothing medicines. The *sardārūj* is thrown on it as with the decoctions but some purgatives do not go into clysters as aloes and the myrobalans. Some of the drugs of clysters do not enter into decoctions—the gentlers and smoothers; they are either softeners used in fevers and swellings of the intestines and dryness of the faeces or they may be taken from things which purge by softening, smoothing, and clearing like violet, marshmallow, thyme,[264] bran, jujube, sebesten, beet,[265] endive leaf, mallow, nenuphar, water-caltrop,[266] flaxseed, licorice root, raisins, and so on.

They are administered with cold damp oils like the oil of violet, oil of nenuphar, almond oil, and sesame oil,[267] with manna and sugar. For cold colic, cabbage,[268] melilot,[269] camomile, and *bauraq* are added to it.

When it is used in cold colic and in similar cold ailments, it is taken from things which purgate by melting and dissolving, and from strong solvents like centaury, rue, southernwood,[270] mint, turpeth, colocynth pulp, violet, melilot, camomile, dill, cauliflower and its leaf, pulp of pounded carthamus, fenugreek,[271] figs and their leaves, raisins, thyme, water-caltrop, hemp [seed],[272] harmel,[237] fennel seed, celery, cumin, anise, marjoram,[274] mashed castor oil plant, and so on. It is administered as a clyster with hot balms like oil of olives, jasmine,[275] yellow gillyflower, bitter almond, oil of the seed [of flax],[276] and also water of honey, sweetmeat, and garum.[277] Turpeth is thrown on it and also pulp of colocynth, Indian salt, opopanax,[278] sagapenum,[279] bdellium, gum ammoniac,[280] and castoreum. These are used according to the need and according to the mildness or severity of the ailment. Also followed are the laws of preparation and the maintenance of the ratios among them.

If [the remedy] is taken for chronic joint ailments, the gentlers are increased such as pyrethrum, ginger, seed of laurel,[281] marum, savin,[282] root of caper, and the purgatives which are specified for it like colchicum and orchis.

For the black bile humors, dodder is added and so on.

If [the drug] is administered for worms, indicated drugs are added as fat, turpeth, Indian salt, natron,[283] juice of the leaves of peaches, that which comes out of the root of mulberry, rinds of pomegranate, special tar,[284] and olive oil.[285]

If [the remedy] is to be used for coldness of wombs and their hardening, then there are added the aromatic drugs as moss,[286] serpolet,[287] nard, and so on with the gentlers and mollifiers.

Such oils are taken as oil of walnut, oil of grain of spurge laurel,[288] the castor oil plant, the olive, the bitter almond, narcissus,[289] and butter. They are administered as a clyster in the beginning and at the end together and with bdellium [290] and so on.

Warm saliva may be administered with these oils for coldness of the kidneys and bladder, and for their hard swellings. In windy colic, it is administered as an enema with balms which calm the wind alone as the oils of rue, jasmine, narcissus, and lily,[291] and with castoreum and those similar to it.

When the humors of the intestines are disturbed or are weak due to coldness, [the remedy] may be administered as a clyster with rose oil and oil of camomile in quantities of ten to twenty dirhams of each of them or both to strengthen the intestines. It may be beet juice and garum to clarify the faeces, and also with the juice of a salt water fish which is called *mānūn*[292] and is found in the breakers.

[The remedy] may be a clyster with salt water only. The enema was first known from a bird with a bent beak which eats so much that he injects sea water from his beak into his rectum. This is when his stomach is full; he continues so until it is emptied.[293]

[In regard to the construction of the clyster], the length of the tube should be that of a small span to a hand span.[294] The width should be equal to that of the small finger. The inside is divided into two parts, a small and a large, their ratios one third and two thirds.[295] The duct of the smaller one allows the air to leave, and the larger permits the clyster solution to enter. The smaller one should not extend to the farthest wide[296] end of the larger but it should be slightly shorter in such manner that when the skin[297] is tied on, the opening of the smaller tube will not interfere with the skin [of the container] but, on the other end, they go together beside each other to the end.[298] The smaller may have another hole on the side of the tube near its top so that the wind may enter into the duct. It may be two holes for if one of them is blocked by something, then the other will take its place. If the large tube has a hole like this, it will be much better and safer [to prevent] obstruction of the enema during the clystering, and the exit will be safeguarded when the straight[299] hole gets something at its entrance or meets compressed matter.[300]

The quantity [of solution] for a clyster is from half to two thirds of a *raṭl*. It is administered lukewarm to warm. The abdomen is given the liquid in such manner that it does not go haphazardly [in any direction]. [The abdomen] should be inclined toward [the site] of the illness and the side of the pain. It may be administered with sticky broths and adhesive balms for fattening[301] the kidneys and for making them lean.

It may be cooked in these broths which are prepared from semolina,[302] and heads, feet, and testicles of roosters, and chick peas—the splendid medicines. To these are added warm balms and then one clysters with it for sexual impotency due to coldness.

Clysters may be prepared by decocting constipating grains as common millet, rice,[303] shelled lentils, and porridge or fried barley in which have been cooked some of the constipating drugs like acorn,[304] gallnut, and pomegranate blossom.

[There is] one clyster with about forty dirhams of it, tending toward lukewarm and thickened with the yolk of a boiled egg in vinegar dissolved in rose oil in the scrapings of intestines after there have been thrown on it gum and starch, both fried, Armenian bole,[305] acacia,[306] ceruse of lead[307]—about three dirhams collected in proportion, and pulverized.

If blood comes from a sore, then a quantity equal to the yolk of the egg is broiled in rose oil until dry. To the dry drugs, there are added yellow amber, burned coral, ashes of papyrus plant, fine powder of frankincense, and dragon's blood plant. If the pain is severe, some opium is mixed with it and a little violet.

For a gentle clyster.

Violet and bran are wrapped together, and white marsh-mallow—unbroken or wrapped,[308] nenuphar—of each a handful, gruel mix of barley[309]—a handful, beet leaves and ivy—of each a bunch, sebesten—twenty in number, figs from Bust[310]—five in number, and jujube—ten in number, are cooked in a *raṭl* of water until one third of a *raṭl* is left. It is filtered and used in a clyster with an ounce each of mucilage of fleawort,[311] balm of vinegar, red sugar,[312] and garum.

A strong clyster.

Centaury	3	dirhams
Fenugreek	1	handful
Mashed core of Carthamus	1	handful
Flaxseed	1	handful
Melilot	1	ounce
Camomile	1	ounce
Rue	1	bundle
Cauliflower and its leaf	1	bundle
Beet leaves	1	bundle
Mountain-mint	1	bundle
Bruised violet	½	ounce
Cumin	1	handful
Fennel seed	1	handful
Figs	10	

All are cooked in five *raṭls* of water until it is reduced to

two *raṭls*. It is then filtered. Two-thirds of a *raṭl* is used in a clyster with the following to strenthen it.

Pulp of colocynth	1½	*dāniqs*
Scammony	1½	*dāniqs*
Indian salt	1½	*dāniqs*
Bauraq	1	dirham
White turpeth	1	dirham
Sagapenum	⅔	dirham
Opopanax	⅔	dirham
Bdellium	⅔	dirham
Fānīd confection	1	ounce
Jasmine oil	1	ounce
Garum	1	ounce

The laxative suppositories which are used to soften the abdomen in colic, the rest of the intestines, and whatever follows are like clysters in softness and severity. Their relation to the purgative clysters is like that of the purgative pills to the purgative decoctions. They are as long as the length of a finger or more so that they may fall into the straight intestines. It is so that the effect will reach to the colon [313] if one desires to treat colic.

If [the remedy] is taken for the ailment of the thigh and the sciatic nerve, it is made into rounded pessaries [314] so that it may remain for a long time in a location near the ailment.

As to the soft ones used in fevers, the softest, coldest, and simplest is the sourmilk [recipe].[315] It is [made from] water of coagulated milk and *nāṭifā* which is made from red sugar if a little pulverized salt is thrown on it at the time of thickening. The "excrement of the mouse" is mixed with *nāṭifā*. All of these may be mixed and strengthened with pulverized Armenian *bauraq*. Marshmallow and violet may be added, both pulverized. It may be administered when the intestines and faeces are dry. The most effective suppository is made with butter firmly frozen in snow.

The strongest of all is the suppository of violet. Its preparation: take five dirhams each of violet, red sugar, and *rikhbīn*; and three dirhams each of scammony, turpeth, and *bauraq*. The latter three are stronger in action and in effect in comparison with the former three so that their quantity is reduced and the others increased. There is also two dirhams of Indian salt. The quantity of salt is reduced since the two reasons for reduction are present; these are the excess of strength and the presence of drugs in the compound which carry out its activity and resemble it in usefulness. Less is administered if all four of them are very strong. Its use is lessened in comparison with it, i.e. the force of purgation. The sugar and *rikhbīn* are dissolved. The drugs are sprinkled on them and made into suppositories.[317]

Acidity is needed in cold colic, for heating the back, and in purging phlegm from its places. The strongest and fastest in purging is soap[318] especially that of Raqqa. If a suppository is made from it, then use it. Or [the soap] is mixed with *fānīd* confection and honey over a fire, and on it are sprinkled pulverized salt, *bauraq*, turpeth, ginger, pulp of colocynth, scammony, and other purgatives similar to these.

The remedy to break the winds resembles black cumin, cumin, castoreum, and others. Or [this remedy] is mixed with hot gums like opopanax, sagapenum, gum ammoniac, and bdellium in the ratio necessary according to the rules of compounding.

Acidic suppository which breaks colic.

Sagapenum
Opopanax
Bdellium
Gum ammoniac
Indian salt
Pulp of colocynth
Bauraq
Scammony
Grain of indigo

[All] are gathered in equal quantities since they are equal to each other in strength and usefulness. The gums are dissolved with juice of rue. The rest is pounded, sieved, and added. It is made into a suppository. One may add to it the shelled seed of the castor oil plant and the *fānīd* confection. It may be mixed with the gall of a cow when it is necessary to acquire more strength and sharpness.

For treatment of the hip.[319]

Cocculus[320]
Turpeth
Sarcocol[321]
Ginger
Root of sow bread[322]
Galbanum
Colchicum
Orchis
Castoreum

One may make a suppository of castoreum and opium in equal quantities to quiet the pain of colic.

Strong suppositories may be taken to warm the kidneys. They are composed of dates, *fānīd* confection, warm pulps, and seeds which give heat.

Constipating suppositories are used to strengthen the stomach and the straight intestines to hold the faeces. Compound [the following]:

Acorn
Pomegranate blossom
Acacia
Tamarisk gall
Sorghum [323]
Rice
Gum

Taken for irritation of the intestines and dysentery.

White lead
Gum arabic
Dragon's blood plant [324]
Saffron
Frankincense
Myrrh
Lycium [325]

When the pain is acute, one may add opium to it. Care should be taken when it is used especially in weakness. It is not used except with acute pain and then only in the needed quantity or less. It is then settled inside in such a way that it does not affect the upper part of the body but in the hope that it will act quickly in calming the pain. This is done by stupefying the feelings and putting the patient to sleep by discharging the spirit which is unwanted.

The preferable way and the best to administer it is to tie it with a string so that it may be extracted when the pain decreases. It may be taken as a pessary or as a suppository to cause the menstruum or hemorrhoids to flow or to block them.

Those which cause flowing and widen the openings of veins.

Root of cyclamen
White hellebore [326]
Mountain-mint [327]
Agaric
Sagapenum

These are gathered together in equal quantities since they are alike in sharpness and strength. They are kneaded with onion juice [328] since it is similar to what is desired. It is administered.

Those which cause retention and which close the openings of those veins.

Kuḥl
Gallnut
Alum
Acacia
Borax [329]
Frankincense
Pomegranate blossom

These drugs are all related in action to each other so that their quantities should be made equal. This is for all except the frankincense because of its warmth. These are all mixed together with gum arabic and made into small suppositories like the seed of the service tree.[330]

Some things that are administered before the pessary will help pregnancy. These are from aromatics, perfumes, gums, and others.

These may be taken as suppositories for worms of the abdomen: pulp of colocynth, kamala,[331] grain of indigo, wormwood,[332] absinth, bitter apricot seed with juice of the leaf of the peach tree[333] dissolved in aloes.

Chapter VI
Emetics

There are many kinds of emetics. One kind causes vomiting of yellow bile and another type is for the black bile.

Those emetics for yellow bile are types of food. They are barley juice, cucumber, and watermelon[334] both ripe in their pulp, broth of soft vegetables like orache,[335] spinach,[336] cultivated mauve,[337] blite, beet leaf, broth of chicken, lamb's feet, fresh fish, soup which is rich with vinegar oil, and manna.

Then there are those which include oxymel, barley water in which kidney beans[338] were cooked, rinds of watermelon and its roots which are pulled and cut,[339] and also the desiccated pulp of the watermelon, beer made from barley flour, seed of orache, and seed of watermelon.

That which causes phlegm to be vomited may be a kind of food as the froth of *kishk* like the *kishk* of wheat with dill, broth of cooked turnip,[340] cooked carrots,[341] cooked radish, cooked fenugreek, oil of Carthamus seed, *ṭarīkh* fish, vinegar sauce[342] like garum, sour infusion of caper, mustard dye,[343] raw olive oil, and honey.

Or, the [emetic] drugs may be honeyed oxymel, onion oxymel with radish juice and aneth juice, and borax, the heart of Carthamus, seed of radish, Indian salt, mustard, and the strength of the white hellebore [344] obtained by its insertion in the radish and then left for one night and removed, and then the radish solution is taken.

That which causes the vomiting of the black bile may be a kind of food like *asfīdbā* and *zirbā*, honey water, and anything which is gentle and is properly dislodging.

Those which are the drug type are honeyed oxymel, honey water, vinegar of caper, sweet wine, emetic resin,[347, 348] *nafṭī* salt, yellow turpeth, and borax. Each of these kinds is used when needed to cast out each of the humors separately. If the humors are compounded, then these kinds are compounded. The edible ones are given priority; then the drugs are prepared according to their need and given to be drunk afterward. The exception to this procedure is if these humors are absorbed by the stomach or they are very thick and viscous. In that case, the drugs are given priority over the edible ones. Certain strong emetics like hellebore, struthion,[349] Mafura of Yemen,[350, 351] and pellitory [352] have been dropped out of use in our time. Whoever wishes to use them must prepare the body and mixture first by wetting the chest and intestines with soft and sweet soup so that they may accept expansion at the height of the movement of vomiting and to yield at that time, to dislodge the humors, to make them gentle by soothers, and quickly to ease their exit.

It is used according to need by those who have the habit of vomiting and whose nature is accustomed to it. The best time for it is in the summer.[353]

A drug which causes the vomiting of phlegm

Aneth seed	1 dirham
Emetic resin	1 dirham
Yellow turpeth	½ dirham

Another [drug which causes vomiting of phlegm].

Borax	1 dirham
Indian salt	1 dirham
Radish seed	2 dirhams

Emetic for black bile.

Barley water	1 *raṭl*
Orache juice	2 ounces
Watermelon root	1 ounce
Cucumber root	1 ounce
Dough salt	1 dirham

It is to be drunk with oxymel and oil of *bakhtaj*.[354]

Another.

Emetic resin	1 dirham
Manna	3 dirhams

They are gathered together and made into pills.

To vomit black bile.

Indian salt	1 dirham
Yellow turpeth	1 dirham
Borax	1 dirham
Khark[355]	1 dirham

Chapter VII
Lohochs

Lohochs are moist having a viscosity like thin sweet jelly. They are taken from a spoon held in the mouth. Whatever dissolves from it is taken little by little to lengthen the period of its passage near the trachea. This is so that it penetrates into it and the lungs by filtering through. It causes gentle flowing of the moistures and adjusts them. [The remedy] removes hoarseness of the voice organs and the breathing and whatever follows it.

Some of them are cold and used to soothe hoarseness when dry coughing occurs, and for intense delicate colds so that it is mixed with them to reduce their acuteness. As for the effectiveness, they provide for the prevention of and take care of swollen conditions. For this, there are the cold mucilages.[356] The mucilaginous and oily matters are such as fleawort, seed of quince, seed of marshmallow, violet [seed], seed of purslane,[357] [seed of] the two cucumbers, lettuce [seed], poppy [seed], mallow [seed], pumpkin seed, almond, and peeled sesame [seed] and their oils, jujube, sebesten, starch, gum [arabic], gum tragacanth, licorice rob, heart of pudding-pipe tree, manna, and so on.

Some are warm and are used to ripen moistnesses, to make them milder, to cut them down, and to get rid of them. These are hyssop, iris, pine [cones], bitter almond, bitter vetch,[358] maiden hair, thyme, pepper, long pepper, root of licorice, saffron, honey, flax seed, fenugreek, and the heart of the cotton seed,[359] squill,[360] dates, figs, raisins, honey, *fānīd* sweetmeat, and so on. It is compounded according to need, especially according to the cough and the particular humors. So the lohochs are prepared. The rules and regulations are retained [in compounding] if the single drugs are not capable of expelling the dangers alone.

Cold lohoch for dry coughing, fever and acute cold in the chest and lungs.

Ten dirhams of the heart of sweet almond, five dirhams each of seeds of cucumber, large cucumber,[361] pumpkin, Jewish mauve, lettuce, four dirhams each of gum tragacanth and starch, three dirhams of poppy seed. All are pulverized and gathered with fifty dirhams of manna dissolved in the juice of Indian watermelon, gummed and made viscous after that, and twenty dirhams of sweet almond oil. The poppy may be added to it when strongly needed to prevent cold. The dose is from five dirhams to an *istār*.[362]

A lohoch which cleanses.

Pine cones	40 dirhams
Shelled bitter almond	45 dirhams
Licorice rob	25 dirhams

[All are mixed with] honey in the required quantity.

Purging lohoch for phlegm.

Ten [dirhams] each [of] flaxseed, bitter vetch, and shelled sweet almond, five [dirhams of] pine cone,[363] seven [dirhams of] powder [364] of crushed peeled lily root, three [dirhams] each of gum and gum tragacanth. These are taken as a lohoch with manna or with crystalline sugar according to the need.

The main purpose of the purging lohoch is that the purge of the bitter almond is exchanged for the sweets, honey, manna,[365] sugar, licorice rob—its dust [sieved part], and a little pine cone. It is gathered in gum and gum tragacanth in contrast to the cleansing lohoch.

This example should be followed and repeated in the rest of the compounded [remedies]. It should be known that getting rid of thick matter from the chest in a coughing ailment cannot be attained by soothers and cleansing agents alone and without mixing them with those which smear and smooth to quiet down the cough. The trachea is coated and whatever follows it.

[The remedy] is prepared by making the important one dominant over the other so that when the humor [of phlegm] is too much and too thick but the coughing is in a measure which does not require too much care, then a strong cleanser is given to [the patient to] drink like iris and agaric compounded with honey and honeyed oxymel. However, if the coughing is severe and continuous but the humor [of phlegm] is not so great and so thick, he is given smoothers which contain the smallest amount of cleanser as flaxseed mucilage, [mucilage] of fenugreek, rob of licorice, "milk" of figs, and grape syrup mixed with gum of the plum, gum tragacanth, and so on. If both of the conditions are the same, then [the oppositely acting drugs] are made equal. Allah knows the truth best.

Chapter VIII
Lozenges

Lozenges are compounded substances prepared for many purposes. It is not expected that they be stored, as are confections, for a long time. They are compounds which, it is expected, will be used immediately and should not be stored long for the future since their strength is quickly lost. They are also affected by changes of the air which enters into them.

Some of them are cold. They are prepared for the hot humor and acute fevers. They are made from seed of endive, lettuce, the two cucumbers, purslane, rose, nenuphar, violet, barberry, sandal, tabasheer, camphor and so on.

Some are hot. These are for opening of the obstruction of the intestines and its hardness as well as for swellings. They are prepared from anise, fennel, nard, mastix, lemon-grass, agrimony, absinth, cuscuta, rhubarb, *lukk*, and so on.

Then there are those which are both hot and cold. They are used in chronic fevers and compounded fevers.

Some of them are lozenges which arrest the blood and constipate the abdomen. . . .[366] is for internal wounds.

We shall write of each kind of lozenge according to its medium, for example, camphor lozenge. This is for acute fevers and heart palpitation with fever. Tabasheer, rose, white sandal, two cucumbers, endive, lettuce, and cultivated mauve in equal parts are gathered and pulverized. With each *mithqāl* of the mixture, half a *ṭassūj* to a *ṭassūj* of camphor is mixed. A grain to a half carat[367] in the weight necessary is kneaded with juice of apples and made into thin lozenges and dried in the shade. They are guarded from being spoiled. The dose is a *mithqāl*.

Again, take sandalwood, rose, tabasheer with their fine seeds,[368] equally since each one of the two classes requires more—one for the abundance of its benefits, and the other for the weakness of its strength. Therefore, the weights are made equal and the camphor is very little because of its strength.

Pearl may be added to it and [then the lozenge] is named for it.

Rhubarb lozenge for cold livers and obstructions in them.

Nard	2 dirhams
Mastix	2 dirhams
Extract of agrimony	2 dirhams
Absinth	2 dirhams
Seed of fennel	2 dirhams
Anise	2 dirhams
Rhubarb	10 dirhams

All are made into a lozenge of [the weight] of one *mithqāl*.

The dose is one. The rhubarb in the liver lozenge is like rose in the stomach lozenge in quantity since this one is specialized for the liver and the other for the stomach. It is like the Vitex[369] in the Vitex lozenge for diseases of the spleen. So take that into account and follow this analogy.

Vitex lozenge for the spleen with accompanying fever.

Vitex	10 pieces of fruit
Tamarisk berries	10
Endive seed	5 dirhams
Cultivated mauve	5 dirhams

All are made into lozenges of three dirhams.

Aloes lozenges for vomiting and diarrhea with coldness.

Frankincense	3 [dirhams]
Rose	6 [dirhams]
ᶜŪdnī	1 dirham
Clove	1 dirham
Sukk	1 dirham
Nard	1 dirham
Isfahan clay[370]	1 dirham
Tabasheer	1 dirham
Cubeb	2 dirhams

[All] are made into lozenges of a *mithqāl* each.

Another for the same thing with hot humor

Tabasheer	1 dirham
Rose	1 dirham
Sumach	3 [dirhams]

Prepared cumin	1	dirham
Coriander soaked in vinegar and fried	2	dirhams
Rind of pistachio[370a]	½	dirham
Mastix	3	[dirhams]
Sūbaq wine[371] of pomegranate seeds	2	dirhams

All are made into four lozenges.

Rose lozenge to strengthen the stomach.

Red rose	10 dirhams
Licorice rob	2 dirhams
Indian nard[372]	1 dirham
Mastix	1 dirham

Another for phlegmatic fever.

Three (?) each of seed of endive, rose,[373] and borage, and a *mithqāl* of agrimony. It is made into lozenges with licorice rob. One may add also anise, bindweed, fennel seed, licorice root, and others.

Whoever notices the differences [in amounts] among these prescriptions and the frequency of them in the *aqrābādhīn*,[374] sees the variations among them, and that each kind is taken for a definite ailment, will realize then that the differences occur because of the variations in the state of the illness. The latter would be in the acuteness, weakness, sharpness, and chronicity; and the variations [among the prescriptions] in the quantity of heat and cold, the state of thickness, gentleness, whether it be compounded or simple, and excessive. It is also according to the different conditions of the patient in strength and weakness, the periods of his sickness to excess,[375] the beginning, decline, and end, and the accidents which happen to the patient during the illness.

The ancients were obliged to prepare different prescriptions for a patient having an ailment each time every day and every hour according to the particular occurrence or disappearance of a symptom. [A patient's] morale is encouraged [by this procedure]. [The physician] adds and subtracts from the prescription according to what he sees fitting. He compounds whatever he wants with an open mind freely, following the rules and regulations.

Rose lozenge is a good useful remedy for stomach ailments especially when [the patient] is weak because of chronic and compound fevers. These are because the stomach has been weakened.[376] [The ailment] does not disappear unless [the stomach] is made strong and its condition is improved. The ratio of rose needed to strengthen the stomach in fevers since it is useful in this condition is like the ratio of the myrobalans to it with no fevers attendant. It is as if the myrobalans are a yeast. The basis for the myrobalans is like that for the rose lozenges. It is so made that the dose of it contains a dirham of rose.

The first thing which must be added to the rose and mixed with it is the licorice root and nard according to the ratio of a half to a fourth. Thereafter, its prescriptions vary according to the differences in fevers. Sometimes more cold medicines promote flowing; sometimes more of the hot are included according to necessity.

Constipating lozenges are made from drugs which thicken the flow of the yellow bile and prevent the flow of phlegm. This is useful for relaxing which occurs in the alimentary organs and arrests the blood. It is useful for sticky itching and to heal wounds.

Those which aid the flowing of yellow bile, very cold constipation, and thin the thick humors are sandalwood, camphor, dry coriander, poppy, seed of lettuce, tabasheer, seed of henbane, rose, wine of pomegranate blossom, grapes, sumach, seed of sorrel,[377] pomegranate blossom, barberry, seed of cultivated mauve, and others.

Those which are good for easing phlegm and all hot obstructions are very dry like frankincense, bishop's weed, cumin prepared with vinegar, sweet Cyperus, rhubarb, and all hot aromatics. It is mixed with strong constipating drugs like pomegranate blossom, acorn, acacia, tamarisk berry, prepared scoria of iron, carob, seed of myrtle, and raisin seed.

Hot seeds which cause flowing are those of bindweed, cumin, and anise. They enter into these remedies to direct the moistness to the urinary organs especially if there are blockages.

Those good for arresting the blood are taken from yellow amber, coral, hematite,[378] sea shells, burned horn of deer, acacia, mimosa,[379] cynomorium, gum, tabasheer, Armenian bole, clay, pomegranate blossoms, seed of henbane, *lukk,* gum tragacanth, and all cold constipators and stickers.

Those good for [colitis] are sticky ones as gum, starch, clay,[380] and all mucilaginous seeds if roasted until sticky.

Those good for internal wounds are sticky ones mixed with healers like frankincense, dragon's blood plant, and others.

Tabasheer lozenges that ease yellow bile with fever.

Red rose	10	[dirhams (?)]
Tabasheer	10	[dirhams (?)]
Sorrel seed	5	[dirhams (?)]
Cleansed sumach [381]	5	[dirhams (?)]

Seed of cultivated mauve	5	[dirhams (?)]
Pomegranate blossom	2	dirhams
Gum arabic	1½	dirhams

They are made into lozenges of two dirhams.

Yellow amber lozenges to ease the blood.

Red rose	3	[dirhams (?)]
Gum arabic	3	[dirhams (?)]
Yellow amber	3	[dirhams (?)]
Starch [382]	2	dirhams
Armenian bole	2	dirhams
Coral [383]	2	dirhams
Tabasheer	2	dirhams
Licorice rob	2	dirhams
Pomegranate blossom	2	dirhams
Acacia	1½	dirhams

All are kneaded in rob of myrtle. The dose is a *mithqāl.*

Coral lozenges for spitting of blood

Gum arabic	5	[dirhams (?)]
Armenian bole	5	[dirhams (?)]
Yellow amber	1½	dirhams
Hematite	1½	dirhams
Licorice rob	2	dirhams
Starch	2	dirhams
Dragon's blood	2	dirhams
Henbane	1	dirham
Chinese cinnamon	1	dirham

[All are mixed] and made into lozenges of three dirhams each. Since the destination of the remedy is distant, seed of henbane and Chinese cinnamon are put in it so that one of them will retain the strength of the medicine holding it up to quiet the cough which is the cause of the spitting of blood. The other makes it penetrate so that it reaches the farthest destination.

Alkekengi lozenge that is effective in kidney and bladder wounds. It has properties of being adhesive, softening, and closing the wound. It reduces the severity of pain and burning while urinating.

Seed of cucumber	10 [dirhams (?)]
Seed of alkekengi [384]	10 [dirhams (?)]
Shelled sweet almond	10 [dirhams (?)]
Licorice rob	10 [dirhams (?)]
Starch	10 [dirhams (?)]
Gum tragacanth	10 [dirhams (?)]
Armenian bole	10 [dirhams (?)]
Gum arabic	10 [dirhams (?)]
Dragon's blood plant	10 [dirhams (?)]
Fresh frankincense	10 [dirhams (?)]
Celery seed	2 dirhams
Opium	1 dirham

They are made into lozenges of three dirhams. The dose is given with violet syrup, celery seed, and opium in a formula which resembles the Chinese cinnamon and henbane [one] in the coral lozenges and for the same reason.

Colitis lozenges.

Red rose	3 [dirhams (?)]
Fried sorrel seed	3 [dirhams (?)]

Fried gum	1½ dirhams
Starch	1½ dirhams
Tragacanth	1½ dirhams

These are made into lozenges with mucilage of fleawort in the size of two *mithqāls*. It is drunk with myrtle rob.

Chapter IX
Powders and Dry Stomachics

Medical powders are compounded according to the weights of their constituents only and not according to their strengths. In their admixture, another mixture is formed. For that reason they are used immediately and for what is mentioned. Another reason is the rapid deterioration [of the powders] because of softness and instability.[385] Most drugs that are used in medical powders are the dry astringent medicines. They are taken by mouth to dry the moistness of the stomach and the intestines. They relieve blockage and retention of urine. Others may be taken as various drugs or powders.[386] But those [powders] taken to astringe the belly and to dry the stomach and intestines and the constipating lozenges are the same as if the latter had not been made into lozenges but taken as powders.

Constipating powders include the stems like those of barley, wheat, rice, and sorghum; Christ's thorn,[387] azarole, service tree, Syrian carob, quince, apple, sumach, barberry, myrtle berries, carob, poppy with its rind,[388] pomegranate, pear,[389] acorn, hard pips of raisins, seed of cultivated mauve, gum arabic,[390] dates, and sugar cane.[391] Gathered with these stems are the stem of *kaᶜk*[392] and white *kaᶜk*. It is sweetened a little with pulverized crystalline sugar and taken as a powder for moistness of the stomach and its deterioration and to give relief.

Clay powder that is useful for abrasions caused by choleric diarrhea.

Twenty dirhams of fleawort; ten each of seed of plantain, cultivated mauve, and grand basil;[393] thirty dirhams each of gum arabic and Armenian bole are taken. The seeds are roasted and the clay pounded. The gum is not made very fine so that it will not slip away from the lining. The seeds are dampened so that the clay and gum will stick. The seed of cultivated mauve is pulverized with the rest but the seed of grand basil and plantain are not pulverized because their stickiness is desired and this will disappear with pulverizing. If pulverized, the fleawort will not be harmed. All are gathered and then three dirhams are administered in the late morning and evening. To swallow, [the dose]is assisted by quince juice or its rob.

Cress[394] powder for the scraping [of linings], fever, and colic.

Fleawort, myrrh, sorrel seed, white poppy seed, seed of purslane, myrtle berry, gum arabic, and Armenian bole in equal parts [are taken]. The seeds except those of sorrel are fried. Sorrel is not since it is not mucilaginous. They are fried[395] until their mucilage becomes sticky and there is not too much dampness so that they may be drier. All are pulverized except fleawort which would cause sharpness [pain] in the belly, and all except seed of myrrh since what is desired [of it] is its external layer. The thick mucilage [when dried] is taken as a powder with the help of quince rob or rob of myrtle if there is coughing.

Seed powders for urine that burns.

Thirty dirhams of shelled seed of watermelon, ten dirhams each of shelled seed of cucumber, of pumpkin, of cultivated mauve, and of poppy; three each of starch, gum tragacanth, and rob of licorice; two dirhams of seed of henbane; and sugar equal to all. Three dirhams of it is taken as a powder in the late morning with violet syrup and rosewater.

Powders which help retain the urine in cases of urinary incontinence without [causing] burning or extreme thirst.

Acorn	50 dirhams
Frankincense	30 dirhams
Dry coriander	10 [dirhams]
Armenian bole	10 [dirhams]
Gum arabic	10 [dirhams]

Three dirhams of it is taken as a dose in the late morning and evening.

Another for the same thing.

Equal parts of cumin, frankincense, myrtle berries, and acorn [are taken]. The dose is three dirhams.

Colchicum powder.

One dirham of colchicum,[396] two dirhams of violet, a *dāniq* and a half each of orchis, cocculus, and scammony, a *dāniq* of anise, a *dāniq* of red rose, and double the amount of all of them of sugar [are taken]. Allah knows best.

Chapter X
Dressings, Coatings, and Cataplasms

Dressings are compounded remedies which have the consistency of electuaries. They are put on exposed members and made to adhere to them. The coatings are thinner in consistency in such a way that if the members are anointed with them, they stick and spread over the surfaces. They do not need to be bandaged or bound on. Coatings are gentler and faster in penetrating and dissolving. The dressings are thicker and more of it stays on the member. They retain the heat longer. That is why they are used mostly for dissolving and ripening.[397]

The cataplasms are either wet or dry. The wet ones are like bladders which are filled with hot water or cloths which are saturated with hot water, then put on the members to warm them and to wet them. With these liquids, medicines may be boiled. Some are relaxants and resolvents like marshmallow, aneth, mallow, melilot, camomile,[398] violet, marjoram, and so on. With these cooked drugs themselves, a cataplasm may be made.

The dry cataplasms are like heated salt, sand, common

millet,[399] bran, ashes, and so on; they are heated and put on the members to warm and dry them. All cataplasms are used to quiet pain. The dry one is better for rheumatic pains and cold matter. The wet one is preferred for stinging pain and sharp matter[400] since, in addition, it opens the pores, dissolves the painful humor, and quiets the sharpness of matter. It makes the member soft and conducive to the distribution of matter so as to hold it and not give it up. In this way [the member] is not injured.

It is prepared from hot drugs and aromatics like cinnamon, wild ginger,[401] lichen, clove, Chinese cinnamon, cardamom, saffron, and so on. The dry cataplasm is pulverized, heated [when] put into a container, and applied to the member. It is used mainly in treatment of the uterus and stomach, for flatulence and the cold humor.

Dressings and coatings are taken from all kinds of drugs for all the types of external and internal ailments or most of them. The exception is the use of the wax and oil mixture. This is specialized and goes under the name of plaster.

Coatings used in warm swellings.

They are made from the two sandalwoods, areca nut,[402] horned poppy,[430] rose, camphor in vinegar, rose water, juice of coriander, and lettuce.

If it is for the liver, it is black nightshade, juice of endive, and juice of quince.

If it is for the spleen, then it is tamarisk berry and borax.

If it is for the chest, use violet, marshmallow, barley

flour, and some soft inhibitors.

If it is for the bladder, a wax and oil mixture is used.

The nerve organs should not be cooled nor should the coatings be devoid of soft matter. The coatings of the important and main members should not be without binding elements and aromatics. There is a special coating suitable for every member such as drugs like colchicum in coatings for the joints, and flours [404] and coriander in swellings of pustules, and lycium in the ointments of ophthalmia, and acacia, lentils, and coriander in swelling of the bloody [matters] and skin of puffy pustules, and plantain [405] in choleric swelling.

The drugs used in coatings of cold swellings are those such as Jewish mauve, camomile, marjoram, southernwood, marshmallow, and dill.

Then, if [the ailment] is in the liver, there are added nard, rhubarb, saffron, myrrh, and so on.

Or, if in the spleen, then there are added rue, borax, gum ammoniac, mountain mint, and root of caper.

Or, in the stomach, there are added mastix, cinnamon, costus, dodder, and lemon grass.

Or, in the testicles or the two breasts, there are added to it cumin, flesh of raisins, flour of fenugreek, and flaxseed.

Or in the rectum, there are added bdellium, camel's hump, marrow fats, and greases.

For whatever is known of ointments for swelling of nervous organs, the neck or types of scrofula, there are added iris, pitch and so on. Every kind of swelling is treated with the ointment which belongs to it as salt, ashes, borax, vinegar, and sweet Cyperus in loose swellings; rue, savin, and cypress[406] in rheumatic swelling; and white lead, washed tutty,[407] juices of cold vegetables, and mucilage for cancer.

As for the ripening of abscesses, this is done by soft, sticky coatings like flaxseed, fenugreek, figs, yeast,[408] and so on.

Constipating coatings are used in diarrhea and include drugs such as myrtle leaves, pomegranate rind, pomegranate blossoms, acacia, myrrh, *rāmik*,[409] frankincense, *kaᶜk* biscuit, sweet Cyperus with the juice of bitter quince, and juice of the ends of vines.[410] In fever, this poultice should not be used since it blocks the pores and retains the heat so that it increases fever.

Those which ease the belly and kill worms are such as indigo seed, cherry seed,[411] borax, black cumin, turpeth, lupine,[412] pulp of colocynth, mezereon,[413] wormwood, scammony, and aloe.

If an application is made with juice of the leaf of the peach, absinth, harmel, and gall of the cow, then this has more effect on children, and likewise for the softness of their skin and for the penetration of the strengths of the drugs to their intestines. Their bellies should be anointed with it and [the skin] covered by thin paper in order that it not penetrate their skin to hurt them.

Those applications which dry the fluid in dropsy and where there is edema in the testicles include sheep dung, cow dung, sweet Cyperus, borax, barley flour, ashes of spadices of the palm tree, and ashes of sea-shells in vinegar.

The application for a fracture, dislocation, and a bruise is made from wild promegranate, cypress, myrtle, flour of the mungo bean,[414] lentil, Armenian bole, acacia, the two sandalwoods, areca nut, glaucium, *būsh,*[415] and marshmallow. It is applied for hot and cold headaches with the applications for hot and cold swellings.

For hot and stupefying things, these are [drugs] such as leaves of poppy, lettuce, mandrake,[416] henbane, and opium. If the pain is severe and cold, then there are castoreum, musk, aloe, euphorbium when there is need for them.

Ointments for skin diseases and their coatings.

For whatever may be attached to the hair, nails, or skin, one uses something which goes with olive oil to make it clear like asphodel,[417] mustard,[418] soapwort, euphorbium, jelly-fish,[419] burned bark of the fig tree, black cumin, thapsia,[420] sesame oil, vinegar, arsenic,[421] *nafṭ,*[422] *qunābarā,*[422a] and so on.

Applications for a scab and an ulcer [on the head].

They are compounded of a hot polisher and a cold obstruent, and something soft and damp for attraction, clearing, for the prevention and removal of the sharpness [of pain],[423] for softening the skin, and moistening the humor. Therefore, there are many of these compounded remedies. They are diversified according to these purposes and the dissimilarities in the need of them according to the humors and their kinds. They are then unknowable [in advance] and infinite [in number]. All are agreeable to anything when put on the proper place.

Application for ringworm.

Aloe	1 dirham
Myrrh	1 dirham
Lycium	1 dirham
Saffron	2 *dāniqs*

Application for hemorrhage of the nose.

Shelled lentils, marshmallow, sandal, an eye collyrium, pure potter's clay, and a little camphor [are gathered]. The forehead is anointed with myrtle juice.

Application for apoplexy.

Mustard and castoreum are pounded with vinegar and applied.

Application for the neck.

Mastix, shell of frankincense, cypress nut and its leaf, myrrh,[424] savin, sarcocol, asphodel,[425] and fish glue [are taken] in equal parts. The glue is dissolved in vinegar and collected with it are seed of lettuce, opium, and mandrake. It is daubed on the forehead. The poppy used is cooked. Allah knows best.

Chapter XI
Balms[426a]

Balms may be compounded with each other like the rest of the drugs either to strengthen their force and quality or to obtain a desired mixture which is acquired by their being prepared together. The balms may be compounded with the strength of drugs by the means of water and fire. The drugs are cooked in water so that the water takes up the essence. Then that solution is mixed with the balm and boiled until the water disappears. The essence remains in the balm.

Or [the drugs], while tender and soft, may be thrown into the balm and placed in the sun until the liquidity acts as a medium between their strength in giving and taking before fading away.

The balms may be compounded with the strength of drugs in the medium of air. This is done by gathering moist aromatics and the oily pulps in leather bags. These [bags] filter them. The tops are tied until [the contents] has withered. Then it is renewed for tender and fresh [material]. That [process] is repeated until the strength is removed and its odor is good. The pulp is pressed when necessary and its oils are taken. This is very weak in comparison with the two previous types.

The [latter] method is preferred in the cold moist balms like the oil of shelled sesame, shelled sweet almond, shelled pumpkin seed, and other similar ones. The moist cold aromatics like violet, nenuphar, and similar ones guard against the power of the heat of the fire and the sun, and the destruction of its moistness that is desirable [to retain]. One is cautioned against rapid putrefaction or its becoming acidic. The pulp also becomes putrid. [However], this takes longer than the time in which the balms become putrid especially the moist balms.

The balms may be compounded with the essence of the drugs. The purpose in compounding the balms is to retain their quality and put their strength in a gentle vehicle which is an effective resolvent penetrating the pores and suitable for the condition of the skin, nerves, and brain. It will be affected by the length of time it comes in contact [with the organs], the longer, the better.

However, the compounded and assembled balms are to be strengthened in their force and their effectiveness by being mixed together. They must resemble the compounded balms like those with violet, nenuphar, Egyptian willow,[426] shelled sweet almond, shelled sesame, white poppy, seed of purslane, two kinds of cucumbers, lettuce, and pumpkin for cooling and moistening; balms with narcissus, lily, jasmine,[427] Egyptian origan,[428] yellow clove, water-caltrop, oil of balsam,[429] oil, olive oil, almond oil, castor oil, Carthamus oil, mustard seed oil, hemp seed, apricot seed, seed of mezereum, walnut, oil of wormwood, absinth, laurel, rue, southernwood, and camomile for heating, dissolving, gentling, and drying; and [balms] with rose oil, quince, henna, and myrtle for strengthening. The compounded ones of these are like those compounded of the hot with the cold, or both of them with a strengthening according to the need.

The balm of the seven pulps[430] is taken from almond, pistachio, sesame, pine, walnut, pumpkin seed, and shelled filbert[431] for headache and earache due to black bile, for elephantiasis and melancholy. When compounded with the strength of drugs by cooking, cooked with it are those hot medicines which are useful for cold diseases. These drugs include costus, nard,[432] malabathrum, elecampane,[433] root of sweet flag, lemon-grass, savin, lichen, cinnamon, wild ginger, ginger, pyrethrum, lemon balm, sweet Cyperus, bastard cumin,[434] marjoram, nard, myrrh, clove, nutmeg,[435] storax,[436] saffron and others.

The drugs may be repeated in some balms and then recooked to extract their strength thoroughly. Or, they may be cooked with constricting medicines which prevent perspiration as myrtle, rose, quince, pomegranate blossom, and others. Or, they may be cooked with hot and cold drugs which strengthen the hair, as leaf of myrtle, myrobalan, flower of anemone, maiden hair, nard, Indian nard, seed of beet, gallnut, Kabul myrobalan, leaf of Christ's thorn, and others.

That which is compounded by exposing it to the sun, i.e. the cold, is oil of violet, nenuphar, Egyptian willow, rose, myrtle, mandrake, and what is taken of greens and cold aromatics.

But the hot is oil of narcissus, lily, jasmine, bush basil, marjoram, wild thyme, yellow clove, eglantine,[437] feverfew, wormwood, and saffron.

The compounded balms with the [solid] matter of the drugs are [those] like castoreum, euphorbium, saffron, myrrh, ginger, pyrethrum, and pepper. It is dissolved in hot oils and rubbed on for epilepsy, atonicity of muscles, glazed eyes,[438] and cold conditions. Ambergris, musk, saffron, Indian aloes, Chinese cinnamon, mastix, cloves, and medical aromatics are dissolved in aromatic oils. It is applied for cold diseases in the main organs—in the reproductive organs and in the womb.

Costus balm is useful for epilepsy.

Costus	1	ounce
Pepper	1/3	ounce
Pyrethrum	[1/3	ounce]
Euphorbium	[1/3	ounce]
Castoreum	1/2	ounce

All of it is dissolved in a half *raṭl* of oil of yellow gillyflower or oil of narcissus. The atonic organs are rubbed with it.

Balm called "the gathered one," is used in all cold diseases and has moderate effects. It does not cause dryness in the member. On the oils of yellow gillyflower,[439] jasmine, terebinth, lily, castor, marjoram seed and laurel [taken] in equal parts are thrown a little castoreum and a little musk. It is boiled lightly and used.

Cold moist balm for hot headaches, vertigo, and dryness.

From pumpkin seed, lettuce seed, cucumber seed, large cucumber seed pulp, pulp of sweet almond, seed of white poppy, and shelled sesame in equal parts, the oils are extracted and used for sniffing and for rubbing. For sniffing, half a dirham is very useful.

Chapter XII
Eye Medicines

These are antimony powders and collyria. Of these, there are coolants, powders, and drops. Then there are dressings and embrocations. The latter two are used at the commencement of eye swellings and the flowing of matter. They are the preventive embrocations. Used are such as the tips of black nightshade, knotweed,[440] purslane,[441] moist coriander, lettuce, flower of pumpkin, poppy, violet, tender rose, or [use] lycium, sandalwood, acacia, glaucium, areca nut, Armenian bole, gum, opium, and so on when the pain is severe. For the best therapy in clearing and removing the matter from [the eye], for some, one may add saffron and aloe.

When there is a necessity for a slight resolvent, one may add to it dry coriander, melilot, flaxseed, and *ka^ck* biscuit; when there is need for greater dissolution where the matter is thicker and the preventive medicines do not quiet the pain caused by thick matter, then the drugs are collected with syrup and it is poured out on their vapors, and the vapors of the liquor of marjoram, camomile, dill,[442] and red fig[443] especially when the weather is cold and the skin is thick. It may be applied with a sponge and hot water or the white of egg and rose-water at the beginning [of treatment].

When the eyes are struck and affected, they are dressed with egg yolk, coriander juice, and rose oil.

For swelling of the veins in the eyes[444] and bulging eyes, pistachio rind, pomegranate pulp, lentils, lycium, and endive [are used].

As to drops, these are the softest eye medicines. They are to be preferred for use in the case of swellings at the beginning [of treatment] and in inflammation. [Their use] cannot approach the hardness of the style[445] and its weight, for the softest of drops are used at the beginning [of treatment] of ophthalmia. The most effective for this is the thin white of the egg[446] to moderate the temper of the eye, to wash it, and to quiet the pain.

Then comes mucilage of fleawort, mucilage of quince seed, a young girl's milk, and whatever is needed for dissolution like water in which dehusked barley is well cooked with the unshelled seed of sweet quince, coarsely ground *jashmīzaj*,[447,448] and a little sarcocol in a double pot and cooked well. Then there are the drops in which the soft eye medicine is dissolved.

As to the drops which are used to ripen pustules, there are mucilage of the seed of origan of Egypt, flaxseed, and fenugreek in milk. It comes next to the [other] drops in lightness of use and for [causing] less pain in the eye.

Powders are used when there is much dirt in the corners of the eye because of their hardness and dryness.

One [powder] is made from large white sarcocol which is preserved in the shade in the milk of a young girl, a little of starch taken from sarcocol, jelly-fish, and sugar, or from sarcocol, glaucium eye medicine, lycium, saffron, aloe, myrrh, and jelly-fish heated more or less if necessary for polishing. However, the important constituent is the sarcocol. The ratio of each one of what is added is as the ratio of a tenth and a third according to its strength and its usefulness and the necessity for it. Opium may be added to it and also camphor with an increase in heat. Myrrh, aloe, and saffron are then lessened in amount and so reduced. More of it is taken for scab [449] and heaviness of the eyelids and their thickness. It is taken from sarcocol preserved in the milk of wild asses for its polishing strength and the abundance of its juice and from celandine since it is very good both for polishing of the eye and the scab, and from myrrh because of its strength in polishing, in dissolving the thick mixture with its contraction, and its stickiness which is good for wounds, from saffron due to its soft, dissolving properties, from eye medicines of glaucium for their strength and preventive properties, from egg yolk dried in the sun for its stickiness, gentle dissolution, and because in anointing the scab of the eye, it acts like the *qīrūṭī* [450] mixture.

The embrocations for the scab are compounded from drugs opposite in nature and action for a diversification of purposes in therapy, as mentioned. It is likewise for the scab of the eye. The sarcocol is increased in weight because of its strong usefulness and abundance in satisfaction in polishing and whatever is sought from this drug. Myrrh and celandine are used as one eighth [of the sarcocol] because of their strength in comparison to it, and the presence of its usefulness in the composition, and glaucium and saffron since they are like moderators for the organ. The weight of egg yolk is made moderate without the intention that it have less usefulness and weakness in its strength. It is therefore used in a quantity half that of sarcocol.

Sharp powders may be taken to be strong in polishing to do away with leucoma;[451] these are lizard dung,[452] borax, jelly-fish, ashes of sea-shell, pearl,[453] shell for glazing,[454] scoria of gold and silver,[455] hematite, and ashes of the wings of the eagle, all preserved in the juice of the sweet flag, celandine and gall of birds. It is all dried and pounded after that.

The drugs of the eye are described by the strength associated with the smallest of their particles. This is caused by bruising them and making them like dust by pounding them; it is for the high sensitivity of the eye, not like the powders which are in need of softness and smoothness with a style. The gentlest of its powders stick to it like the *kuḥl* powders. Also, they are not pounded because of their hardness as are the collyria.

The use of coolants is like that of *kuḥl* powders. This is except for the pomegranate coolant which is used in the form of drops. It is used mainly to quiet the eye with inflammation and to repel strong drugs. Those taken are from flower of the violet, burned coriander, starch, gum, and gum tragacanth, all preserved in vinegar; and from scoria, preserved sarcocol, burned lead,[456] jelly-fish, and opium. It is like the pomegranate coolant and the saffron coolant.

If it is made from drugs which are sharp, polishing, and burning to the eye as in the treatment of lippitudo of the eyelids[457] and pterygium,[458] and so on, it should not be made of camphor and opium. It is called coolant in contradistinction to others of the hot *kuḥl* powders.

Kuḥl powders. Since most of these are used in strengthening the eye, washing it, and polishing it, and the eye is a moist organ and most of its weakness is from moistness, then the drugs which polish it and keep it healthy should be dry [459] *kuḥl* powders.

As to the collyria,[460] they are used in diseases of the eye for polishing and strengthening. They are compounded variously for different purposes. It is necessary to use them like the embrocations and dressings, and prepared to keep their strength ready for administration and anointing by the style. Though the eyes are highly sensitive and cannot take strong drugs, nevertheless they are muscular, and weak drugs do not affect them when used in softening thick matter and dissolving deep rooted foreign matter in them.

Drugs cannot be put on them as they are on other organs. Embrocations and dressings are applied since they are more acceptable in comparison. It is also because they move continuously. Thus the *kuḥl* powders and collyria may be made strong and used for long periods so that both elements are satisfied—the hardness of the eye layers and [the eye's] receptiveness to mineralogical drugs.

Most of the drugs are made from them because their retention is desired. Drugs good for strong polishing in *kuḥl* powders are those such as tutty and stibnite [461] which are soaked in rainwater and preserved in fennel juice, marjoram juice, scoria, marcasite,[462] pearl, coral, hematite, burned copper,[463] "sea crab" [464] which is washed and soaked, Indian malabathrum, saffron, ginger, white pepper, jelly-fish, lycium, glaucium, pepper, long pepper, celandine, camphor, yellow myrobalan, musk, Andarānī [465] salt, nard, and lichen.

The chelidonium [466] and [other ingredients] are good

to make eyelashes grow. They are burned seed of dates, smoke of frankincense, Indian nard, grain of balsam, lapis lazuli,[467] burned shell, burned chelidonium, acacia, burned ink,[468] juice of onion, leek,[469] tutty which is good to stop tears, scrapings of yellow myrobalan, aloe, pepper, long pepper, ginger, Indian salt, jelly-fish, celandine, saffron, *kuḥl*, marcasite, pyrethrum, calcined sea-shells, sal ammoniac, and juice of unripe grapes.

The weak eye collyria are taken from white lead, gum arabic, gum tragacanth, starch, preserved sarcocol, jelly-fish, lizard dung, glaucium, saffron, camphor, rose, opium, and scoria.

The strong eye collyria are taken from green vitriol, pepper, verdigris,[470] malachite,[471] hematite, arsenic, sal ammoniac, jelly-fish, borax, gum ammoniac, sulfide of mercury,[472] sagapenum, agaric, colocynth pulp, long pepper, ginger, Indian spikenard, scoria, Indian salt, burned shell used for glazing, lizard dung, excrement of bats, egg shells, and gall.

Strong medicines should not be void of weak drugs which reduce the strength like starch, gum tragacanth, gum, and white lead in quantities necessary to subdue the strength and protect the eye from its heat and harm. It is better that its action be weakened, to slow the effect, and prolong the time of its use. In this way, it is safer rather than to damage the eye and pain it severely. The eye is thus exposed to the pouring of matter into it but the eye collyria which are used in eye wounds are those taken from drugs which polish and dry without burning. This is because the eye is strongly sensitive and its wounds are subject to swelling and severe pain.

Thus, it requires ameliorators and those which normalize. By the former is meant those which polish and dry without burning such as tutty, "burned lead,"[473] burned lead, *qalīma,* shell for glazing, hematite, washed pearl, *kuḥl,* clear and unclear frankincense, preserved sarcocol, and dragon's blood plant.

Those which quiet and are normalizers are such as glaucium, starch, gum tragacanth, gum, seed of rose, saffron, opium, henbane, and mandrake.[474] The physician must compound according to the condition of the wounds and their time, gradually and cautiously. He must assemble the mild eye collyria and the strong one equally or by priority. He must dilute the eye collyria at the beginning of ophthalmia and for pustules in milk to reduce and moderate the effects of any opium and camphor. Also in the final stage [of treatment it is] diluted in water so that it does not harm and that its strength may weaken to become milder to dissolve the remnant of ophthalmia.

Dressing for itching. [Take] tender seed of endive for which two cloths[475] are prepared. The dressing is smeared with it and with rose oil.

Another is shelled lentil, sumach, red rose, and pulp of pomegranate. It is mixed[476] and dressed.

Embrocation for inflammation and swelling of the eyelids. [Take] rose collyrium, glaucium, acacia, lycium and chelidonium. [The mixture] is embrocated with egg white.

Drops that are useful for all kinds of ophthalmia.

Sarcocol	2	dirhams
Seed of sweet quince	20	grains
Pure saffron	½	*dāniq*

Celandine	2	*dāniqs*
Kishk of barley [477]	20	grains
Fenugreek	5	grains
Coriander	20	grains
Sugar	½	dirham
Gum tragacanth	1	*dāniq*

It is cooked in clear water in a glass vessel, then decanted.

Coolant useful for redness of the eye and to reduce its heat.

White lead	5	[dirhams]
Juice of marcasite	3	[dirhams]
Gum arabic	3	[dirhams]
Hematite	3	[dirhams]
Pearl	3	[dirhams]
Burned copper [478]	4	[dirhams]
Musk	½	*dāniq*
Camphor	½	*dāniq*

It is pounded and used.

Powder for leucoma.

Glazing shell	1	dirham
"Indian crab" stone	1	dirham
Scoria of gold	1	dirham
Jelly-fish	1	dirham
Lizard dung	1	dirham

White camphor collyrium.

White lead	3	dirhams
Gum tragacanth	7	dirhams

Gum arabic	7	dirhams
Silver scoria	5	dirhams
Sarcocol	5	dirhams
Starch	7	dirhams
Jelly-fish	7	dirhams
Camphor	½	dirham

Kuḥl for epiphora.[479]

Indian tutty	10	dirhams
Coral	2	dirhams
Yellow myrobalan	2	dirhams
Aloe	2	dirhams
Pepper	1	dirham
Long pepper	1	dirham

Another for epiphora.

Indian tutty and shavings of yellow myrobolan are pounded in juice of sour grapes.

Chapter XIII
Aromatic Powders and Salves[480]

As for salves, they are made from drugs which make the flesh grow, close up the wounds and ulcers, heal, cicatrize, and dissolve the extra flesh, eating it away.

As for that which makes the flesh grow, it is the one which dries without burning, in all degrees of drying, according to the need for it that is required by the body members, and the condition of the ulcers. It smooths as [does] Aristolochia, iris, frankincense, aloes, scoria of silver, tutty, bitter vetch, sarcocol, pitch, celandine, litharge,[481] and white lead. Those [salves] which close [the wound] are those which have them.

Adhesive and binder which returns the slowing blood to a normal state.

It adheres like dragon's blood plant, pine resin,[482] gum, galbanum,[483] mastix, gum ammoniac, resin of terebinth, opopanax, frankincense, and myrrh.

The healer is the one which hardens the flesh of the

ulcer. It dries [the ulcer] in moderation and when it cicatrizes, it strongly dries the surface which becomes even with the surface of the skin. It makes [the ulcer] like the skin in dryness. That is why it is called "cicatrizer."

Those drugs which perform these two actions, more or less, are the astringents like pomegranate blossom, rose and its seed, rind of pomegranate, leaf of licorice, gallnut, dill, burned yellow vitriol,[484] *kuḥl*, red lead, washed burned copper,[485] aloe, and burned copper.[486]

Those which eat the extra flesh away and dry ulcers are such as verdigris, sal ammoniac, arsenic or quicklime.[487]

If [the remedy] is used as a salve then it is like the non-astringent drugs such as litharge, or burned sea shell when used concentrated.

The drugs which eat and dissolve the flesh may accidentally become healers. They dry moderately if a small quantity is used with oil and wax as a salve.

From these drugs the salves are made up. The method of compounding is according to the types of ulcers. Since the ulcers are mostly in need of all these properties, i.e. making flesh grow, binding, healing, cicatrizing, polishing, and dissolving, poultices are so compounded from all these kinds and degrees depending on their different requirements. They may be gathered in one single remedy for two or more purposes so that most salves are useful for that reason.

The dry remedies may not adhere to moist ulcers nor may powders or saturated compounds so that their strength does not penetrate into the pores and in depth. This is especially true of minerals which are in balms and salves when used as dressing to lengthen the time of application. The oils penetrate with their strength, cut down sharp [pain] and moderate it. They do not allow drying or harm because of any coarseness. It is as though they were put together with water to be agreeable to the muscles, nerves, and skin with their particular viscosity and mildness.

The oils which are used in poultices are olive oil, pure oil,[488] wax, [fat from] the hump of a camel,[489] oil of rose, myrtle, violet, nenuphar, clove, fat of chicken and duck, marrow of the leg of the cow, and butter. All of these are taken according to the need for cooling and moistening, astringing, heating and dissolving, and for mucilages to ripen the hardened parts. The latter mucilages are such as those of fenugreek, marshmallow, fleawort, and myrrh. The gums may be dissolved in some of them when one desires dryness. To break the heat, it is done in vinegar. Some are [dissolved] in wine for warming, dissolving, washing, and polishing. Litharge is used for its moderateness in heat and coldness, its astringency, and its slight drying which is suitable for boils. It is introduced into many therapeutic salves and made in large quantity since it is so very useful and because of the weakness of its force.

Salve with wonderful action in making the flesh grow and in cicatrization if ulcers are not serious.

One ounce if litharge is pounded like *kuḥl* and three ounces of olive oil is poured on it. It is cooked and stirred until it dissolves. Then two dirhams each of frankincense, sarcocol, dragon's blood, galbanum,[490] and dry pitch are pounded and thrown on. It is cooked until it becomes a thick salve which makes the flesh grow. It is used in summer and whenever it is hot.

Five dirhams of litharge is pounded like *kuḥl*, then pounded in vinegar until it dissolves and softens. Then rose oil is poured on it until it thickens. It is soaked in the vinegar once and then in the oil until it swells and becomes a salve. Then five dirhams of white lead is thrown on it and a little camphor.

Salve good for fistulas, to cleanse any filthy, dirty ulcer, and to eat the dead flesh.

Verdigris	1 ounce
Sarcocol	½ [ounce]
Gum ammoniac	½ [ounce]

All are pounded in vinegar and then kneaded in honey.

Another cleansing salve [is made] from pounded sarcocol and the same honey.

The powders are preferred to the salves for one of three [uses] as for closing up ripe soft wounds. These do not require anything except to be closed up and to be held together. They are made up of aloe, dragon's blood, acacia, bark of frankincense, sandarach,[491] yellow amber, "stone of Khwārizm,"[492] sarcocol, myrrh, pig skin, and pine tree both pounded, gum of the oak and so on.

For the drying of moist ulcers with much dirt and pus, one uses resin of frankincense, pomegranate blossom, litharge, burned paper, henna, dry coriander, bark of elm,[493] rind of burned dry pumpkin, rind of acorn, licorice leaves, lily root, Aristolochia, jelly-fish, rind of pomegranate, dill, gallnut, barley[494] flour and its hull, red anemone, and so on.

For the burning of spoiled, putrefying flesh, and cauterizing it to get rid of it, one uses sharp cauterizing drugs like green vitriol, verdigris, sal ammoniac,[495] arsenic, quicklime, *qalī*[496] soda, soda,[497] distilled, killed mercury,[498] alum,[499] and strong, dry astringents like iron scales,[500] burned copper, gallnut, burned meerschaum (?),[501] acacia, and so on. One should be careful in using it to keep it away from healthy flesh. After using it, ghee must be used to make the dry scab[502] fall off and quiet the burn and pain there. These are the two proofs that the bad flesh has sloughed off and that the remedy has reached the healthy flesh.

Powder for cicatrization.

Frankincense
Sarcocol
Meccan myrrh
Dragon's blood

Equal parts [are taken]. [The remedy] is known as the "four drugs."

Powder which dries.

Litharge	1	part
Licorice leaf	1	part
Rind of myrobalan	1	part
Gallnut	1	part
Pomegranate rind	½	part
Celandine	½	part

Powder which consumes.

Burned yellow vitriol
Gallnut[503]
Verdigris
Sarcocol

Equal parts [are taken].

Chapter XIV
Dentifrices

Since the teeth are bony and of dry temper, the proper thing is that [the dentifrices] must be according to a dry humor. In spite of that, they are classified with the dampness of the mouth, the esophagus, and drink. They are subjected to changes in the external, misty vapors of respiration, in the vapors of thick humors, and by the food which rises from the stomach. It is a necessity that the health [of the teeth] be maintained by powders. These are dry drugs pounded and sprinkled on them to clear away the extraneous matter of moistness. [The dentifrice] is fastened and stuck to them by heat. Further it dries them.

The polisher with which the teeth are rubbed clears them of discoloration [504] of the teeth and tartar.[505] It is made from pearl, coral, Syrian glass, jelly-fish, dross of glass,[506] salt burned in honey, green polishing clay, *qalī* soda, meerschaum,[507] Aristolochia, ashes of shells, burned hair, borax, burned aloe, and so on.

Dry astringents are sprinkled on them and their roots

to move and to loosen whatever surrounds the teeth near the gums, and for their support.

When cold, and there is an absence of redness and heat in the gum, then one takes burned antler of deer, sweet Cyperus, tamarisk gall,[508] Indian spikenard, exterior of acorn, savin, pomegranate blossom, nard, dill, lemon-grass, gallnut, cinnamon, rose, aloe, acacia, iris, pyrethrum, musk, mastix, and clove.

For loosening of the gums due to heat, their reddening, swelling, and bleeding, take tabasheer, rose seed, sumach, cynomorium,[509] acacia fruit juice, sandalwood, blossom of the vine, areca nut, camphor, dry coriander, shelled lentil, rind of sour pomegranate, tamarisk berry, myrobalan, belleric myrobalan, emblic myrobalan, acacia, pomegranate blossom, sealing clay, flour of bitter vetch, and so on.

From every nature, it is compounded according to the need for the best polisher, best astringent, the hottest and coldest product, and the need for all dentifrices of compounded strengths and actions. This is when all these are together according to the interest and care for each one of them.

Dentrifices which polish the teeth and remove cavities.

Syrian glass
Meerschaum

Equal parts are strongly pounded. The teeth are rubbed with it while taking care of the gum.

Another.

Jelly-fish

Darānī salt [510]
Earthenware
Ashes of sea shells
Burned barley
Ashes of roots of cane
Round Aristolochia

All [are taken] in equal parts.

Dentifrice which strengthens the gums and [holds] the teeth firm.

Burned deer horn	1	part
Darānī salt	1	part
Yellow myrobalan	1	part
Pomegranate blossom	½	part

Allah knows the truth.

Chapter XV
Gargles

Gargles are either to make gentle the thick humors in the head and to ease them down by way of the mouth, or to prevent the thin ones from coming down by thickening them and narrowing the duct. They are also [used] to reduce swellings in the throat.

Also, they are for ripening so that the one used to gentle the thick humors and make them descend from the brain is hot and sharp. It is made from such drugs as pyrethrum, ginger, thyme, barberry,[511] sweet flag, mustard, mountain-mint, rind of the root of caper, iris, borax, pepper, marjoram, serpolet, *iyārij*, juice of honey, and garum,[512] or oxymel of sugar, of honey, or of onion.

That used to prevent colds is any cold astringent cooked in water and then gargled, as rose, pomegranate blossom, carob,[513] lentil, grain of myrtle, poppy, and so on.

Those used for swellings of the throat and at the beginning of hot swellings are juices of repelling cold greens like black nightshade, lettuce, moist coriander, endive, and so on; and juices of cold fruits like the Syrian mulberry, sour pomegranate, sumach and so on; and cold mucilages like that of fleawort, plantain, bush basil, grain of quince, and so on; and that which comes out of the cold, astringent drugs like pomegranate blossoms, rose, acacia, tamarisk berry, dry coriander, and so on.

At the beginning [of treatment] and at the time for the need of the solution there is that which comes from hot vegetables like celery, cabbage, fennel, cuscuta, and so on; that which comes from hot fruits like figs, raisins, purging cassia, jujube, and so on; hot mucilages like those of fenugreek, flaxseed, myrrh, garden cress,[514] and so on; that which comes from hot drugs like licorice root, lily, marshmallow, fennel root, costus, and so on; from those which ripen swellings of the throat as *al-khamīr*[515] soaked in milk or in sesame oil with fig, *maïbakhtaj*[516] in cabbage juice, and the juice[517] of compounded barley; and that uncompounded with the scales of the cassia tree.

Chapter XVI
Preserves[518]

The purpose of robs is preservation in the storing of some fruits like myrobalan, emblic myrobalan, citron, apple, quince, and so on; some blossoms like rose, violet, nenuphar, and many from trees as the rose of quince, and so on; and also roots of plants as ginger, secacul,[519] carrot, turnip, and so on. Though soft, its moistness is retained. [That which is to be preserved] is prepared by putting it in honey and leaving it [there] because [honey] is the best [substance] in which moist things may be kept from change and decay. It adds gentleness and penetrativeness and makes [the preserve] agreeable to the temper.

The rules for preserving fruits are concerned with the removal from them of bitterness and any strong elements in them by soaking and boiling them. They are put in a quantity of honey which is not too excessive. It is then put in the sun but covered from it.

The flowers and blossoms are prepared by taking them after the blossoms have been cleared completely from the stalks. Each *raṭl* is put in four *raṭls* of honey and put in the sun thus.[520] Instead of honey, juice [521] of cane may be used or honey of manna and melted *fānīd* confection as much as is desired. It may be taken from crystalline sugar by pulverizing it and putting it in the sun.

When it is desired to use [a preserve] in hot ailments and tempers, then do [522] to the roots of the plants whatever is done to the fruits. They are sweetened to the extreme even by boiling them in salt water, washing them many times, cutting them into pieces, splitting them, and putting them into honey in the same manner as the fruits. This may be carried out with the preservation of the aromatics as saffron, clove, cinnamon, cardamom, and so on and then pounded.

Chapter XVII
Sniffing Medicines, Sternutatives, Fumigants, and Odorants

The drugs which are used as fine powder in the nose are snuff medicines. They may be used as drops or they may be hot and dry and are injected to get rid of phlegmatic remnants from the brain, open blockages of the head, heat its humor at the end of cold diseases like epilepsy and migraine, for distortion of the mouth, cold hemicrany, and so on.

[The snuff] is taken from those like castoreum, sal ammoniac, turpeth, black cumin, harmel, aloe, garum, opopanox, borax, thyme, peppers [including black and white peppers],[523] asafetida, gum ammoniac, euphorbium, musk, pyrethrum, Indian salt, bur-reed,[524] thapsia,[525] gall of a bird, and others; urine of the camel, onion juice, marjoram, rue, beet, vinegar, oil of bitter almond, narcissus, lily, and so on.

For a moist cold snuff to cool the brain and to moisten it in dry, hot diseases like hot hemicrany, vertigo, and so on, one takes from the juices of lettuce, endive, black nightshade, cucumber, pumpkin seed, rose, and opium; camphor, tabasheer, and so on.

Sternutatives are used in a blower[526] to open the nostrils to smell and to get rid of cold remnants from them. They are hot medicines like struthium, sow-bread, black cumin,[527] borax, castoreum, euphorbium, Aristolochia, seed of the balsam, pyrethrum, musk, dried urine of camel, peppers,[528] rue, thyme, barberry, hellebore,[529] mustard, aloe, marjoram, sal ammoniac, ginger, and gall.

Some of them are fumigants as incenses, either moist or dry. The hot moist fumigants are used to open the nostrils and to soften the [dried] mucus. They are taken from such as marjoram, wild thyme, wormwood, southernwood, melilot, camomile, absinth, fennel, mint, hyssop, dill, rue, thyme, cabbage, and so on.

[The fumigants] are also used to open the orifice of the ear to loosen the matter and dirt, and to dissolve the [ill] odors. [The materials in the fumigants] are cooked in a gourd bottle. Its spout is held near the nose and the ear. Or [the fumigant] may be poured on directly. Salt and vinegar may be added according to the need.

The fumigant may be used with syrup and with preserves by sprinkling it on the hot millstones.

The moist cold [fumigant] may be used to cool the brain and to moisten it by retention to guard against the heat and dryness of the brain. It is prepared from violet, nenuphar, moist coriander,[530] lettuce, mallow, Jewish mauve, Egyptian willow, cucumber, leaves and rind of pumpkin, poppy and its rind, rose and its flower, bush basil, sempervivum,[531] plantain, marshmallow, bruised barley, and so on. It is cooked and milk is poured on it as well as violet oil and other oils. Heated stones are thrown in it. Its fumes are received from a distance so that the head is not heated but the vapors reach it lukewarm.

Fumigation may be used with vinegar by sprinkling it on heated stones and leaning over them.

Dry fumigants are smokes which strengthen the head and brain like musk, aloe, sandalwood, costus, ambergris, and *sukk*.

For rheum and to prevent acute catarrh, there are bran of white meal soaked in vinegar and dried after that, and flour of barley, flour of bean,[532] white sandalwood, rose, violet, gallnut, camphor, crystalline sugar.

For the cold rheum and cold catarrh, there are frankincense, dry storax, costus, sweet Cyperus, sandarac, paper, aloe, ambergris, and others. [The fumigant] may be taken for very moist coughing with sulfur,[533] costus, galbanum, myrrh, cinnamon, saffron, cubeb, Aristolochia, frankincense, and red arsenic using a tube in the mouth.

For a fumigant to force the birth of a child and to expel the placenta, one may use opopanax, sulfur, myrrh, galbanum, and gall of the ox by a funnel in the vagina.

Odorants which are hot are used to moderate the humor of the cold brain. They are either aromatic plants like jasmine, narcissus, eglantine, and others; perfumes like musk, ambergris, saffron, and others; grasses from wormwood, southernwood, wild thyme, thyme, and others; non-grasses like castoreum, storax pounded with vinegar and roasted; or fruits like citron, coconut,[534] watermelon, and others.

Some [odorants] are cold and used to quiet the heat of the brain. They are either aromatics like myrtle, violet, nenuphar, and others; perfumes like sandalwood, camphor, rose, and others; or grasses and drugs [535] like mandrake, bark of the camphor tree, and such as wine or fruits like apple, quince, mandrake and others. They are used singly or compounded from the various species according to the need.

Sniffing remedy for acute hemicrany.

Oil of violet
Nenuphar
Seed of pumpkin
Egyptian willow
Milk of women
Juice of lettuce
Endive

Equal parts [are taken].

Sternutative for epilepsy, apoplexy, and distortion of the mouth.

Struthium
Black cumin
Euphorbium
Pepper
Castoreum
Aristolochia
Seed of balsam
Musk
Pyrethrum

These, in equal parts, are pounded, and blown into the nose.

Vapor for cold hemicrany.

Marjoram
Mountain-mint
Camomile
Melilot
Southernwood
Aneth
Wormwood
Wild thyme
Laurel
Watermelon

One leans over it.

Vapor for hot hemicrany.

Violet
Nenuphar
Stems of marshmallow
Bruised shelled barley
Rind of pumpkin
[Rind] of watermelon

It is all poured in a basin; then a little violet oil is thrown on it. One leans over it.

Vapor for cold rheum to prevent flowing [of mucus]

Costus	½ dirham

Frankincense	½ dirham
Sandarac	½ dirham
Aloe	½ dirham
Liquid storax	½ dirham
Sugar	½ dirham
Black cumin	½ dirham
Cumin	½ dirham
Thyme	½ dirham

It is pulverized and made into balls the size of chick peas. One uses its vapor.

Allah knows best.

Chapter XVIII
Aromatic Baths[535a]

Aromatic baths are made of drugs which are volatile under ordinary conditions, hot or cold, cooked in water, filtered, and poured on the head from a distance. They are for certain diseases. The vapors and their dissolving drugs must not be prepared from astringent sternutatives because of the importance of the brain and its significance in order to keep its strength and its functions from weakening.

The drugs are cooked in flasks whose tops are covered to retain the gentle parts[536] which penetrate the pores quickly. The aromatic baths are preferred for this rather than others.

Sedatives[537] may be mixed with [the aromatic bath] such as leaf and rinds of poppy, mandrake, lettuce and its seed, coriander, the tips of black nightshade, and henbane in heat and dryness. If the pain is severe, then one may use hot sedatives like tarragon, dill, saffron, storax and others.

When the pain is severe with coldness attending, then

there are mucilaginous matters from plants like marshmallow, leaf of sesame, mallow, purslane, and from seeds like fleawort, seed of origan of Egypt and plantain when very dry. It may be anointed with oils and milks, pouring it on or running it on. The head should be washed and cleaned of it, after it has dried,[538] with beet juice, water of bran, marshmallow, and so on of whatever cleans. This is so that its heat will not decay the brain, block the pores, and divert the heat and vapors to it. Then the danger would increase and the case become critical. The calamity is thus doubled.

Aromatic bath useful for lethargy and cold hemicrany.

Camomile
Aneth
Wild thyme
Marjoram
Mountain-mint

[All] are cooked, filtered, and used to wash the head.

Aromatic bath that moistens and puts one to sleep.

Violet	1 handful
Nenuphar	1 handful
Root of marshmallow	1 handful
Leaf of lettuce	1 handful
Leaf of Egyptian willow	1 handful
Rind of pumpkin	1 handful
Black nightshade	1 bundle
Mallow leaf	1 bundle
Sebesten	1 handful
Red rose	1 handful

White poppy leaf	1 handful
Barley dough	1 handful
Watermelon	1 handful

[All] are cooked and used to wash the head after filtration.

Chapter XIX
Medicines for the Hair

Some of them make it grow. These are varied according to the reasons which prevent growth.

Some of them are drugs for falling out of the hair or coatings which dissolve and make gentle the thick humor and which open the pores like garlic [539] and onion when they are rubbed on and coated with mustard, thapsia, cabbage, euphorbium, burned filbert nut, burned wormwood, borax, rue, hellebore, arsenic, excrement of mice, rind of burned lupine, Aristolochia, jelly-fish, ashes of cane, burned bitter almond, pyrethrum, and ashes of southernwood. These are compounded and anointed once with oil, and once with vinegar according to the cause of the falling out of the hair. One starts with the weakest and goes to the strongest.

Some help to retain whatever remains of falling hair and attract nutrition to the roots of the hair. They are drugs which exert retentive power, have heat, elasticity, and softness; and are oily like myrtle and pine and their seeds, ladanum,[540] China tree,[541] leaf of sesame, leaf of pumpkin, Kabul myrobalan, maiden hair, flax, leaf of hemp, belleric myrobalan soaked in milk, red anemone, nard, mastix, seed and juice of beet, acacia, gallnut, ashes of the inner bark of the pine, seed of marshmallow and its roots, mucilages and oils used of them according to the heat or coldness of the humor of the brain and the moistness or dryness of the organs of the head. [The head] is rubbed and coated with that made [from the above simples].

The basis on which the therapy depends is knowledge of the humor of the brain and the organs of the head so that one may choose of the hair drugs whatever antagonizes the humor which prevents the growing of hair. If it causes the nature of the organs of the head and its compounded [natures] to return to temperateness even if it does so by other than hair medicines, then the hair will grow and become long. The humors thus must return to a tempered condition.

[There are drugs for] the protection of the hair, strengthening of its roots and the attraction of nutrition to them. [These are] drugs for the hair which are "fertilizing" medicines.[542]

As to the black [dyes] other than those which [cause] the skin to peel, they are all astringent and hot oils which strengthen the prevention of heat of that which hinders the nutriment from going to the roots of the hair. These would be like oil of myrtle, emblic myrobalan, lily, narcissus, costus, ben nut oil,[543] red anemone, oils from colocynth, black cumin, and mustard.

Then there are the hot drugs which coarsen [the hair] and prepare the way for acceptance of the black dye to which [the hair] is exposed. [Examples of these drugs] are ladanum, nard, clove, aneth, juice of walnut shell, emblic myrobalan, burned copper, scoria of iron, red anemones, fenugreek, gallnut, sweet Cyperus, costus, malabathrum, saffron, beet seed, maiden hair, celery seed, acacia, and ashes of the bark of the pine.

The darkeners which cover are the dyes and drugs. These are green vitriol, gallnut, litharge, quicklime, henna, and leaves of indigo. As to the knowledge of their compounding and the ratio of one to the other, this is known by the dyers of wool and hair.

As for women, the indigo leaf [544] and henna are enough for them. They use them according to the condition of their hair. Some confine themselves to henna and are satisfied to make [the hair] red, and some use only wood leaves and are satisfied with brightening [the hair]. Some gather them together or use them one after the other successively.

A dye with which we finish the book.

Gallnut [545]	1	*manna*
Red vitriol [546] brought from Kashgar and broken up	1	*istār*
Sal ammoniac	1	*istār*
Rind of emblic myrobalan	5	*istārs*
Scoria of copper	5	*istārs*
Gum tragacanth	½	*istār*

The gallnut is put into a new iron pot. This is then put on hot ashes. The top of the pot is covered by a felt lid. It is stirred every hour until it is so well roasted that it is almost burned. Then it is placed on a [piece of] flat felt prepared for it and the edges of the felt are turned over on it quickly. It is stamped by foot and pressed until the reaction in it dies out while covered. It is removed and pulverized. The rest is added to it pulverized. They are all pounded and mixed well each with the other, ground finely by a millstone [used for] saffron. It is dissolved while hot to make it slightly thick. The hair is covered with it quickly before it grows cold and is left until it dries. If necessary, this is repeated. The gallnut may be replaced by *barghand*[547] if pitch blackness is not sought.

Allah is the most omniscient of the right and to him is the returning and retreating. Praise be to Allah, the Lord of the worlds. Prayers and peace to the best of His creation, Muhammad, and his relatives, and all his friends. With the help of Allah, this was accomplished in the city of Baku on Tuesday, the third of the month of *Rabīᶜa Awwal* in the year of 857[H].[548]

Notes and Comments on the Translation

1. The subtitle refers to the *Aqrābādhīn* and two other texts which are also on the subject of medicine and bound in the same volume.

2. Gloss: "Praise be to Allah who oriented us to this; if he had not done so, we would not have been so directed. M. b. ᶜAlī b. ᶜUmar al-Samarqandī."

3. Abū Jaᶜfar, known better as al-Manṣūr, reigned as Caliph from 754–775, founded the city of Baghdad and in its suburb of Karkh a great hospital. Other hospitals were organized later in this city so that it remained for hundreds of years an important center of Arabic medicine. It is of interest that al-Samarqandī had evidently studied the medicine then prevalent in Baghdad and had himself made this observation. *Cf.* M. Levey, *Journ. of the Albert Einstein Hospital* ***10***, 120–127 (1962).

4. In Arabic, *Mithrūdītūs.*

5. "Disease . . . originates from want or misdeed or from misfortune." From "*Tibb-ul-Nabbi* or Medicine of the Prophet," by al-Suyūṭī, fol. 7, translated by Cyril Elgood in *Osiris 14,* 52 (1962).

6. I.e., composed of many simples.

7. *Qarābādhīn.*

8. *Aqrābādhīnāt* (plural).

9. *Jalā',* also "clearing."

10. *Tamlīs,* also "a smoothing."

11. *Taḥlīl,* also "opening," or "dissolution."

12. For heart ailments since camphor penetrates the heart. Camphor is *kāfūr, Cinnamomum Camphora* Nees & Eberm., or called *Laurus Camphora* Linn., of the Dryobalanops family. *Cf.* al-Kindī (no. 118), Levey, M.A.B. (17). For chemical properties, *cf.* Gstirner (55 ff.).

13. Cinnamon, *dar ṣīnī,* is *Cinnamomum ceylanicum* Nees, or sometimes another species is meant. *Cf. al-Kindī* (no. 54) for the ancient uses. It is still used today in Egypt, India, Iran, Iraq, and in other countries as part of the native pharmacology. *Vide* Levey, M.A.B. (17, 18). In Chinese, it is called *jou-kouei, juh-kwei, yuh-kwei, jou-kouei-pi,* and is used for the kidneys and nerves, and to facilitate menstruation (Sobeiran 154–155).

14. Haematite is *sādhanaj* or *shādhanah.* It has many uses in present day medicine in Egypt internally as a desiccative and externally for the eyes. It is considered as an astringent for haemorrhage. *Cf. al-Kindī* (no. 234), Maim. (96).

15. *Turbid. Ipomoea turpethum* RBr. = *Convolvulus Turpethum* L., a tropical Asiatic vine found throughout India.

In Sans., it is *trivṛit,* Hind. *pitohri,* Tam. *shivadai;* in India, it has long been used as a cathartic. Most of the turpeth in India consists of the aerial stems or mixture of stems, plus the root, and not only of the roots which alone are rich in the purgative principle (Chopra 185–6).

Loew FJ (462) states that the Arabic *turbid* comes from the Sans. given above which means "three sided," from the appearance of the plant. Heb. is *turbad* and Syr. *torbed. Cf.* also Loew AP (410) for Gr. ἄλυπον and τουρπίττη from the Arabic.

IB (407) quotes ibn Sīnā that this drug is good for nerve disorders. This drug is given as *turbud* in Achundow (174–5). As an Indian element in Persian pharmacology, *cf.* Laufer (584).

Today, in Egypt, the root is employed as a purgative, in powders, pills, decoctions, and in electuaries (Ducros 28–29).

16. Verdigris is *zinjār.* It is used today in the Near East for eye ailments. In ancient times, it was known in India, Egypt, and in Babylonia. *Cf.* Levey M.A.B. (21).

17. Castoreum is *jundubādastur.* Cf. al-Kindī (No. 117). This is a dry secretion from the prepuce of the *Castor fiber* L. It is sold today in the bazaars as a resolvent, antispasmodic, stimulant, and antihysteric.

18. *Ufiyūn,* opium, is considered as a universal panacea in the Near East (Ducros (8, 98). It is usually taken as a paste or sweet known as *maᶜjūn* or *manzūl. Cf.* Levey M.A.B. (47).

19. A gloss in the text has "a kind of wax and oil mixture." *Qīrūṭī* is from κηρωτὴ (Diosc. I 19). It generally means "cerate" or "salve used medicinally."

20. This last phrase is omitted in the Leiden MS, fol. 159a.

21. Gloss in Leiden MS, fol. 158b. "The strength of the illness, for example from drinking many poisons is like that from the poison of snakes and scorpions. It requires the poison of snakes which cools, and the poison of the friendly scorpion. There is no one remedy which counteracts it so that one is obliged to compound. If a hot illness takes place, for example, in the second degree, the therapy requires that which cools it in two stages. To satisfy that qualification, that which cools in three stages when compounded with a hot drug in the first degree will result in the second [cold] degree. The differences in the conditions of an illness are the determining factors. When the single drug does not fulfill the therapeutic requirements, then compounding is necessary."

22. Gloss: "The Persian word, '*jawārishnāt*' means stomachic." "It is used most of the time for confections composed of condiments, of the three varieties of pepper, and of ginger." P. Sbath and C. D. Avierinos, *Deux Traités Medicaux*, Cairo, 1953, p. 47.

23. Probably a sudden fever.

24. "Water is the King of drinks in this World and the Next." From "*Tibb-ul-Nabbi of Maḥmūd bin Mohamed al-Chaghhayni*," translated by Cyril Elgood in *Osiris 14*, 187 (1962).

25. Oxymel is *sakanjubīn* and *sakanjubīn sādaj* is malabathrum oxymel. Al-Kindī uses oxymel in an ointment for baldness. Ibn Sīnā found it useful for the stomach. *Sakanjubīn* is from the Pers. *sirka-anjubīn*. *Cf.* al-Kindī (no. 223) and Levey M.A.B. (12).

26. Honey is *ʿasal*. Al-Kindī uses honey in a polish for teeth. *Cf.* al-Kindī (no. 21) and al-Kindī G. (175). IB (1542) states that some physicians use honey for intestinal and stomach disorders. Honey was probably used mainly as a vehicle for distasteful drugs but also as a purifier in Achundow (233–4) and to remove phlegm (*Muntakhib* 22b). Honey was also important in industry such as in compounding ink, making gold *līqs* and sizes, and in the preparation of alcoholic drinks (Levey M.A.B. 9, 24, 27, 29, 46).

27. More vinegar is used for thickness and more honey is used if the humors are putrid.

28. *Piyāz ʿunṣul*. Gloss reads "wild onion." In Pers., this is the sea-onion, *Squilla maritima, Piyāz* by itself is "onion," *piyāzi dashtī*, "wild onion." *Baṣal* also means "onion" and requires an adjective to give it a specific meaning. *Cf. baṣal* in the index. For *ʿunṣul, cf.* Maim. (60). In *Al-Muʿtamad* (341), it is equated to the "genuine onion."

29. Gloss: "That is to say the hot seeds are used with the cold seeds.

30. Endive is *hundabā'*, *Cichorium Endivia* L. The Arabic word, according to Loew FJ (I 433ff.) is from the Syr. *anṭūbiyā*, in turn from Gr. ἴντυβος. This plant is indigenous in Egypt and in the East Indies. In earlier times, endive was used for the heart, stomach, gout, scorpion bites, and for the eyes, all of these unknown to al-Samarqandī Cf. al-Kindī (36, 74).

31. *Khiyārain* is "two kinds of cucumber." It is a mixture of cucumber and musk-melon. The seeds are generally used. This mixture is of Persian origin. Steingass (490).

32. Celery is *karafs*. It may also be smallage or parsley. Probably *Apium graveolens* L. In al-Kindī A (103b), celery is used in a poultice for the stomach. There are many types of celery given by Maim. (196). *Cf. al-Kindī* (no. 122).

33. Anise is *anīsūn*. Usually the seed of *Pimpinella anisum* L. *Cf.* Paul of Aegina (621, 630, 659, 710, 725) for various *Pimpinella* species. Al-Kindī A (116a, 127a, 138b) uses anise in an electuary for the liver, for the kidneys, to enrich the urine, in an eye collyrium, and in a stomachic also good for the rheums. Al-Samarqandī continues to use anise for some of these purposes. *Cf.* al-Kindī (13). Anise fruit is used in present day Egyptian medicine as a carminative, stimulant, and emmenagogue.

34. Fennel is *raziyānaj*, *Foeniculum vulgare* Mill. or other species. Fennel was probably known in Babylonia. Diosc. (III 70) has it, μάραθον, to expel menstrua, for dog bites, and for the sight.

In India, it is *madhurika, methica* in Sans., *bâdi* in Bom. and Hind., *sopu* in Tel., *shombu* in Tam. It is commonly cultivated in India but is a native of Europe. In India, the fruit is used as a diuretic, purgative, stimulant, and emmenagogue. The root is also purgative (Nadkarni 557–559).

Maim. (351) gives synonyms as *shamār* in Egypt, *and bisbās* in the Maghrib.

In Persia today, fennel is *rīshah-i-raziyānah* (the root of fennel). It is important in that it is one of the five "opening roots" of the ancients; the others are parsley, celery, asparagus, and butcher's broom. The roots, with *Carum copticum* Benth. and Hook. are given for flatus. Alone, it is given in infusions for toothache and pains after childbirth. (Hooper 119–120). Ducros (77) gives the modern Egyptian usage as an aperitif, stomachic, diuretic, emmenagogue, carminative, and aphrodisiac.

35. *Ghāfit* is agrimony and some kinds of elecampane. *Agrimonia Eupatoria* L. and others. It is used today in the Near East and in the Maghrib today as a detersive and astringent for the throat and

intestines (Ducros 171). It is used in al-Kindī A (115b) in an electuary for compound fever of jaundice and phlegm.

36. Rhubarb is *rīwand or rāwand.* Probably *Rheum Rhaponticum* L. *Cf.* Loew AP (170; Loew FJ (I 356–7).

Diosc. (III 2) has rhubarb, ῥᾶ, for sciatica, the kidneys, bladder, liver, asthma, dysentery, fevers, and animal bites.

Achundow (210) states that there are two kinds of rhubarb, the Chinese and that from Khorasan. On the other hand, Laufer (547 ff.) believes that there is only one kind, the one from Persia having been brought to China in the tenth century. In 1154, al-Idrīsī mentions rhubarb as a product of China growing in the mountains of Tibet. (*Vide* W. Heyd, *Histoire du Commerce du Levant,* Leipzig, 1885–6, II, p. 665–667). That the Chinese did not know the rhubarb from time immemorial is indicated by the composite name *ta hwań* "the great yellow one," or *hwań liań* "the yellow good one." For all genuinely ancient plants there is a root word of a single syllable.

In India, the rhubarb is not too well known in the interior (Ainslie I 343). The most common rhubarb in India is the *R. emodi* Wall. found in the Himalayas. In Sans., it is *amlåvetasa*; Hind. and Punj. *revand-chini;* Bom., Mah., and *ladakirevanda-chini*; Tel. *nattu ireval-chinni*; Tam. *variyattu.* It is used with ginger as a laxative for children. It is also used when teething, for chronic dysentery, for catarrh of the biliary ducts with jaundice, and in certain skin diseases (Nadkarni I 1056–8).

IB (1018) devotes one of the longest sections in his book to rhubarb. Al-Rāzī is quoted as having used it for the stomach. The *Tuḥfa* (355) states that Chinese rhubarb is imported from the Orient. Al-Razzāq (774) gives *rāwand* as a stomachic, carminative, and febrifuge.

The *R. palmatum* L. is known in Persia today as *rīvand-i-chinī.* In Teheran, it is used as a paste for syphilitic ulcers (Hooper 163).

37. Sugar is *sukkar.* Sugar cane was grown in India and China in very early times. Red sugar is crude and has its color from an impurity. Al-Kindī uses red sugar in a clyster. *Tabarazd* sugar is crystalline and considered to be the most refined. This is found in a drug used by al-Kindī for pain of the gums and throat (al-Kindī A (124a, 108a).

38. Caper is *kabbar, Capparis spinosa,* L. Al-Kindī (no. 116) employs caper root rind in a poultice for the spleen. It is used in Egypt today for ulcers and scrofula, and also as a carminative and aphrodisiac (Ducros 30). In Iran, the root and bark are used in intermittent fever and rheumatism (Hooper 94).

In Sans., it is *kakadani,* and in Hind. and Punj. it is *kabra.* It is used in palsy, dropsy, gout, and rheumatism in India (Nadkarni I 267).

39. Purslane is *farfakh, Portulaca oleracea* L. Achundow (159) gives this as a synonym for *baqlat al-mubārak* and *baqlat al-hamqā*. It is probably from the Persian *perpehen* through the Syr. *farfaḥīna*. It is good for the stomach and teeth.

Maim. (59) gives the Gr. πέπλιον (*péplion*). Ducros (14) states that it is originally from India. In Egypt today it is mainly a vermifuge. In modern India, the seeds are a refrigerant and used in diets for scurvy and liver diseases. It is also a vermifuge there. Some synonyms are Sans. *loni, lonīka*, Hind. *khursa*, Tam. *parukire* and *parpukire*. It is abundant in India and Ceylon.

40. *Lukk* is Gummi laccae. It is probably the gum obtained from various botanicals. Achundow (265) states that the best is gum arabic and is good for the liver. That it is gum arabic is highly doubtful.

Loew AP (413) gives Aram. *lakā*. Lac is originally Indian but, at present, comes from Bengal, Siam, Assam, and Pegu. It was used in ink at the beginning of the eleventh century (Levey M.A.B. 19). In Sans., it is *lakṣa; lākh* in Hind.; *lakha* in Guj. in Ayurvedic medicine, it is used for haemoptysis; in Yunani medicine, it is a tonic for the liver, stomach, intestines, and kidneys. It reduces fat in adipose persons and is a haemostatic in India (Nadkarni II 150).

41. *Idhkhir* is lemon-grass, *Andropogon Schoenanthus* L. *Cf.* al-Kindī (no. 94). In al-Kindī G. (nos. 38, 59, 62), lemon-grass is employed in perfumed oils.

Loew FJ (II 295) states that Schoenanthus oil was well known in Syriac. Loew AP (25, 168, 187–8, 346, 411) discusses lemon-grass oil. Aram. is *adqīr*.

Dutt (271, 294) gives the Beng. vernacular as *gandhabinā*, Sans. as *bhustrina*. Chopra (87) gives *rohisha* as the name in Bombay, *rousaghas* in Hindi. The plant is used today in India as an aromatic stimulant and febrifuge. The oil is applied in rheumatism and neuralgia. It is grown in the warmer areas of India from the Punjab to Burma and south to Travancore.

42. *Faqad* is Agnus-castus, *Vitex Agnus-castus* L. Achundow (163) has it equivalent to *banj-angusht*. Al-Kindī A (133b) uses this chaste-tree with other simples to cure insanity, the stroke of madness, and epilepsy. Al-Kindī calls it *banjakusht*. *Cf.* al-Kindī (no. 34).

In Egypt today (Ducros 44), this botanical is used as a calming agent in hysteria.

43. *Mishkatarā mashīr* is dittany, *Origanum Dictamnus* L. This name is Syriac and is also *miskiṭrā mashīᶜ* (IB 2138). Maim. (242)

gives this name as *miskiṭrāmashīr*. *Faudanaj* may be related to dittany. *Cf.* al-Kindī (no. 62).

43a. *Afithīmūn* is dodder, *Cuscuta Epithymum* L. It is probably the Akk. *kiššatu,* Syr. *Kĕsûthâ* (DAB 187). Diosc. (IV 177) gives *ἐπίθυμον* (*epithymon*) as good for melancholy, phlegm, and black choler when given with honey. The Gr. word comes from *πέιθυμίς*, a name for thyme (Carnot 120). Cf. Paulos (642). Ḥunain (106) considers the dodder as a drug to relax the black bile. IB (112) quotes ibn Sīnā that dodder is for epilepsy. Syr. *kasyōn* is given in Budge (II 720).

Al-Ghāfiqī (80) states that this is not the real epithymum but is imported from the land of the Berbers. It is a kind of cuscuta (*kushūth*).

This plant is a parasite which grows on some thyme plants and so their association in the literature. It is also called *kushūth zanjī, aflanja, sikār ᶜAlī,* and *shan* in Pers., and *eftīmūn* in Turk. The *Tuḥfa* (32) believes it to be the parasitic plant, *sidr*. Loew FJ (I 453) discusses this plant in Mishnaic and Talmudic times.

C. planifolia Ten. and *C. hyalina* Roth are grown today in Iran to be used for rheumatism, and with other drugs in a remedy for excessive salivation (Hooper 110–111).

44. The Leiden MS (160a) states that the juice of pomegranate is used here.

45. Gloss: "If the fruits and vegetables are pressed, the juice taken from them is called the "extract." If that juice is made viscous by cooking in the sun, it is called a "rob" and, if sugar is added to it, it is made more viscous and then it is called "syrup." It may be dried in the sun and so a flat cake is made. It is related to what is taken from, for example, the wormwood, and others."

46. To cool the humors.

47. *Safarjal* is quince, *Cydonia Vulgaris* Willd. Al-Kindī A (116b) has quince seed in a myrtle drug for coughs, and as a dentifrice. Quince seed, in modern Egypt, is used as an emollient, lubricant, and refresher (Ducros 26). Ibn Bādīs (1025) uses quince to test henbane (Levey M.A.B. 50). Cf. also al-Kindī (no. 228).

48. *Ḥiṣrim* is verjuice, "juice of unripe raisin" (*Tuḥfa* 181).

Cf. also Diosc. (V 6) giving *ομφακίον*, which is considered good for the eyes, dysentery, mouth, ulcers, and fistulas.

In Arabic, it is also *ghazz al-ᶜinab*. In Pers., it is *ghūra fashraj* which means "rob of verjuice." It is useful for the intestines and other ailments (*al-Muᶜtamad* 97).

49. *Rummān* is the pomegranate, fruit of the *Punica Granatum* L. *Cf.* Levey CCTM (51, 108, 112) and Levey M.A.B. (16, *passim*). *Ramān* (Ar.) may have come about by a metathesis of *nurmū* (Akk.)

and *NU.ÚR.MA* (Sum). This tree grows from Persia to Northwest India (Bailey 2861). In Indian languages, it is, Sans. *dadima-phalam, kuchaphala;* Hind. *anar, dhalim;* Ben., Mah. *dalimb;* Sind. *anar-dakum;* Arabic in India *shajratur-rumman;* Pers. *gulnar;* Tam. *madalam;* Burm. *sale-bin.* The fruit is used after diarrhoea; the bark is used as an anthelmintic; the flowers are for haematuria (Nadkarna I 1031 ff.). For chemical properties, *cf.* Gstirner (220 ff.).

50. *Kumathrā* is pear, pear tree, *Pyrus communis* L., etc.

Maim. gives the synonym as "the plum" (*ijjāṣ*) in the Maghrib. Achundow (246) claims it strengthens the stomach. Loew FJ (III 235 ff.) and Loew AP (208) give the Syr. as *kumtĕrā.*

The Akk. for pear is uncertain but Thompson gives *kameššaru* as possibly *Sorbus domestica* L. but the designation of *P. communis* for the Akk. word is unlikely (DAB 305). The Chinese pear, *kumathrā ṣīnī* is probably the *P. chinensis* Roxb. or *P. sinensis* L. (Bailey 2869).

51. *Līmū* for *līmūn.* Lemon, lime, and others. *Citrus Limonum* Sp. Risso, *Citrus Limetta* L., etc.

IB (2055) states that the rind, pulp, and seeds are used. The juice is probably meant in this text.

The above species grow in India. The lemon tree is *limpaka* in Sans.; *jambira* in Hind. and Duk. The lime is *madhu-karkita* in Sans. They are used as stomachics and in fevers. The citron is also a species of *Citrus.* Cf. Dozy (563); *Al-Muᶜtamad* (465).

52. *Anbarbārīs* is barberry, *Berberis vulgaris* L. *Cf.* abū Ḥanīfa (22). *Ambarbārīs* is given in al-Ghāfiqī (15) where al-Rāzī is quoted to the effect that barberry is good to confine the bowels, and helps the inflamed stomach and liver. This plant was not known to the Greeks. In Arabic, it is also called *barbārīs* and *ᶜūd al-rīḥ;* in Pers. *zirishk;* in Turk. *qadīn tuzlughy,* and in Ber. *ārghīs* for the bark of the roots. *Cf.* IB (146). This drug was unknown to al-Kindī.

53. *Rībās* is ribes or rhubarb-currant, *Ribes rubrum* L. or *Rheum Ribes* Gronov. It grows from Asia Minor to Persia (Bailey 2928).

Maim. (350) gives the synonym as *ashṭiyālla* in Sp. (*Achethiella* is from Lat. *acetosella*). *Rībās* comes from the Pers. *revās, rīwās, rīwīz, rīwāj* (Vullers II 88, 99, 100). IB (1072) gives it as rhubarb-currant.

Loew FJ (I 357–360) states that ribes was unknown to the Greeks and Romans. *Cf.* Loew AP (171), Nabāt (326).

In Persia today, it is *gul-i-livās* used as a purgative (Hooper 164).

54. *Āss* is myrtle, *Myrtus communis* L. Sum. *GIR* and Akk. *āsu* are myrtle. Myrtle grows in the Mediterranean region. Medicinally, it was used in ancient Mesopotamia in a poultice for the stomach, internally "when a man's saliva comes from his mouth," in an enema

for strangury, and in fumigation for the ears. The oil of myrtle was well known. A powder of myrtle was used for blains. The bark, *KUŠ.GIR*, was also used. Ibn al-Waḥshīya has myrtle wood used for its bark. Myrtle was not very popular (DAB 300–301).

Diosc. (I 112) notes myrtle, *μυρσίνη*, for its binding power, using mainly the juice of green myrtle. It is good for the stomach and as an antidote for a scorpion sting. It assuages eye inflammations. Beaten leaves are used in plasters for ulcers. Theophrastus (I 14, 4) uses the same term for myrtle, *μυρσίνη* is a variant for *μύρτος*. The Indo-Eur. is *smer* "to anoint" (Carnoy 183–184).

Galen (VII, XII, 81) considers myrtle as a good desiccative, as earthy and cold.

Myrtle occurs often in Aram. as *'āsā*. Its etymology is uncertain. The Pers. *mūrtus* is from the Gr. The South Ar. is *ḥadas, hadas, khaḍes, and khaḍer*. The Heb. is *hades*. *Cf*. Loew FJ (257–274). The Syr. is *asā*. The Talmud (Loew FJ 268) notes that people dancing in front of the bridal procession held myrtle in the hand. It was believed that roses and myrtle were to be found in paradise.

Al-Ghāfiqī (9) quotes al-Rāzī that when fresh myrtle wood is put on the little finger of a man who is suffering from swelling in his groin, it soothes the pain. This is a doubtful quote since al-Rāzī was not superstitious. Other synonyms are *mirsīn* in Turk., *mūrd* in Pers., and *myrtus* in Lat. In the *Yu yaṅ tsa tsu, asa* is given for myrtle but is confused with myrrh (Laufer 460–461).

Ducros (4) gives Ar. synonyms as *mersīn* and *riḥān*. In South Arabia, it is still known as *hadas*. The leaves are employed today as an astringent in decoctions, in cataplasms, and in oily applications on ulcers and haemorrhoids.

In India today, it is called in Hindi and Punj. *vilayiti mehndi*. The leaves are used in India also as an astringent, and the drug is believed useful in epilepsy, and in stomach and liver diseases. A decoction is employed as a mouth wash in cases of aphthae. Its fruit is carminative, and useful for diarrhoea, dysentery, internal ulceration, and rheumatism. Sometimes the leaf is used for a scorpion sting (Chopra 173).

55. *Summāq* is sumac, *Rhus coriaria* L. Al-Kindī uses sumac in a drug for gum and mouth pustules (al-Kindī A 105b). In Egypt today, sumac is used as an astringent, antiseptic, and antihaemorrhagic (Ducros 28). *Cf*. al-Kindī (no. 263). Mediaeval Arabs used it also for polyurea, pain of the gums and teeth, eyes, and for contusions. *Cf*. Levey M.A.B. (24).

56. *Firṣād* is white mulberry, *Morus alba* L. IB (434, 1679) quotes al-Rāzī that it is a stomachic. *Cf*. Levey M.A.B. (20 for *tūt* as mulberry. This tree is very common in China where there are many

species of *Morus*. In Chinese, it is *sang, sang-pi, san-szu, sang-chou,* and *sang-ken-peh-p'i* (Soubeiran 140–141). In China, it is used for the nerves and rheumatism.

In India, it is *toola* in Sans. and in Tam. *kambilpuch*. It is a purgative and anthelmintic there (Nadkarni I 816–817).

57. Leaves of white mulberry boiled with leaves of black fig and of vine in rainwater produce a liquor which dyes hair black. A gloss under the word reads, "*tūt*."

58. *Zaᶜrūr* is azerole, probably *Crataegus Azarolus* L.

Achundow (212) gives the Pers. synonym as *azdaf* stating that it is good for the stomach and yellow gall. Maim. (132) gives synonyms as *al-ijjāṣ al-shitiwī* "winter plum," and *al-mushtahā* "the appetizing," *shajārat al-dubb* "the tree of the bear," and *al-nulk* which is the medlar tree (Frey. IV 336; Vullers I, 458). Loew FJ (III 244 ff.) gives Mishnaic *ᶜozrār*. *Cf.* Loew AP (25, 286, 288). IB (1112) gives the Sp. as *mushtahī*. The azerole grows in North Africa and Asia Minor (Bailey 887). *Cf. Tuḥfa* (152); *Al-Muᶜtamad* (204).

59. *Nārsinjid* is equated to azerole in the text. *Nār* in Pers. is pomegranate, teat; *sinjid* is the jujube tree or its fruit.

60. *Tabāshīr* is tabasheer, a species of *Bambusa*. Al-Kindī A (104b) has tabasheer in a prescription for mouth pustules and for protection of the soft gum from heat. In Egypt today, it is used in dry collyria as a tonic (Ducros 148), and in Iran in cardiac cases. *Cf.* Achundow (231).

61. Gloss: "That is to say with the juices of the fruits."

62. *ᶜŪd hindī* is aloeswood, *Aquillaria Agallocha* Roxb. and *A. malaccensis* Lemk. In al-Kindī A (114a), aloeswood is employed in a prescription to remove the decayed part of teeth, to treat bad breath, and to polish the teeth. In al-Kindī G. (2b, 5b, 9b, 12a, 12b). this simple is a part of various perfumery products.

In Egypt today, aloeswood is used as an astringent and fumigant (Ducros 167). In India, it is known as a stomachic aperient (Ainslie I 583) and is used in vertigo and palsy (Ainslie I 479–481).

63. *Maṣtaka* is mastix, probably from *Pistacia Lentiscus* L. *Cf.* the note on the testing of blue bdellium in Levey M.A.B. (50). In the Arabic period, mastic gum was used as a stomachic, for obstructions, and to combat nausea (IB 2139).

63a. *Qāqulla* is greater cardamom, *Elettaria major* Smith. It is probably *qāqūlā* in Akk. (B. Meissner, ZA *6,* 293 (1891). In al-Kindī A (105b, 107b), it is used for gum and mouth pustules, and for throat pain.

This plant grows in Southeast Asia, Ceylon, and on the Malabar Coast. It is used as a stomachic in India (Ainslie I 52).

64. *Qaranful* is clove, *Caryophyllus aromaticus* L. Al-Kindī A

(114a) uses clove in a dentifrice to treat rotting teeth and bad breath. *Vide* also IB (1748). Ducros (184) notes that clove is used in present day Egypt as a carminative, aromatic, and condiment. In al-Kindī G. (no. 90), clove is a constituent of perfumes. Bayān (22) has clove in heart preparations for palpitation. *Cf.* Levey M.A.B. (48), Achundow (245).

65. *Zaᶜfarān* is saffron, *Crocus sativus* L., sometimes the root of *Curcuma longa* L. Al-Kindī G. (no. 130) uses saffron in a musk perfume and in many other perfumery products. Al-Kindī A (92b, 94a) has saffron in an Indian electuary to raise the spirits, and in a nasal medicine for scrofula. Saffron comes from an ancient Akk. word *azupirānu*. Saffron is a stimulant and antispasmodic. The dried, red stigmas are used as a coloring agent in Ayurvedic and Yunani remedies today. *Cf.* al-Kindī (no. 302); Levey M.A.B. (22); Levey, M., *Journ. Hist. Med.* 16, 402 (1961).

66. *Barānīyye* is unknown. It may be a geographic term.

67. *Fustuq* is pistachio, probably *Pistacia Terebinthus* L. It is not mentioned in al-Kindī but is in al-Kindī G. (no. 28) where it is employed in aromatic salves. *Cf.* Levey M.A.B. (26).

68. *Utrujj* is citron, *Citrus medica* Risso var. *cederata*. It may be the Akk. *khaṣkhallatu* "sour juice," Sum. *A.AM*. It is used externally only (DAB 313).

Diosc. (I 115) gives μηδικὰ μῆλα which came into Ar. as *tuffāḥ mā'i*. *Utrujj* is from Pers. *turunj* (Vullers I 439) which is from Sans. *mātulaṅga* or *mātuluṅga* (Laufer 581). In Afghan, it is *turanj*; in Baluchi *trunj*. *Utrujj* is cognate to Heb. *ethrōg* which is *Citrus medica* L. *lageniformis* Roem. There are many different species, according to ᶜAbd al-Laṭīf (Maim. 1). *Cf.* Clément-Mullet, J.-J., *Journ. asiatique* VIᵉ ser., *15*, 17–41. For *ethrōg* and Syr. *ethrūngā*, *cf.* Loew AP (46). The Talmud discusses the *ethrūgā* or *ethrūngā* (Gitt. II 44b).

In India, *Citrus medica* is probably *Mithá nebu* as described by Roxburgh. It is called *madhukarkati* and is used in carminative medicines for dyspepsia. It is good for intoxication and narcotics (Dutt 126). *Nimbuka* is the name in Sans. In the Hindi and Beng. vernaculars, it is *kágjinembu*.

Al-Kindī G. (nos. 38, 49, 53–55, 59, 60, 62, 63) has citron in various recipes for many drugs with and without perfumes. In no. 79, he discusses the distillation of citron juice. *Utrujj* is not found in al-Kindī.

Al-Ghāfiqī (11) states that the blossoms are like narcissus flowers but thinner, and quotes Galen that a small dose of it strengthens the stomach and promotes digestion. Synonyms are *citrea* in Lat. (Pliny), and in Gr. περσικὰ μῆλα.

IB (16) quotes ibn Sīnā that the acidity of the citron strengthens the heart, is difficult to digest, and causes colic.

69. *Khashkāsh* is poppy, *Papaver somniferum* L. In Sum., it is *UKUŠ.RIM,* and in Akk. *irru*. In Babylonia, it was used for the stomach, urinary trouble, the head, and for swellings.

Diosc. (IV 64) has it for inflammations, sleeping, pain, headache, and eyes.

Achundow (195) mentions the white and black poppies; the uses are essentially those of the Greeks and Babylonians. Al-Kindī and al-Kindī G. do not mention poppy. Maim. (401) gives the white one as *al-nuᶜmān al-abyaḍ*, and the wild as *ṭārakhīrā*. IB (794–797) mentions the same uses.

Ducros (55–56) states that opium from the poppy is used in Egypt to put children to sleep. It is used in ophthalmia and for inflammations. Hooper (147) gives it as *kavl-a-kūknār* or *tukhm-i-khash khash* in modern Persia.

Ufiyūn, or opium, is *chasa* in Sans., *apini* in Tam. and Tel. The Indians, in the eighteenth century, used opium for the pulse and to augment the heat of the body, in small doses (Ainslie I 272–3). In the last century and earlier in China, opium was employed for leucorrhoea, dysentery, diarrhoea, spermatorrhoea, and other ailments. Some of its names were *yn-tsee-chou, yn-tchou-hoa, yin-shu, yang-yen,* and *ying-sze-shu* (Soubeiran 214 ff.).

70. Gloss: "That is, the barley used by the chemist."

71. *Nailūfar* is nenuphar, *Nymphaea caerulea* L. and *N. lotus* L. var. *alba*. This botanical is not mentioned in al-Kindī's works. The Arabs used this simple for insomnia due to heat, for pleural disturbances, and the lungs. The flowers are not much used today. The testing of the nenuphar is discussed in Levey M.A.B. (49).

72. *Lisān al-thaur* is borage, especially *Borrago officinalis* L. The Ar. is a translation of the Gr. βούγλωσσον. Diosc. (IV 127) considers it efficacious for abscesses. Achundow (265) has it for heart palpitation and the lungs. Maim. (211) gives synonyms as *al-kuḥailā', al-ḥumāḥim,* and *al-ᶜalīs*.

In modern Egypt (Ducros 118), borage is used as an emollient, diuretic, and sudorific.

73. *Badranj-būya* is balm, mountain balm, and sometimes balm-mint, *Melissa officinalis* L. The Pers. name means "odor of citron." Theoph. (VI, I, 5) lists this plant, μελισσόφυλλον, among the spineless ones and as an "undershrub." Diosc. (II 104) gives synonyms as μελίτταιον, μελίτταιναν, μελίφυλλον, and others. It is considered good for bites, dysentery, dysmenorrhoea, ulcers, gout, and poisonous mushrooms. *Cf.* Berendes (334). Achundow (160, 347) lists this simple as good for the heart, especially palpitations, the eyes, stomach, and

liver. Maim. (40) gives synonyms as *bādranbūya, bādranjūya, ḥabāq turunjī,* and *al-turunjān.* In error, Maim. also calls it *marmākhūr.* Al-Ghāfiqī (145) calls it *al-lāʿiba al-naḥliyya* "furnishing juice to the bees." It is good for scorpion stings, bites of dogs and tarantulas. *Cf.* also IB (221). Loew FJ (75) gives melissophyllon as the Syr. *gagulā.*

Tuḥfa (72) gives another synonym as *bādarūj,* and the Kabyle as *tizizouit* (*al-Razzāq* 123). In Persia today, this simple is used as a carminative and tonic (Hooper 114). Hooper (89). gives *bād-i-ranjah-būyah* as the *Asperugo procumbens* L. in present day Iran.

74. Gloss: "To prevent the mixture of anything burned with that not burned so as not to spoil the latter in the second boiling."

75. *Zūfā* is hyssop, *Hyssopus officinalis* L. The original cognate is *zūpu* in Akk. Al-Kindī A (115b) uses hyssop in a remedy effective for quartan fever, jaundice, and the fever of every second day. Bayān (34) considers hyssop as a drug for asthma, chronic coughing, and pain of the side. *Cf.* al-Kindī (no. 315).

76. This is to loosen the mucus in the bronchi and trachea.

77. *Khiṭmī* is the marshmallow, *Althaea officinalis* L. Al-Kindī G. (no. 50) uses marshmallow in distillation processes to obtain perfumes. *Cf.* also al-Kindī (137).

In Egypt today, the mallow is used for the chest, in bladder ailments, and as an emollient in tuberculosis (Ducros 99). It is generally used in the Near East for coughs to facilitate expectoration.

78. *Zabīb.* Raisins are not often described in the literature since the product is so omnipresent. *Zabīb* is given in *Al-Muʿtamad* (193–4). The latter states that if one eats raisins with the seeds, then they are fattening, and if eaten without the seeds, then they tend to make one thin. Al-Kindī A (102a) uses raisins for ear swellings.

79. *Khūlanjān* is galingale, *Alpinia officinarum* Hance. Al-Kindī A (139a) employs galingale root as a stomachic, and for the effects due to excessive intercourse. The Ar. word comes originally from the Chinese *kao-lian-kian,* according to Hance. Laufer believes it is from Sans. *kulañja.* This simple is not found in al-Kindī G. *Cf.* al-Kindī (no. 138); Levey M.A.B. (31). In the latter it is used in a colored ink for holy books.

80. *Sūsan* is lily or iris, any of the many species of *Liliaceae* and *Iridaceae.* The blue lily is *sūsan āsmānjūnī.* In al-Kindī (102b, 119a), it is used (i.e. the oil) for swelling of the ears and pus in them, and in a remedy for haemorrhoids. In al-Kindī G. (no. 110), white lily is used in making drugs which also contain sesame oil and rose water. *Cf.* al-Kindī (no. 267).

81. *Parsīya wushān* is maiden hair, *Adiantum Capillus Veneris* L. Theoph. (VII 14) has maiden-hair, ἀδίαντον as useful to prevent

falling out of hair of the head. Diosc. (IV 134–5) has this plant for asthma, dyspnoea, for bites, for the stomach, alopecia, and makes cocks more hostile.

In Hind., it is called *hansraj* or *mubaraka*. The juice is used in Southern India for all kinds of fever and for chronic cough (Chopra 562). It is also used as a tonic (Ainslie II 215). Paul of Aegina (610) thought it good for swellings and the lungs.

Al-Kindī G. (Recipes 53, 54, 56) has *barshnān* in perfumes. IB (256, 388, 1155, 1324, 1440, 1934) quotes ibn Sīnā that this drug is used for fistulas and ulcers. Some synonyms given by the author are *shaʿr al-jabār* "hair of the giant," *shaʿr al-arḍ* "hair of the earth," *liḥya al-ḥimār* "beard of the ass," *al-sāq al-aswad* "black leg," and *kazbarat al-bīr* "coriander of the well." In Maim. (182), Meyerhof gives the translation of the Pers. *parr-i-Siyāwushān* as the "hair of the (Persian hero) like Siyāwush. The *Tuḥfa* (65) spells it as *barshiyaushān*.

This plant is found today in Iran, Afghanistan, Western China, and in the Northwestern Himalayas. The root is used as an expectorant, to relieve respiration, and for spasms in whooping cough (Hooper 81). Ducros (115) gives the uses in present day Egypt as a diuretic, for rheums, bronchitis, and alopecia.

82. *Sabastān* is sebesten, *Cordia Myxa* L. Al-Kindī A (92b) has sebesten in a remedy to lift the spirits of a patient, and to strengthen the stomach and liver. It is used today in Iran, Egypt, Syria, and other neighboring regions for bronchial and pulmonary affections.

In Hind., it is *chakargand*, in Ben. *buhul*, and in Tam *naruvali*. It is fairly common in South India where it is used as a mild tonic (Chopra 478; Nadkarni I 380). *Cf.* al-Kindī (no. 223).

83. *Laban* is milk. *Cf.* Achundow (178). Al-Kindī A (97a, 129a) has sour milk in a remedy to be applied to leprosy. The milk of the ass is used in ophthalmia, leprosy, and skin fissures.

84. Gloss: "White."

85. *Ṣandal* is sandalwood, *Santalum album* L. When the white type is meant, the adjective is often missing. In al-Kindī A (94a), this simple is used with others in a poultice for the liver and spleen. Al-Kindī G. uses sandalwood often in perfumery operations (*cf.* fol. 18b, 26a, 26b, 58b ff., 63a–63b, 70a–70b). Al Akfānī (4a) uses sandalwood in a prescription for a swelling. It is used today in Iran for its antiseptic action in the genito-urinary tract. In Egypt, white sandalwood is used as an aromatic and for gonorrhoea.

86. *Tamar hindī* is tamarind, *Tamarindus indica* L. In al-Kindī A (135a), tamarind is used with other simples to prepare a diluent. *Cf.* also al-Kindī (no. 274). The tamarind is indigenous in India, and is used in Egypt as a mouth wash and for thrush, and in Iran, the

seeds are used in a plaster for boils (Hooper 175). In India, it is used as a collyrium and laxative, sometimes for jaundice (Ainslie II 327). *Cf. Munatakkhib* (30a).

87. Gloss: "Not maggoted."

88. *Kuzbarah* is coriander, *Coriandrum sativum* L. Al-Kindī A (96a, 135a) has coriander in a prescription for headache due to heat, and in another recipe for a diluent. Dry coriander indicates the dried leaf. Ibn Bādīs in Levey M.A.B. (29) has coriander in a kind of ink product. In Egypt, it is used as a stomachic (Ducros 199), and in Iran for toothache and headache (Hooper 106). It is also a stomachic in India (Ainslie I 92). The Ar. word is originally the Akk. *kusibirru* (Meissner, B., *ZA* (1891) 294).

89. *ᶜAdas* is lentil, usually the *Lens esculente* Moench. Al-Kindī G. (no. 4) has peeled lentils in a musk recipe. In al-Kindī A (108a), it is used in a drug for toothache.

90. Gloss: "Dozen."

91. Leiden MS (160a) has "seed."

92. Gloss: "Like the viscosity of oxymel."

93. This title does not conform with the author's table of contents although the subject matter corresponds.

94. "The word *iṭriflāt* (sing. *iṭrifl*) signifies confections made of the three kinds of myrobalans, chebulic, emblic, and belleric myrobalans." (Sbath,P. and C.D.Avierinos, *Deux traités medicaux,* Le Caire, 1953, chap. 1 of Sahlān ibn Kaysān's *Mukhtaṣar fī al-adwiya al-markaba fī akthar al-amrāḍ.*).

95. Gloss: "Because the meaning of *iṭri fwakehufil* is 'three' in Indian."

96. *Amlaj* is emblic myrobalan; *balīlaj* is belleric myrobalan; *halilaj kabūlī* is Kabul myrobalan. For a fuller description, *cf.* Levey M.A.B. (44); al-Kindī (no. 9). Al-Kindī G. (7a, 7b) has emblic myrobalan in musk recipes. In al-Kindī A (92b), it is in a prescription to make one happy, to strengthen the heart, and stomach. It is good for the liver also. Bik. (3b) uses it for the intestines. In Egypt, it is still used as an anti-diarrhetic and light purgative (Ducros 10); in Iran, it is employed to stimulate the appetite (Hooper 150). In India, from where it comes today, it is used as a vulnerary and eccoprotic (Ainslie I 239).

Laufer (378) gives the Chinese names of the three myrobalans: *ho-li-lo* is chebulic; *p'i-li-lo* is belleric (in Sans. *vibhītaka;* Pers. *balīla*); *a-mo-lo* is emblic (in Sans. *āmālaka;* Pers. *amola*). Tou Kin of the Sung in "Treatise on Wine" *Tsiu p'u* states, "In the country *Po-se* (Persia ?), there is a congee made from the three myrobalans.

97. Above this a gloss reads: "Like the stomach, intestines and liver."

98. I.e. the excrements.

99. Gloss: "A place in India." Baṣra was a popular name for a city, sea, swamp, and desert, from Morocco to India.

100. I.e. the weights of each of the first three.

101. Gloss: "That is, for the strength of dryness."

102. Gloss: "It is rancid and it stinks."

103. *Shirāmulaj* is a Persian remedy of belleric myrobalan soaked in milk. It is from *shir* "milk" plus *amlaj*. The latter is from Pers. *āmala* or *āmula* (Laufer 581) which comes from Sans. *āmālaka*. IB (264, 1273) states that it is a milk mixture. *Cf.* Maim. (374), and note 96 earlier.

104. Gloss: "Of Kabul, black and yellow."

105. Gloss: "Kabul myrrh."

106. *Muql* is false bdellium. It is a resin which may come from various species as *Hyphaene thebaica* Mart., *Balsamadendron africanum* Arn., *B. Mukul* Hook, etc. (Maim. 230). Al-Kindī A (136a) has this simple in applications for the lungs and head. In Iran and Iraq, false bdellium is applied in a plaster for muscular rheumatism (Hooper 103–104). Cf. al-Kindī (147) for blue bdellium.

107. *Kahrabā* is yellow amber, the resin of *Populus nigra* L. Al-*Kindī* A (138b) uses this simple for nosebleed and as a haemostatic agent. Al-Kindī spells it *kārabā*.

The buds are used in India as a depurative, and the bark for colds (Nadkarni I 1005).

108. *Jullinār* is pomegranate flower, of the *Punica granatum* L., a wild species. Al-Kindī G. (14b) uses this in a recipe for a substitute for saffron. Al-Kindī A (99b) has it in a poultice for the liver and stomach, and to relieve pain of the spleen and to strengthen it. Pomegranate flower is used in ink by ibn Bādīs. Levey M.A.B. (26). *Cf.* al-Kindī (113).

109. *Kharmāzaj* is tamarisk gallnut. It is not found in al-Kindī's works.

110. *Nānakhwāh* is Royal cumin or bishop's weed, probably *Ammi Copticum* L. Al-Kindī A (134a) uses this simple in a prescription for haemorrhoids. Ducros (230) states that the fruit is used in Egypt today as a diuretic and stomachic. In Persia and India, it is used in cases of cholera (Hooper 95). *Cf.* also IB (2202); Maim. (259). *Al-Muᶜtamad* (512 ff.) gives the seed of this plant as a diuretic.

111. Gloss: "It is that which is soaked in vinegar and dried after that in the shade."

112. Gloss: "The *bustad* is coral." The gloss spells coral as *basad*.

113. Gloss: "That is, its weights are less than what they were before when haemorrhoids were present."

114. Gloss: "That is, reduce the honey."

115. *Maqarr,* perhaps "rectum" or "anus."

116. *Zanjabīl* is ginger, *Zingibir officinale* Rosc. Al-Kindī A (125b) and abū Ghālib Ansāf (?) have this in a collyrium for the eyes. In India today, ginger is employed for gout, and in paralytic and rheumatic disorders. *Cf.* Levey M.A.B. (49). For the etymology, *cf.* al-Kindī (no. 306).

117. *Filfil* is pepper, probably the black type, *Piper nigrum* L. The white is *filfil abyad.* Al-Kindī A (107b) uses black pepper in a prescription for pain of the gum and throat. In India today, it is used as a stomachic (Ainslie I 303–5). Al-Rāzī has it in use for intestinal ulcers. For the etymology of the word *filfil, cf.* al-Kindī (no. 65).

118. *Dār filfil* is long pepper, *Piper longum* L. Al-Kindī A (114b) has long pepper in the preparation of a syrup. In Chinese, it is *py-po-ly, pi-po, pi-pa, pih-poh,* and *pi-po-tze,* and it is used in China as a stimulant, stomachic, and astringent. *Cf.* al-Kindī (no. 52). The Chinese and English came originally from the Sans. *pippali.* Cognates are found in Hind., Guj., Ben., Ar., Tel., Tam., and other languages. In the Ayurveda, it is used to cleanse ulcers, etc. In Yunani medicine, it is for the liver, spleen, gout, epilepsy, paralysis, and the stomach (Nadkarni I 965–969).

119. *Sanā* is senna, leaf of many species as *Cassia acutifolia* Del., *C. angustifolia* Vahl., and *C. obovata* Coll. (Nadkarni I 282 ff.). Al-Kindī A (135a) uses a Meccan senna in a prescription for a diluent. The species *C. senna* Wood. is much used in India as a purgative. For Indian senna, *cf.* Chopra (87 ff.): it is called *hindi-sana* in Hind.

120. *Siracost* is a type of manna. According to Steingass, it comes from *shīr khist,* the manna of *Atrophaxis spinosa.*

121. *Shābīzaj,* a Persian word for mandrake fruit, of *Mandragora officinarum* L.

The Akk. is *pi(l)lū,* and according to one writer a cognate to *luffāḥ,* an Ar. synonym for mandrake (DAB 217). *Pilu* "egg" fits the mandrake; Diosc. (IV 164) writes of a male and female. The Syriac mentions its two little balls "like the testicles of a man" (Budge 708) when referring to the *kahīnā* root. In Semitic, the word for egg is equivalent to that for testicle as Ar. *baiḍ.* Another Ar. synonym is *yabrūḥ.*

In India, it is called *putrada, raktavindu* in Sans., *lakmani, bhagener* in Hind., *mardami* in Pers., *katavjate* in Tam. It is sedative, anaesthetic, narcotic, and cholagogue (Nadkarni I 764).

For etymology, *cf.* al-Kindī (no. 158); Loew AP (188).

122. *Qishmish* for currants is a Persian word.

123. *Ghārīqūn* is agaric, *Agaricus officinalis* L. Al-Kindī A (115b,

135a) has agaric in a preparation for quartan fever, jaundice, stomach, and liver. It is used in India as a styptic and cicatrizing agent (Ainslie I 6).

124. *Cf.* Maim. (65). For etymology of *basbāyij*, *cf.* al-Kindī (no. 41). The root of the common polypody is usually used today for rheumatic pains, for digestion, and as a purgative for bilious disorders.

125. *Ifsintīn* is wormwood, *Artemisia Absinthium* L. Various species of Artemisia grow in the Near East but it is difficult to determine their ancient names. One may be the Akk. *sīḇu* which is cognate to the Syr. *šīḇā, A. Judaica* L. In Babylonia, it was used for swellings, bruises, in clysters, for fumigation, and as a stomachic (DAB 361, 362). Theoph. (VII, 9, 5) mentions wormwood, ἀψινθίον, as having a sweet smell but deadly. Diosc. (III 23) states that it grows on Mount Taurus in Cappadocia and that it purges bilious humors from the stomach. Al-Ghāfiqī (27) quotes Galen that wormwood is imported from Pontus.

Maim. (3) gives *kashūth rūmī* as an Ar. synonym, and the Sp. as *yerba baṭra*. Other synonyms are *shiḥ, shiḥ al-rabīᶜ, daqn al-shaikh,* and *shaiba* in Ar., *tāshtalt* in Ber., *afsintīn* in Pers., and *pelin* in Turk. IB (113) gives *damsīsa* as the Egyptian name of wormwood. Loew FJ (I 379) gives many *Artemisia* plants well known medically in the Near East.

A. Indica Willd. was used in seventeenth century India as a stomachic, deobstruent, and antispasmodic (Ainslie II 194–5). In Persia today, *A. vulgaris* L. is grown and used as a stomachic tonic (Hooper 87–8). The *Indica* species was known in nineteenth century China and earlier as *yin-tchin-kao, in-czen-chua,* and *yin-ch'in-hau;* it was used for the stomach, and for catarrh, fever, and jaundice (Soubeiran 164).

Al-Kindī A (93a) uses wormwood in a dressing to reduce swelling of the spleen.

126. *Usṭūkhūdūs* is lavender, *Lavandula Stoechas* L. Diosc. (III 26) gives lavender, στοιχάς, as good in a decoction for ailments of the thorax, and also in antidotes. Cf. also Ber. (281–282).

Lavender is used by Jābir (175b) in a preparation for the bite of a mad dog. This plant is not mentioned in al-Kindī's works. It has not been recognized as an article in Sino-Iranian commerce of ancient times.

In Syriac medicine (Budge 275), lavender is found in a prescription for diseases of the chest; this text is, of course, almost entirely Galenic. The compounded medicine is called in Syr. *metdōrīṭōs*.

Maim. (6) gives the synonyms as *washa'iᶜ ash-shaikh, arshanīsa, sunbul al-ahāniya*. The Ar. *usṭūkhūdūs* comes from the Gr. as given by Dioscorides; Syr. is *lebōnthā* and Heb. ēzibyōn. The Gr. probably came from the word for "in line" referring to the order of the small flower (Carnoy 254). *Tuḥfa* (13) gives the Ber. as *tāymerzā*. An Ar. synonym given is *al-ḥalḥāl*.

In India, lavender juice (of *Lavandula Carnosa* L.) was squeezed from the leaves, then mixed with pounded sugar candy, and prescribed by native practitioners in cases of cynanche. With gingilie oil and other simples, it was used as a cooling liniment for the head (Ainslie II 144–5).

Loew FJ (II 73–4) gives *azōvyūn* as Mishnaic, and *stycados* from Albertus Magnus. In the Heb. literature, lavender is sometimes confused with marjoram.

Al-Ghāfiqī (28) quotes Galen (VIII, XII, 136) that lavender fortifies all the inner organs. Other Ar. synonyms are *liḥlāḥ* and *kammūn hindī*. The Pers. is *ustūkhūdūs* (from the genitive of the Gr. word). Turk. is *husāme, lavanda otu, qarabash otu,* and others. Bīrūnī gives *dahār* as known in Sind. In Hind., it is *dharu*. (al-Ghāfiqī 38).

IB (62) quotes al-Rāzī that lavender helps epilepsy and melancholy, and is used as a purgative. Ibn Sīnā uses it to help evacuate the black bile humor from the head and the heart.

In India today, lavender is used as a resolvent and carminative. (Chopra 151).

Ducros (6) gives the synonyms as *muwaqaf al-arwaḥ* and *mumisk al-arwaḥ*. It is used (that is, the flowers) internally today in the Near East as a stimulant, tonic, and antispasmodic.

127. Gloss: "Fine."

128. Gloss: *"Halīlaj, balīlaj, amlaj."*

129. Maim. (200) has *kazmāzak* instead of the text's *kazmāzaj*.

130. *Khabath al-ḥadīd* is scoria of iron. Al-Kindī A (94a, 101a, 118b) uses scoria of gold in a nasal medicine for scrofula, scoria of silver for a boil and for haemorrhoids. *Cf. al-Kindī* (no. 133) and *Al-Muᶜtamad* (116). In the latter, scoria of iron is noted as the strongest drying agent; it also dissolves swellings.

131. Gloss: "Chronic."

132. *Kundur* is frankincense, especially from *Boswellia Carterii* Birdw.

In Sans., it is *kapitthaparni, salakhi, kunduru*. In Hind., it is *lobhan* after the Ar. *lubān* (Nadkarni I 211). In India, it is used as an emmenagogue, ecbolic, aperient, diuretic, and alterative (Chopra 469).

Al-Kindī (123b) *lubnā* is used in a clyster to protect the patient against certain humors, and in another prescription of the same work (137b), it is in a preparation to eradicate the worm, and to purify the air which spreads epidemics. *Kundur* which is Pers. is a synonym of *lubān* (Semitic). *Cf.* Maim. (188).

133. *Suᶜd* is sweet cyperus, *Cyperus longus* L. Al-Kindī A (107a, 114a) has sweet cyperus in a drug for canker, ulcers, and decaying of the teeth. It is used to polish the teeth and for bad breath. It is used in Egypt today as a stomachic and emmenagogue; in Iran it is a dentifrice (Hooper 112). For etymology, *cf.* al-Kindī (no. 259).

134. *Sunbul* is nard of which many species are possible. The Indian nard is *Nardostachys Jatamansi* D.C. Al-Kindī A (92b, 104b) has nard in a prescription for pustules in the mouth and for protection of the soft gum from heat. Wild nard is used in a drug to make one happy. In al-Kindī (138b), Indian nard is used in a stomachic developed by al-Kindī himself.

The Indian nard is used today; in Egypt for epilepsy, convulsions, and hysteria (Ducros 130), and in Iran and Iraq for nervous ailments (Hooper 143).

135: The text has *"fanjanush"* instead of *"penjanush."* In Pers. *penj* is "five," and *nush* comes from *nushiden* "drink," to mean "five drinks." It is an electuary which contains iron filings, wine, almond oil, and other simples.

136. *Qarᶜ* is pumpkin, gourd, *Cucurbita maxima* Duch. (pumpkin) or *C. Pepo* L., *Lagenaria vulgaris* Sér. (calabash). Al-Kindī A (91b, 121b) has the long gourd in an electuary for cold affliction of phlegm, black gall, nervous conditions, rheumatism, and for an ointment effective for the limbs, bladder, and kidney. *Cf.* al-Kindī (no. 199) for etymology.

The *qarᶜ* is still used in Iran and Iraq today for chest complaints internally (Hooper 108).

137. *Khass* or *khash* is lettuce, *Lactuca sativa* L. In Akk., lettuce is *ḫassu*, in Sum. *ḪI.IṢ*, and was used for inflammations and burns. Loew AP (75, 175, 181) gives the Heb. as *khasā*.

Achundow (193) has it for the head, eyes (also Thābit b. Qurra), and sleep. IB (792) quotes ᶜAwwām that lettuce excites the appetite and calms the bile. Al-Rāzī believes that care must be exercised in prescribing lettuce. Cf. al-Dīnawarī (155–6 Ar.).

In Persia today, it is called *tukhm-i-kāhū*, and is prescribed for fevers.

In al-Kindī A (132b), this simple is employed with ass's hoof for quartan ague fever.

138. *ᶜAnbar* is ambergris. The Sans. is *ambar-sugandah* (Chopra 544). Al-Kindī A (107b) uses ambergris in a preparation for pain

of the throat. Al-Kindī G. (*passim*) employs ambergris frequently in perfumery products. *Cf.* Levey M.A.B. (47) where the testing of crude ambergris is described.

139. *Khiyār shanbar* is purging cassia tree, *Cassia Fistula* L. Maim. (387) gives *al-qiththa' al-hindī* "Indian cucumber," and *al-kharrūb al-hindī* "Indian carob" as synonyms. IB (836, 1742) quotes ibn Sīnā that it is effective for gout.

The pudding pipe or purging cassia tree is known in Sans. as *nripadruma, aragbhada, arakvadam;* in Hind. as *sonhali, amulthus;* in Duh. as *kirvali, amaltas;* in Guj. as *garmala;* in Tel. as *kondrakayi;* in Tam. as *konai, konraikkai.* It is common throughout India and Burma.

In Ayurvedic medicine, it is used as a mild laxative and for diseases of the heart. In Yunani practise, it is used in liver disease, intestinal ulceration, as a laxative, and in children's chest ailments. Externally, it is used for gout, rheumatism, and ringworm (Nadkarni 285-286). *Cf.* Chopra (473) for uses in rheumatism and snake bite.

In Chinese, it is *tchang-ko-tsee, chang-kwo-tsz-shu,* and *tchang-ko-tze,* used as a purgative (Soubeiran 280).

In modern Egypt, it is used as a purgative (Ducros 58) as it is in Iran (Hooper 96). In Iran, it is called *fulūs.*

140. *Milh hindī* is Indian salt or perhaps some other Indian mineral. Indian salt is red, according to *Alaune* (121 ff.) Cf. Levey M.A.B. (32).

141. *Rubb al-sūs* is licorice rob, rob of *Glycyrrhiza glabra* L. Al-Kindī A (115a) uses licorice root in an electuary for coughs resulting from catarrh, and the leaves (94a) in a coating for scrofula.

The licorice plant is indigenous in Arabia, the Persian Gulf coasts, Afghanistan, Turkestan, Asia Minor, and Siberia. In Yunani medicine, it is used as a nerve tonic, to correct purgatives, and for diseases of the liver, bladder, and lungs (Nadkarni I 582–584).

142. Gloss: "The *ṭassūj* is 1/24 of a drachma or 1/4 *dāniq* or 2 barley grains of weight."

143. *Sūranjān* is colchicum, *Colchicum autumnale* L. Al-Kindī A (136b) has colchicum in a drug to lift the spirits. The important colchicum in India is *C. luteum* Baker species which grows in this country and in the Mediterranean area. It is called *hiranya-tuttha* in Sans.; *surinjan* in the vernacular, *haran* in Hind., and *surinjan* in Kash. It is used chiefly in rheumatism and gout. *Cf.* al-Kindī (no. 65); (Nadkarni I 369–370).

144. *Būzaidān* is orchis (?), perhaps *Orchis Morio* L. The Pers. is *būzīdān* from *abū Zaidan,* according to al-Ghāfiqī (140–141). Maim. (56) gives a synonym as *khuṣā' al-thaᶜlab* "testicles of the fox." Al-

Ghāfiqī repeats the statement of ibn Juljul that it is an Indian remedy. Al-Bīrūnī is quoted as saying that *būzīdān* is Pers. and the Sindī name is *shadhwār*. The kind which comes from Baghdad is *al-mustaᶜgila* which is fattening. The Turk. is *sehleb*.

Achundow (167) considers it good for the nerves and rheumatic pains especially with rose honey. *IB* (373, 1330, 2130) quotes ibn Sīnā that *būzaidān* is an antidote. Hooper (186) claims that *būzīdān* in Iran today is the shrub *Withania somnifera* Dunal. Some confusion exists as to its properties.

145. *Mīzamiraj* is uncertain. It is possibly *miyūfizaj* (Pers.) which is stavesacre, *Delphinium Staphisagria* L. Al-Kindī A (105b, 133b) uses stavesacre in rosewater for paroxysmal fever. *Cf. Tuḥfa* (258).

146. *Kammūn* is cumin, usually the seed of *Cuminum Cyminum* L. and others. Al-Kindī A (122b) has cumin in a rubbing preparation for rheumatism in the knees and other joints. For etymology, *cf.* al-Kindī (no. 120).

Cumin, in modern Egypt is used as a carminative and emmenagogue (Ducros 202). In Iran, the seeds are prescribed for pain after childbirth (Hooper 109).

147. *Shīṭaraj* or *sīṭaraj* is pepperwort or rose colored leadwort, *Lepidium latifolium* L. It may also be *Plumbago rosea* L. Al-Kindī A (96a) has pepperwort in a drug for leprosy. This simple is used in the Middle East for medicinal purposes today as a sudorific (Hooper 155). For etymology, *cf.* al-Kindī (no. 254).

148. *Ṣaᶜtar* or *saᶜtar* is thyme, origan, and savory. There is much confusion as to the identification of this plant. *Cf.* Maim. (157, 319). Achundow (227) gives various translations. Al-Kindī A (96a, 103b) uses thyme for erysipelas, and in a poultice for the stomach.

In Iran, thyme leaves are used as a carminative (Hooper 178). For chemical properties, *cf.* Gstirner (531 ff.).

149. *Ḥinna'* is henna, *Lawsonia alba* Lam. Al-Kindī A (96b, 99b, 113b) employs Meccan henna for ulcers and in a tooth medicine. Al-Kindī G. (219) has henna in perfumery products. For etymology, *cf.* al-Kindī (no. 90).

In Egypt today, it is used as an astringent and in unguents (Ducros 91). In India, the henna leaves are used as a dye. In Iran and Iraq, it is used for skin diseases, boils, and leprosy (Hooper 134–135).

150. *Juljulān. Dozy* (205) gives one possibility as sesame. Loew AP (377) gives it as a maghrib word under *Sesamum orientale* L. According to *Al-Muᶜtamad* (71), "It is sesame of which there are two kinds, white and black. The Arabs call it *duhna al-sallīṭ*." *Cf.* IB (499, 1218).

151. Gloss: "Fifteen dirhams."

152. *Saqmūniyā* is scammony, *Convolvulus Scammonia* L. It is a gum resin obtained by incision of the living root. The gum emulsifies in water while the resin does not. DAB (13) claims that scammony is *abukatu* in Akk. but this uncertain.

Diosc. (IV 170) gives it as σκαμμωνία: it is from *sqam* (Carnoy 236). The Ar. word comes from the Syr. which comes from the Gr.

Maim. (281) gives the synonym as *al-maḥmūda*. *Cf.* Loew FJ (I 451 ff.) and Loew AP (143); also Achundow (220, 377).

Today, in Egypt, it is used as a drastic purgative (Ducros 122). For chemical properties, *cf.* Gstirner (444 ff.).

153. *Lauz* is almond, probably *Amygdalus communis* L. Al-Kindī G. (no. 61) has *lauz*, more likely the sweet almond, together with jasmine oil, costus, and sandalwood in a salve. The sweet almond grows in northwestern Persia. In mediaeval Arabic times, almond oil was used for the stomach and intestines, and to increase the sperm. The bitter almond was much more popular as a remedy. *Cf. Al-Muᶜtamad* (461).

154. Gloss: "That is to say, it has the strength of constipating and the force to ease."

155. That is, weakly purgative plus two other constituents weakening it and preventing it from full activity, and the third strengthening it.

156. *Janṭiyān al-rumī*, Greek gentian, *Gentiana asclepeadea* L. is diccussed in Diosc. (III 3), γεντιάνη, as good for animal bites, convulsions, liver, and stomach. It is used in ulcers and in collyria.

Maim. (77) gives the synonyms as *kūshādh*, in Sp. as *bishlishku* (*basilisco*), and also *dawā al-ḥayya* in Ar. "remedy of the serpent." The Pers. is *gūshādh* or *kūshādh*. Al-Ghāfiqī (204) quotes ibn 'Imrān, "There are two different kinds of gentian, one is a herb that grows on mountains, and in cold, wet, and snowy places; this is the Greek (*rumī*). The other is the *Jurmaqān*." The latter is the one mentioned by Dioscorides. The first kind is the Pers. *kūshādh*, in Gr. βασιλίσκον, *basiliskon*. The latter is the *G. lutea* L. IB (515) also quotes ibn 'Imrān about the two species. Al-Rāzī writes that gentian is an important antidote.

Loew FJ (I 653) gives the Syr. as *jentiana*, from Galen, as an antidote. *Cf.* Vullers (I 246) and *Al-Muᶜtamad* (75). This simple is still used in modern Egypt (Ducros 37), especially the *G. lutea* L. plant.

157. *Ghār* is sweet bay, *Laurus nobilis* L. Al-Kindī A (123b, 137b) uses the oil of sweet bay in a clyster to warm and dry the kidneys. The seed is used in a recipe to eradicate the worm and to purify the air during epidemics.

For etymology, *cf.* al-Kindī (no. 68). *Ghār* usually refers to the seed.

158. *Zarāwand ṭawīl* is greater Aristolochia, *Aristolochia longa* L. In al-Kindī A (94a), it is used in a recipe for a coating for scrofula. The round species, *A. rotunda* L., in al-Kindī A (122a) is employed in the preparation of an oil of wild cucumber for the binding of sinews, pain in the back, perspiration of women, and for all pains of rheumatism.

159. *Qirṭim* is carthamus, especially its seed, from *Carthamus tinctorius* L.

This plant, also called safflower (*ᶜaṣfūr*), is still sold today in Egyptian bazaars for dyeing, and as a laxative and carminative (Levey M.A.B. 30). The red florets are used in Afghanistan, Iran, and Syria as a dyestuff and cosmetic (Hooper 84).

The Aram. is *qurṭĕmā* (Loew FJ I 394 ff.) and in Heb. *qôrṭem* (*Cf.* Maim. 300). The word *qortom* is used today for the flowers.

In present day India, it is used for jaundice. It is called *kusum* in Hind. and Ben. (Chopra 472).

160. *Kattān* is flax, *Linum usitatissimum* L. Flax was well known in ancient Babylonia (Levey CCTM 87). In Sum., it is *KAT,* in Akk. *kitū,* Various species of flax are found in the Near East (Loew FJ II 209; DAB 113). The Syr. is *kettānā*. The Gr. word comes from the Semitic. *Cf.* Loew AP (171 ff.); flax for paper (Levey MAB 10).

161. *Jawārashnāt.* Mainly stomachic confections.

162. *Hīl* is lesser cardamom,, *Elettaria Cardamomum* Wh. & Matern. Sometimes *hāl.* In al-Kindī A (92b, 114a, 135b), it is employed to lift the spirits, for bad breath, and for rotting teeth. For etymology, *cf.* al-Kindī (no. 71).

163. *Bisbās* is mace, *Myristica fragrans* Houtt. In al-Kindī A (135b), mace is a simple in a compounded remedy to strengthen the spirit. *Bisbās* is equal to *bisbāsah*. Etymology is in al-Kindī (no. 46).

In Egypt today, mace is a tonic, stomachic, liniment, and internal and external aromatic (Ducros 37). In India and Iran also, it is used medicinally (Hooper 142).

164. *Kabbābah* is cubeb, *Piper Cubeba* L. In al-Kindī A (105b, 108a), cubeb is used for the gum and mouth pustules. Achundow (251–252) claims that it purifies the throat and is good for the kidneys.

It is called *sungadha-muricha* in Sans., tailpepper in Engl., *valmilaku* in Tam. It is used as a diuretic in India (Nadkarni I 400 ff.) as it is used in modern Egypt and Iran (Ducros 195; Hooper 151–152).

165. *Misk* is musk. There are many recipes for musk perfumes in al-Kindī G. (pp. 271–274) and various kinds of musk. Musk is mentioned as one of the principal aromatics in Māsawaih's small work

translated by Levey; it is called *Kitāb jawāhir al-ṭīb al-mufrada* (*Mukhtaṣar fī maᶜrifat ajnās al-ṭīb ilḥ*) (*Journ. Hist. Med.* XVI, 398–399 (1961). Māsawaih describes the major types of musk. Al-Nuwairī (d. 1332), in his *Nihāyat al-arab fī funūn al-adab* follows Māsawaih's ninth century work. *Cf.* Wiedemann 49 (1917). Musk is a secretion found in a vesicule at the prepuce of the male *Moschus moschiferous* found in lower Tibet. Masᶜūdī, in his *Murūj al-dhahab* (I 353) states that the Tibetan variety is better than the Chinese since the Chinese must go through a harmful sea journey. *Cf.* ibn Qurra (826?–901) in his *Al-dhakhīra fī ᶜilm al-ṭibb*, ed. by G. Sobhy, Cairo, 1928, par. 53, 185, 300. In India, it is used as a stimulant and antispasmodic. It is also used in dyspepsia, typhus, and in dysentery (Ainslie I 228). *Cf. Talmud Babli, Barochat* 45; *Yerushalmi, Barochat Per.* 6.

166. *Salīkha* is cinnamon, *Cinnamomum aromaticum* Nees. It is equivalent to *dār ṣīnī* (Maim. 95). This bark is used in al-Kindī A (92b, 114a, 136b) in the *nosh-darū* electuary which makes people happy and strengthens the stomach and liver. It is also used in prescriptions for the spirits, and for dental medicines. Achundow (218) states that it is a red dye, and is good for the stomach and liver.

Salīkha may also be the *C. cassia* Blume which is indigenous in Ceylon, southern India, and Burma. In Yunani medicine, it is a stomachic, deabsorbent, diuretic, aphrodisiac, demulcent; externally it is used for palpitation, melancholia, dropsy, liver, diarrhoea, and hiccough. The *Ayurveda* has it for many diseases. The Sans. is *gudatvak, thwak;* Pers. *saila-myah;* Tel., Tam., and Mal. *lowanga-pattai;* Punj. *kirfa* (Nadkarni I 328 ff.). *Cf.* IB (1205).

167. *Sādaj* or *sādhaj* is malabathrum, *Laurus Malabathrum* L. or *Cinnamomum malabathrum* L. Loew AP (269) gives Aram. *sadag* and Gr. μαλάβαθρον=φύλλον=Aram. *fīlōn.*

Achundow (221) considers Indian malabathrum as good for the sight and heart. It is a diuretic and good for jaundice. Hunain (168, 158) uses it in ophthalmia.

The Gr. word for malabathrum probably comes from the Sans. *tamala,* a kind of tree, and *pattra,* meaning "leaf." The Sans. is also *tilaka;* Hind. *jangli-dalchin;* Tam. *ilavangam.* It is native to the Konkans and Malabar Coast. Its seeds are used in India for children in dysentery and coughs. The dried buds are used with other drugs in diarrhoea, dysentery, and coughs (Nadkarni I 332).

168. *Ushna* is lichen, moss. Perhaps *Alectoria usneoides* Ach. It is used in al-Kindī A (93a) together with galanga for fistula. In the same MS, (125a), it is found in a collyrium for the eyes.

169. *Qīrfah* is an inferior kind of cinnamon. Many species are

possible. In various prescriptions in al-Kindī A (92b, 105a, 114b), it is used to dissipate sadness, to tighten the uvula, for loss of hearing, and for a stiff neck.

170. *Nāramushk* is the ironwood tree, *Mesua ferrea* L. Maim. (250) gives synonyms as *al-nāghabashk, muzz, mushk al-rummān.* The latter two are doubtful, however. *IB* (2205) quotes al-Rāzī that it is called *nārqāssīs,* and has the properties of nard. *Tuḥfa* (287) gives *jullanār al-rummān.*

In Sans., it is *nagkesara, champeryah;* Hind. and Tel. *nagakesara, gajapushpam;* Tam. *cheru-nagapu;* Can. *nagasampige;* Burm. *kengan, gungen;* Ar. in India *narse-kaisar.* The term *al-nāghabashk* seems to have come from the Sans.

In Ayurvedic medicine ,it is used for many disorders. In Yunani practise, it is a tonic for the heart, expels wind, antispasmodic, diuretic, emmenagogue (Nadkarni I 792 ff.). The buds, flowers, leaves, bark, and root are used. *Cf. Nabāt* (19); Levey M.A.B. (26) gives *nārmishk* as an astringent in present day Egypt (Ducros 65).

171. *Falanjamushk* is basil (?), perhaps *Calamintha officinalis Mön.* Achundow (239) considers it good for digestion. Maim. (47) has synonyms as *baranjmashk, al-qalthamān,* and *aṣābiᶜ al-fatayāt.* IB (1676) has *faranjamishk.* It may also be a Thymus plant.

Laufer (589–590) gives Middle Pers. as *palangamushk,* and New Pers. as *palangmishk.* This plant may also be of the *Ocimum* genus. *Bulan* is a Sogdian word and so *bulan ralak* is "aromatic basil." The Sans. is *surasī* or *surasā.*

172. That is, the excess dampness.

173. *Qaulanj,* colic.

174. *Sadhāb* is rue, especially *Ruta graveolens* L. Al-Kindī A (91b) has rue gum with other simples in an electuary for phlegm, black gall, rheumatism, and nervous conditions. In al-Kindī G. (49b, 99b, 181b) rue is employed in antidote prescriptions for many kinds of poisons. For etymology, *cf.* al-Kindī (no. 225). *Cf.* Levey M.A.B. (29). This drug is known in India as an antiseptic, stimulant, emmenagogue, irritant, and abortifacient. In Sans. it is *sadapaka, somalata*; Pers. *satap*; Ben. *ispand*; Tel. *sadapaka*; Tam. *arvada.* It is cultivated in Indian gardens (Nadkarni I 1081–1082). *Cf.* Achundow (217); ibn Īsā (308–309).

175. *Bauraq* is a mixture of carbonates and/or a borate. *Cf.* Levey CCTM (122) for *bōrīth* cinders (Malachi III:2; Jeremiah II:22). Syr. *burka* is probably related to Akk. ᵘ *ṭābtu barikatu.* The Pers. is *baura* or *būra.* In most cases, it may be translated as impure natron. In al-Kindī (111a), it is used in a dental remedy to arrest deterioration of the gum and for canker in the mouth and elsewhere. *Cf.* al-Kindī (no. 42), Levey M.A.B. (23, 29).

176. The froth was generally considered to contain the impure constituents and so it was discarded.

177. *Ishāl* is diarrhoea.

178. Gloss: "Strengthening it."

179. *Cf.* V. Minorsky, transl., *Ḥudūd al-ʿālam*, Oxford, 1937, p. 142.

180. Gloss: "That is, the Iraqi, not the Syrian carob."

181. *Kharnūb nabaṭī* is the Nabataean carob, *Anagyris foetida* L. Its synonym is *yanbūt*. *Cf.* Maim. (180).

182. That is, the organs of digestion.

183. Perhaps, lessening of intercourse.

184. Gloss: "It is an electuary since it soothes."

185. *Shaʿīr* is barley, *Hordeum sativum* L. For etymology, *cf.* al-Kindī (no. 244). In al-Kindī A (113b), barley flour is employed in a dental medicine to sweeten the breath and to strengthen the gums. In earlier Greek works, barley is important for inflammation, leprosy, the joints, and the abdomen (Diosc. II 86).

In Iran today, it is thought of as an important nutritional element in the diet (Hooper 126).

186. Gloss: "In purity."

187. Gloss: "Bottles."

188. That is, they retain their properties or characteristics as seen on the surface where rapid oxidation would generally take place.

189. *Iyārij*.

190. Gloss: "Which are needed."

191. Gloss: "That is, all the medicines after kneading."

192. *Kathīrā* is gum tragacanth, from *Astragalus gummifer* Lab. and others. Levey M.A.B. (29) has the gum in a white *līq*. Al-Kindī A (103a, 115a) has this simple in prescriptions for strengthening the limbs and in an electuary for a cough due to catarrh. For etymology, *cf.* al-Kindī (no. 132). The *A. hamosus* L. is used in Iran today as a suppurative and astringent (Hooper 90).

193. *Nusakh* (pl.) means copies, recipes.

194. *Anṭākī sāqmūnīyā* is Antiochan scammony, probably *Convolvulus* scammonia L. This plant is found in China and Syria. In China, *C. arvensis* L. was used as a laxative (Soubeiran 186). Laxatives are described early in the Arabic medical literature. Yūhannā ibn Māsawaih, the personal physician to the Caliphs from Hārūn to al-Mutawakkil, is listed as having written two texts on the subject, *Kitāb al-adwiya al-mushila* and *Kitāb iṣlāḥ al-adwiya al-mushila* (IAU I 176; ibn al-Qifṭī 381).

195. *Ḥanzal* is colocynth, *Citrullus colocynthis* Schrad. The pulp, *shaḥm* is used. Al-Kindī A (101b) has colocynth for that under the skin which causes itching. *Abdāl* (187b) uses this simple for the liver and spleen.

In modern Egypt, it is a purgative and astringent (Ducros 93), and in Iran and Iraq it is a drastic hydragogue cathartic (Hooper 100–101). *Cf.* al-Kindī (no. 80) for synonyms.

196. *Cf.* Galen, Kühn, vol. 13, p. 129 for ἱερά πικρά.

197. That is, seed.

198. Gloss: "That is, not soft."

199. *Shīramaraj* is unknown.

200. *Khīr bawwā* is lesser cardamom, *Elettaria Cardamomum* White and Matern. This is equivalent to *hāl-bawwā* and *jar-bawwā*. It is the small *al-qāqulla*. It is *al-shashīr* which is Pers. (Vullers II 479). *Cf.* IB (1722), Loew (III 499 ff.).

In India, this simple is *ela, truti, kapita* in Sans.; *choti* in Hind.; *elachi* in Guj.; *elakaya* in Tam.; *palah, bala* in Burm.; *kakilahi-khurd* in Pers. It is cultivated in western and southern India, Ceylon, and Burma. It is used for impotency in Ayurvedic medicine. In Yunani practise, it checks nausea, vomiting, headache, is good for the heart, digestion, and hepatic colic. (Nadkarni I 475–476).

201. Nīl is indigo, probably *Indigofera tinctoria* L. Levey M.A.B. (23) gives the Pers. as *līlanj* and the Akk as *lalangu*. In India, it is used for hepatitis and nephritis. It is used mainly as a dye today. It is frequently confused with woad, a dye obtained from *Isatis tinctoria* L. *Cf.* Levey CCTM (105).

202. Gloss: "Narrowness of breathing."

203. *Irīsā*. *Cf.* IB (216) and an earlier note above.

204. Gloss: "Musk of the pomergranate." *Cf.* IB (2205) and earlier note above. The flower has small structures on it which appear like the seeds of the pomegranate. Some are red and some are yellow. It is acerbic and aromatic. Al-Rāzī thought it to be the flower of a tree called *nārqāssis, Mesua ferrea* L. It yields nagkassar oil. It is from the balsam tree family.

205. Gloss: "The weight of each one is from one to two *dāniqs*."

206. *Sukk* is a confection of dates, gallnuts, and Indian astringents and aromatics. There are many different *sukk* compositions. *Cf.* Jābir (187a) and Wiedemann, E., *Arch Med.* 8 (1914) 83 ff.

Laufer (551) states that ibn Sīnā wrote that *sukk* was originally a secret Chinese remedy containing emblic myrobalan. Achundow (211) gives *rāmik* as a constituent of *sukk*. Al-Kindī G. (p. 331) has it in perfumes. The *sukk* confection is somewhat similar to *ghāliya* (*Cf.* Jābir 219). *Sukk* is often a perfumed remedy containing *rāmik* as a base together with gall apples, raisins, dates, aloeswood, sandalwood, and others (Wiedemann, *loc. cit.*).

207. *ᶜUdnī* is an aloe.

208. *Mishmish* or *mushmush* is apricot, *Prunus Armeniaca* L.

In Babylonia, it was probably *armānu* in Akk. and *MA + GUNU KUR.RA* in Sum. The Syr. is *ḫazzūrā armĕnāyā* (= *ḫašḫura armannu*) (DAB 304). The Gr. μῆλον αρμενιακόν is similar to the Akk. and Syr., "Armenian apples."

Maim. (233) gives the Ar. synonym as *al-tuffāḥ al-arminī* "Armenian apple." IB (2136) states that apricot is good for the stomach (from Diosc. I 115). The word *mishmish* comes from the Aram. (Vullers). *Cf.* Loew AP (150).

209. *Lisān al-thaur* is borage.

210. *Falanjamashk,* in this case.

211. From Pers. *gul* "rose" and *āb* "water."

212. Hermes Trismegistus was the moon god, the special deity of medicine, like Apollo in Greece. He was first mentioned in a papyrus of the third century A.D. from Hermopolis (Garrison 55).

213. Rufus flourished in the first half of the second century under Trajan in Rome and in Egypt. He was a Greek anatomist and a physician highly regarded by the Muslims.

214. Aḥmad ibn al-Ḥusain al-Mutanabbī (d. 354 H.).

215. Gloss: "Which was given to Galen and others."

216. *Lūghāziyā* is a kind of aperient. Dozy has *lūghādhīyā,* a medicine compounded of many ingredients.

217. *Khubbāzī* is mallow. The genus and species are uncertain. Maim. (229, 390 gives *khubbāzī barrī* as the wild mallow. *Cf.* al-Kindī (no. 137), *Nabāt* (163, 167). The latter gives the family as *Malvaceae* and genus as *Malva. Malva sylvestris* L. var. *mauritiana* Boiss. is known in Teheran as *gul-i-panirak,* and is imported into Iran and Iraq today. It is used for coughs and as a purgative (Hooper 138). *Cf. Al-Muᶜtamad* (115–116). In Egypt today (Ducros 99), the mallow is used for coughs, bladder ailments, and in tuberculosis.

218. *Ṣabir* is aloe, *Aloe vera* L. and *A. Perryi* Bak. Al-Biṭrīq (89a, 89b) uses aloe for jaundice, phlegm, and the stomach. Al-Kindī A (101a) has this in a prescription for a boil.

Aloe is still used in Iran and Egypt, in the former as a purgative, and in the latter as an emmenagogue, desiccative, and detersive (Ducros 141, Hooper 83). For chemical properties, *cf.* Gstirner (13 ff.).

219. Gloss: "A maximum of two months."

220. Gloss: "Hot cake."

221. Gloss: "That is, powdered and not kneaded with honey."

222. *Wajj* is sweet flag, *Acorus calamus* L. In al-Kindī A (114a), sweet flag is used for bad breath, to polish the teeth, and to remove the decaying part of teeth. *Abdāl* (188a) has sweet flag in use for the stomach and to strengthen the liver. The sweet flag is of Indian origin. In India and Iran, it is still used as a tonic, for rheumatism, insecticide, and for aromatic vinegar (Ainslie I 417–419). In the

Near East, it is used as an aphrodisiac and carminative, and in ophthalmia (Ḥunain 166, 158). *Cf.* al-Kindī (no. 298).

223. *Qusṭ* is costus, *Auklandia Costus* Falc. Al-Kindī A (98b) has costus in a remedy for the kidneys and bladder, and (124a) in a clyster introduced into the penis for the dripping of urine, its odor, and for calculus. Al-Kindī G. (no. 94) has costus in *khalūq* salves. In Levey M.A.B. (48), the test for costus is given. *Cf.* also Achundow (243). In mediaeval Arabic times, costus was used for impetigo, quartan fever, alopecia, and in other illnesses (IB (1785), *Tuḥfa* (350), Maim. (338)).

224. *Shīṭaraj. Vide* note 147 above.

225. *Fūwwa* is madder, *Rubia Cordofolia* L. or *R. tinctorum* L. Madder has been found on the cloth of an Egyptian mummy (Lucas 172 ff.).

Diosc. (III 143) considers madder, ἐρυθρόδανον, as a diuretic, good for the spleen and for the expulsion of the secundine.

IB (1710) gives madder as a tonic and diuretic.

Indian madder is *R. Cordifolia* L. in Sans. and Bom., it is *manjista* used as an emmenagogue and diuretic (Nadkarni I 1075–6). In Iran today, it is *rūnās* and *rūniyās*, and is used as a dyestuff and medicine (Hooper 166–167). In modern Egypt, *R. tinctorum* L. is found in the bazaars to be used as a tonic and for dysuria. It is imported there from Asia Minor. *Cf.* Loew AP (311) who gives Aram. and Syr. as *pūtā*.

226. Gloss: "Seed of Greek celery."

226a. *Dūqū* is wild carrot, mainly *Daucos carota* L. in India, it is called Sans. *shikha-mulam*; Sind. *pitai gajar*, Hind., Mah., Guj., and Ben., *gajar*; Tam. *gajjara-kilangu*. It is indigenous to the western Himalayas and Kashmir. The root is used for ulcers and worm troubles. It is also an aromatic, stimulant, and carminative (Nadkarni I 441–442).

227. *Nigella sativa* L.

228. *Karawiyā* is caraway, *Carum Carvi* L. This plant name is not yet known in Akk.

Diosc. (III 57) considers it, καρώ, good for the stomach and in antidotes. *Cf.* Paulos (181).

Achundow (248) claims it is a diuretic and stomachic. Maim. (195) gives synonyms as *al-kammūn al-armīnī* "cumin of Armenia," *qarunbād*. "*Al-qardama* is the wild caraway." IB (1913) quotes Galen that caraway juice is not good for anyone. Al-Rāzī believes that it is a good stomachic and carminative. The *Tuḥfa* (340) gives *karawiyā* as a synonym of *qardamānā*.

Loew FJ (III 437 ff.) and Loew AP (207, 348) discuss caraway in detail.

In India, it is called *shiajira* in Hind.; *shimayi-shombu* in Tam.; and *jīra* in Ben. It is used as a stomachic and carminative (Nadkarni I 279). In modern Egypt, caraway is used for the same medicinal purposes (Ducros 114). Laufer (383–384) gives the Chinese as *ši-lo, zi-la* for cumin and caraway. The Sans. is *jira*, and Middle Pers. *zira*. In Pers. caraway is *shāh-zīre* "cumin of the Shah." or *zire-i-rumi* "Byzantine cumin."

In al-Kindī A (122b), cumin is in a rubbing preparation for rheumatism in the knees and other joints. For etymology, *cf.* al-Kindī (no. 120).

229. *Futrāsāliyūn* is parsley, *Apium graveolens* L. Achundow (241, 246). It is equivalent to *karafs*. In al-Kindī A (103b), celery is in a poultice for the stomach. The cognate in Syr. is *paṭrāselīnōn* (Budge 326). *Cf.* Diosc. (III 64) for σέλινον κηπαῖον.

In Persia today, this simple is used as a carminative, aromatic, and tonic. The drug is heated in boiling water so that its vapor may be inhaled for headache (Hooper 86).

The word *karafs* is of Semitic origin. This word is still used in Egypt where celery is used for diuresis and as an emmenagogue and carminative (Ducros 31).

230. *Kashūth* is dodder, *Cuscuta Epithymum* Murr., etc. In Akk., it is the *kishshatu* to which Syr. *kĕshūthā* is cognate (Loew AP 171, Loew FJ 456).

Diosc. (IV 177) lists it, ἐπίθυμον, as effective for phlegm and melancholy. Maim. (186) gives synonyms as *kushūthā*,

The *Cuscuta* is well known in India, in Sans. as *amaravela*; Punj. *nilathari*; Hind. *akasbel*. It is regarded as a purgative and anthelmintic (Nadkarni I 419–420).

231. *Marw* is origan of Egypt, *Origanum Maru* L. In Pers., it is *marmāḥūz* or *marmākhūr*. Al-Kindī A (97b) has this simple in the preparation of a poultice for a swelling where formation of an abscess is feared. *Cf.* Maim. (40, 235), Loew AP (97, 252). *Marw* is frequently used for perfumery products in al-Kindī G. (*passim*). This drug is used today in Egypt as a diuretic, expectorant, and antiasthmatic (Ducros 172, 218).

232. *Hashā* is thyme, *Thymus vulgaris* L. In al-Kindī A (93a, 93b), it is used in dressings for the liver, stomach, and spleen. Earlier, in the same sentence, al-Samarqandī (fol. 16a) uses the wild thyme (*ṣaʿtar*). The latter may be various species (*cf.* al-Kindī 273). Thyme is very popular today in the Middle East for many ailments.

233. *Marmāḥūz. Vide note* 231. In the same sentence, al-Samarqandī (fol. 16a) refers to the seed of *marw* and the herb *marmāḥūz*. In the Ar. literature, these plants are usually equivalent but it is evident that al-Samarqandī thinks otherwise. *Cf.* IB (2109, 275, 781, 2061).

234. *Qanṭūriyūn* is centaury, *Erythraea Centaurium.* It is Pers. and refers to the small centaury. The great centaury is *Centauria Centaurium* L. and is often meant when *qanṭūriyūn* is used. Al-Kindī A (122a, 138a) uses centaury to destroy calculus, and for general rheumatic pains. Cf. al-Kindī (no. 196), Achundow (243).

235. *Cf.* IB (388). *Vide* note 81 above.

236. *Fautanaj* is mint or mountain mint, *Mentha Pulegium* L. and others. Sometimes, the mountain mint is called *fautanaj jabalī.* Al-Kindī A (93a, 93b, 99b, 122a) uses various kinds of mint for the spleen, liver, and stomach.

For related species and their uses, *cf.* al-Kindī (no. 62).

The *M. piperita* L. is used in Egypt today as a stomachic and antispasmodic (Ducros 233). *M. sylvestris* L. is used today in Iran and Iraq for rheumatism, dysentery, and other ailments (Hooper 140).

237. *Falanjamushk. Cf.* Laufer (589), IB (1676).

238. *ᶜAnab* is jujube, *Zizyphus vulgaris* Lamk., *Z. Jujuba* Lamk., *Z. Lotus* Lamk. The first is found in the Mediterranean and in south and east Asia, the second in China, and the last in North Africa.

Jujube is used in an erysipelas application in al-Kindī A (96a). Many of the *Z.* species bear an edible berry-like drupe. The fruit is suppurative, expectorant, and used as a blood purifier in India (Nadkarni I 1318).

The vulgaris species is well known in India where it is known in Sans. as *soubira*; Punj. *sanjit,* and in Pers. *sinpo-i-Jilani.* It grows in the Punjab, Himalayas, Kashmir, and Baluchistan.

239. Gloss: "And it is liquid."

240. Gloss: "That is, it attracts the chyme depositories." The word "chyme" is used here as some kind of catalyst or catalytic element or agent.

241. *Khaml.*

242. *Sardārūj* is unknown. *Sar-dārū* is the name of a Pers. medicine (Steingass).

243. Gloss: "It is what is added to the decoction after it has been cooked and filtered for strengthening and purging some of the humors."

244. Text has *basfanij*; it should read *basbāyij.* In al-Kindī A (136a), common polypody is used with *iyārij* and various simples for an undisclosed ailment. The common polypody is *Polypodium vulgare* L. The *P. taxifolium* L., in India, is used as an emmenagogue and to bring on abortions (Ainslie II 486). The *P. repandum* L., *hou-soui-pou-tsao,* in China is used for the kidneys and to help the knitting of bones, and for the teeth (Nadkarni I 1001).

245. *Saudā'* is also "melancholy," a result of excess of black bile.

246. *Ghāfit* is agrimony and some kinds of elecampane, *Agrimonia Eupatoria* L. and others. In al-Kindī A (115b), agrimony is in an electuary for compound fever of jaundice and phlegm. *Cf.* al-Kindī (no. 67).

247. *Shirabakht* is perhaps Pers. *shīr pukht* "Oil of sesame." In this case, it is probably the seed of sesame since it is not measured in volumetric terms. The diacritical mark is missing from the *bā*.

248. *Taranjubīn* is manna, probably *supalu* in Akk. and *RIM* in Sum., perhaps from the *ᶜāqūl*, the camel-thorn, *Alhagi Maurorum* Tourn. In Bukhara and Basra, it is used as a substitute for sugar (DAB 270). *Tarangubīn* in Pers. is "Honey of the rose," a sugary exudate of certain desert plants. It may be found on a variety of plants. *Cf.* Alfred Kaiser, "Der heutige Stand des Mannafrage," Suisse, 1924. In Maim. (166, 386), the synonyms are given as *mann* and *rizq*.

Today, the Arabs call it *al-ḥāj*. Ducros (128) gives its use as a vermifuge and laxative. Hooper (81) gives this plant as *Alhagi camelorum* Fisch. He states that the camel's thorn or camel-thorn (*kār shūtur* in Pers.) is a thorny shrub found in the deserts of Iran, Syria, and Egypt. A saccherine exudation forms on the plant; it is shaken off the branches and collected. In Iran, it is employed as a laxative and expectorant. *Vide Al-Muᶜtamad* (50) and in *Al-ṭibb al-nabawī* by Ḥāfīz Abī ᶜAbdallah M. b. a. al-Dhahabī (d. 748 H.), Cairo, 1961, p. 38.

249. *Turāb*, possibly *turābu'l-qai'*, literally emetic earth, a resinous matter used in Persia as a vomitive.

250. *Tarkhūn* is tarragon, probably *Artemisia Dracunculus* L. Achundow (230) considers this good for digestion. Paul of Aegina states that it is not good. It cleanses the brain of moistness, is good for fever, epilepsy, and the intestines. Maim. (173) writes, "Some say these are the leaves of pyrethrum (*ᶜāqir qarḥā*) but this is not confirmed by recent authors. The latter say, on the contrary, it is a species of celery (*karafs*)."

Tarkhūn is Pers. (Vullers I 433) which, perhaps, comes from Gr. δράκων or δρακόντιον (Maim). Today, it is known for its pungent aromatic foliage that is used in making pickles. IB (1459) states that it is a legume well known in Syria but rarely found in Egypt. Ibn al-ᶜAwwām believes that there are two species, Babylonian and Greek. The *Tuḥfa* (200) says that it is called *maᶜdnūs* in Algiers and Tlemcen, in the extreme Maghrib *al-barshīl*. Loew AP (77) and Loew FJ (I 380) give the various species of *ṭarkhūn*.

251. That is, where the esophagus joins the "cardiac end" of the stomach.

252. *Milḥ nafṭī*. *Napṭu* in Akk. is a kind of naphtha. The *nafṭī* salt has the smell of nahptha, is somewhat black, and is

found near naphtha wells. This salt is used in a drug for the spirits (al-Kindī A 136b). The word naphtha here does not refer to a specific modern chemical. The salt was probably derived from this strong smelling flammable liquid (used by the Muslims in Greek fire) by distillation.

253. *Shāhtiraj* is fumitory, *Fumaria officinalis* L. Al-Kindī A (134b) has fumitory in an original diluent. *Cf.* al-Kindī (no. 247). Fumitory has many medicinal uses in the Middle East today.

254. *Māhīzahraj* is cocculus, *Anamirta paniculata* Colebr. Diosc. (IV 164) gives τιθυμάλλον. The Pers. word above is equivalent to *māhīzahra*. Maim. (178) gives the names of related plants as *yuttu^{c}*, *labaniyya, kabwa, shubrum, lā^{c}iya, māhūbdāna,* and *^{c}ushar*. It is listed in Achundow (277) for poison treatment, rheumatism, and to catch fish by stupefying them. IB (2057) states that the Pers. *māhīzahra* means "fish poison." Leclerc thought it to be *Menispermum Cocculus* L.

255. *Ijjāṣ* is plum, probably from *Prunus Armeniaca* L. Theoph. (I, X, 10) calls it κοκκύμηλον. *Prunus domestica* is a native of China. It is mentioned in the *Ši kin, Li ki,* and in *Moṅ-tse*. The Sino-Indian word is given in the *Fan yi min yi tsi* with the translation *li* (Laufer 216). IB (21) quotes Galen that it is good as a laxative. There are two types, the larger being less astringent. The plum tree in Syriac medicine is used in compounded remedies to produce coughing and to check abscess (Budge, fol. 111b). Al-Biṭrīq (74b) uses this simple for fever, yellow gall, and the stomach. Al-Kindī A (135a) uses it as a diluent. For etymology, *cf.* al-Kindī (no. 96).

256. *^{c}Inab al-tha^{c}lab* is black nightshade, *Solanum nigrum* L. Al-Kindī A (96a, 132b) uses nightshade for erysipelas. This plant is a common bazaar medicine in India today. The black berries of the plant are used as a diuretic and diaphoretic in heart disease attended with oedema. It is called *kakamochi* in Sans.; *munna-takali-pullum* in Tam.; *kanchi-pundu* in Tel. (Chopra 595). For the etymology, cf. al-Kindī (no. 98).

257. *Nulk* is of the medlar, probably the dessicated fruit of *Mespilus Azarolus* L. (?). Maim. (132) gives *za^{c}rūr* as a synonym, from Semitic sources. There is uncertainty as to a possible difference between the two synonyms given above. *Cf.* Loew FJ (III 244) where this problem is left unsettled because of lack of sufficient evidence. Also *cf.* Loew AP (486, 488).

258. Gloss: "*Al-wujah*. It is the medlar tree. The best one is the very red. The yellow is the thickest, and is for the abdomen. It is cold and sour."

259. *Shirkhist* is siracost. In Pers., it is "dry sugar," a kind of manna. Achundow (355) states that it comes especially from *Atraphaxis spinosa* Hausskn. It comes mainly from Afghanistan.

260. Gloss: "One of the contrary purgatives should be more or follow the siracost for the decoction since the juice of sour pomergranate and the rosewater should not be put together according to the well known rule. The purgative should not be put together by squeezing but by softening. The purifier depends on this rule. Thus, it is generalized."

261. Gloss: "For the swellings."

262. *Liblāb* is ivy, probably Hedera Helix L., and equivalent to *lāghiyah*. It was known to al-Kindī. *Cf.* Achundow (283).

In Hind. it is *lablab*; Punj. *banda*, and Kash. *karmora*. *Cf.* Nadkarni (I 608), Chopra (494).

263. Gloss: "That is, strengthened by *sardārūj*."

263a. Gloss: "Thickened honey."

264. Gloss: "*Shaᶜtar*." The text has *saᶜtar*.

265. *Silq* is beet and others. It may be various species of *Rumex* and *Chenopodium*. In Achundow (217, 376), *silq* is considered to be *Beta vulgaris* L., and good for the spleen and liver. Al-Kindī A (131b) uses beet leaves in a poison to kill mice. The word *silq* probably comes originally from the Akk. *silqa,* or it may come from the Gr. σικελιωτικός. *Cf.* Levey M.A.B. (17) where *silq* is mixed with ink.

266. *Ḥasak* is water-caltrop, *Tribulus terrestris* L. Al-Kindī A (91b) has it in a remedy good for black gall, rheumatism, and nervous conditions.

It is used today in Iran as a diuretic, and its oil for gonorrhoea (Hooper 180). In Egypt, it is also a diuretic today (Ducros 83).

267. *Bakhtij* is a decoction or a kind of oil. Elsewhere in the text, a gloss gives "Oil of sesame." *Bakhtij* is from the Pers. *pukhta* whose plural is *pukhātij* (IB 251).

268. *Kurunb* is cabbage, *Brassica oleracea* L. var. *capitata.*

Diosc. (II 120) considers it, κράμβη ἥμερος, as a binder, antidote, anthelmintic, and for inflammations, and oedemata. The Ar. comes from the Gr.

Achundow (246) and Maim. (184) discuss *kurunb*. The latter gives synonyms as *baqlat al-anḍār,* and *al-qannabīṭ*. These may be, however, different species. Loew AP (213 ff.) gives Aram. as *kĕrūbā*. *Kurunb* is used in an ointment for ulcers which discharge into the abdomen in al-Kindī A (102a).

In India, it is *kobi* in Hind.; *kovipu* in Tam.; *panjoli* in Guj., and is used as an anthelmintic (Nadkarni I 217–218).

269. *Iklīl,* probably for *iklīl al-malik,* is melilot, *Melilotus officinalis* L. It is used by al-Kindī A (93b) for the liver and stomach, and in a relaxant. For etymology, *cf.* al-Kindī (no. 97).

270. *Qaiṣūm* is southernwood, *Artemisia Abrotanum* L. *Artemisia* is also *shīḥ*. The cognate to this is *sikhu* in Akk. (DAB 233).

Diosc. (III 24) gives southernwood, ἀβρότονον, as good for sciatica, convulsions, dysuria, and as an antidote.

Maim. (337) gives synonyms as *miswāk al-rāᶜī* "shepherd's toothpick," Sp. *sharrin,* and Ar. *ᶜubaīthārān*. *Cf.* Loew AP (78 ff.), Loew FJ (I 379 ff.).

Many species of *A.* are known in India but not *Abrotanum* (Narkarni I 141 ff.). The *A. maritima* L. is the best known in India and Iran. In the latter country, it is called *darmanah* (Hooper 87).

In China, *A. Abrotanum* is called *yn-tchin-kao, in czen-chua, yin-ch'in-hau,* and is used for dysuria, catarrh, and fever (Soubeiran 164).

271. *Ḥummāḍ* is sorrel, a *Rumex* species. Maim. (150) gives the synonyms as *al-baqla al-khurāsāniyya* "vegetable of Khorasan," *al-silq al-barrī* "the wild beet," Sp. *al-labāṣṣa,* Ber. *ṭāsamāmt.* Ar. is *al-qaṭaf*. Ducros (90) writes that Cairo druggists sell *ḥummeḍa* as a stomachic and blood tonic. *R. conglomeratus* L. and *R. obtusifolius* L. are known in Teheran as *tukhm-i-ḥummāz. R. obt.* is given for pyorrhoea (Hooper 167).

272. *Shahdānaj* is hemp, *Cannabis sativa* L., from *shah-dāna* (Pers.) "royal grain."

It is probably *A.ZAL.LA* in Sum. and *azallū* in Akk.; likely the *C. Indica* Lam. The Akk. *azallū* is cognate with Syr. *azal* "to spin." It is found in a "drug for grief," for the stomach, swelling, impotence, and fumigation. Hemp was also used in ancient Egypt. It is *kanfa* in Syr. and Aram. (Loew FJ I 255; Loew AP 348).

Diosc. (III 148) gives hemp. κάνναβις ἡμέρον, as good for the ears and genitals (*cf.* Berendes 359). There is also a wild hemp in Diosc. good for oedemata. Origin of the Gr. name is unknown.

In India, hemp is known as *vijaya, siddharpatri, ganjika, bhanga, hursini* in Sans; *ganja, charas* in Hind.; *kanja* in Tem.; *segujav* in Burm. The plant is a native of Persia, Western and Central Asia, and almost all of India. When grown in hot regions, the female plants yield a resin having intoxicating properties. In Yunani medicine, it is employed as a retentive, anaesthetic, and astringent; in Ayurveda and Siddha, it is an aphrodisiac and has narcotic properties (Nadkarni I 256 ff.).

There is a *Cannabis chinensis* in China known as *ko-ma-jin, mo, ma, ta-ma, cho-ma, hwang-ma,* and not listed as an anaesthetic but for its value as a diuretic, emmenagogue, and anthelmintic (Soubeiran 144–145).

In Egypt, hemp is *tīl* for exciting one to delirium (Ducros 40).

Achundow (223) has hemp as good for headache and ears. Maim. (348) gives *qinnab* as hemp. The synonyms given are *al-shahrānaj, shahdānaj al-barr* "wild hemp," *ḥabb al-samna* "grain of grease." *Qinnab* comes from the Gr. It is not mentioned in al-Kindī.

273. *Ḥarmal* is harmel or wild rue, *Peganum harmala* L. Harmel is used by al-Kindī A (133b) for insanity and epilepsy. In Egypt, harmel seeds are used as a diuretic and vomitive (Ducros 22); in Iran, the seeds are considered an aphrodisiac (Hooper 148). *Cf.* al-Kindī (no. 82).

274. *Marzanjush* is marjoram, probably *Origanum Majorana* L. In al-Kindī A (93b, 98b, 103b, 117a), marjoram is used for the liver, stomach, kidneys, bladder, and middle ear, especially in poultices. For etymology, *cf.* al-Kindī (no. 168).

274a. *Khirwa*ᶜ is castor oil plant, *Ricinus communis* L. It was well known in ancient Egypt (L. Keimer, *Die Gartenpflanzen in alten Aegypten*, Hamburg, 1924, I, p. 120) and in Mesopotamia. Ricinus is *AG.PAR* in Sum.; *šagabegalzu* in Akk. It was used in Babylonia for the stomach, dysentery, purgation, cough, and in poultices.

Theoph. (I 10) and Diosc. (IV 161) list the castor oil plant, κρότων for plasters, candles, purging, sunburn, erysipelas, oedemata, and the stomach.

Hunain (155) uses it to open pores of the skin. Maim. (396) gives synonyms as *tartaqa* (Sp.), κίκι, *rijinu* (*ricino* Sp.). The Chinese ricinus, *al-khirwa*ᶜ *al-ṣīnī* as al-dand. Κίκι comes from Egyptian *k*ᶜ*k*ᵒ, similar to Heb. *qiqāyōn*.

The castor oil plant was originally native to India. In Sans., it is *eranda, vatari;* Hind. *endi;* Sind. *ayrunkukri;* Punj. *arand, erand;* Pers. *bedanjir;* Tel. *eramudapu;* Tam. *amanakhu;* Burm. *kesusi*. In Yunani medicine, it is used today as a purgative, for paralysis, tremor, asthma, cough, colic, and as an emmenagogue (Nadkarni I 1065–70).

Cf. al-Kindī G. (233) for its use in perfumery. Also Loew AP (352, 407).

The *R. communis* L. in Persia today is *garchak farangī* and is used as a safe purgative. It is *kurwa* in Iraq. Chinese ricinus is used in Egypt today (Laufer 403–404).

275. *Zanbaq* is jasmine, *Jasminum officinale* L. or *J. Sambac* Aitch. In al-Kindī A (99b), jasmine oil is used for haemorrhoidal pain. This use is not mentioned in al-Samarqandī. In the latter (19a), it is in a purgative, in a remedy for cold colic, for coldness of the womb, and hardening of the womb.

276. Gloss: "*Kittān.*" This is flax.

277. *Murrī* is garum. IB (2111 bis) quotes Galen that garum is

good for ulcers, and al-Rāzī that it is good as a collyrium for small-pox. *Tuḥfa* (276) states that garum is made of numerous simples as a syrup of roots and that its properties are multiple. The Syr. is *mai keṭme* (Budge 721).

Dozy under *murrī* states that it is derived from the Gr. αλ-μυρίς. Renaud and Colin (*Tuḥfa* 133) give it as the γάρος of Diosc. (II 32) made from salt fish, and used for bowel ulcers.

ᶜAbd al-Razzāq (217) give it as a plant preparation mainly of barley and wheat macerated in salt.

278. *Jāwashīr* is opopanax, odorous resin of ***Opoponax Chironium*** Koch. It is used in al-Kindī A (91b) for rheumatism, phlegm, and black gall. In al-Samarqandī (19a), it is used in a clyster for cold colic and chronic arthritis.

In India, it is used as an antispasmodic and emmenagogue (Ainslie I 280); in Egypt today, it is an antispasmodic and laxative (Ducros 62).

279. *Sakabīnaj* is sagapenum, the root of ***Ferula persica*** Willd. or *F. Scowitziana* D.C. For etymology, *cf.* al-Kindī (no. 229). In al-Kindī A (98b), it is used for the kidney and bladder. In Iran, it is used in a plaster for rheumatism, and in Egypt as a purgative and aphrodisiac (Hooper 119, Ducros 126).

280. *Ushaq* is gum ammoniac, aromatic gum resin mainly from *Dorema Ammoniacum* L. The Akk. word is not yet known for this product (DAB 339); the ancient Mesopotamians surely knew it, however.

Diosc. (III 84) mentions a gum ammoniac which was probably from *Ferula tingitana* L. from North Africa.

Gum ammoniac was not too well known in India since it had to be brought from Persia. Ainslie (I 158–160) states that it is from *Heracleum Gummiferum* Willd. In southern Arabia, the tree which yields this simple is called *ṭurthuth*. The Persians call it *darukht ushuq*.

Loew FJ (III 457) states that this resin was known to the Syrians as *ōshaq*. Al-Nuwairī (Wiedemann 49, 21, 46) gives *wushshaq, 'ushshaq, wāshaj, liṣāk al-dhahab* as synonyms for the tree, and for gum ammoniac *kalkh* and *'ushshaq*.

In India, it is used as a resolvent for scrofulous tumors.

Maim. (124) gives an interesting synonym as *qātil nafsihi* "suicide."

Syriac medicine (Budge II 58, 100, 454, 470, 506, 698, 716) uses gum ammoniac with other simples for headache, hemiplegia, for scars, jaundice, spleen, worms, in a plaster for wounds. IB (83) quotes ibn Sīnā that it is desiccative and a good aperitive.

The gum ammoniac of Morocco comes from the *F. brevifolia*

(Bailey; C 1228). In Cairo today, the gum is called *ushaq kadhab* and *fassukh*. It comes from Persia and Morocco to be used as a laxative and abortive internally (Ducros 174).

In the bazaars in India, gum ammoniac is sold for catarrh, asthma, liver, and spleen ailments.

281. *Ghār.*

282. *Abhul* is savin, *Juniperus Sabina* L. and other species.

This term is obviously not cognate to the terms for other species of juniper as the Sum. *ZA.BA.LAM, DUP.RA.AN,* and the Akk. *zabalum, daprānu* (DAB 268).

Diosc. (I 76) gives *βράθυ* as good to mitigate inflammation and ulcers. Applied with honey, it is effective for all blackness and foulness, according to Diosc.

The juniper genus is native in Europe and Western Asia and is not found in Indian materia medica as a rule.

Abhul is cognate to Turk. *habhel* which is the *drupacea* species. *Cf.* Loew FJ (III 37), Loew AP (82).

In ibn Waḥshīya (14b), large juniper berry is administered with other simples for opium poisoning. *Cf.* Siddiqi (126) for use of juniper in Persian medicine. It is also employed in Syriac medicine in a compound medicament for spongings which are effective for protracted hardness and tumidity of the spleen (Budge II 468).

Al-Ghāfiqī (5) quotes ibn Waḥshīya from his *Kitāb al-filāha al-nabaṭī* that there are four kinds:

1. Indian, called *dībadār,* from Sans. *devadāru* but it is not a true juniper.
2. Has leaves like the tamarisk and a pungent smell.
3. Like the cypress with a pungent smell.
4. Broad but not tall, has no fruit.

The *dībadār,* often taken for juniper, is "tree of god" in Sans., and has the same meaning in Ar. *shajarat Allāh*. Ar. synonyms are *al-ᶜirᶜar* and *barāthwā* (Maim. 22). The latter is from Syr. *barūthā*. Other synonyms are Turk. *qara ardij;* Pers. *sarw-i-kūhī*. *Cf.* Issa (102) for other names.

Juniperus communis L. is sold today in Egypt as a diuretic, tonic, and stomachic (Ducros 41).

283. *Naṭrūn* is natron. *Al-Muᶜtamad* (525) gives it as Armenian *bauraq;* the best is found in Wādī Naṭrūn, Egypt. It is useful for colic. Maim. (51) gives the synonyms as *bauraq* and *bauraq arminī*. The word *naṭrūn* comes originally from hieroglyphic Egyptian *n.t.r.y.* from which the Gr. *νίτρον* also comes. Interestingly, the Akk. *nitiru* and *nitru* are similar (DAB 255, Levey CCTM 172, Issa 319). *Vide* index for *bauraq* and its uses.

284. *Qiṭrān* is tar. Maim. (341) states, "It is an oil which one

extracts from cedar (*al-sharbīn*) which one calls *shabīn* in the Maghrib." It may be from the cedar, pine, cypress, and other woods. It is procured by dry distillation, *Cf. Tuḥfa* (150).

285. *Duhn al-zait* is olive oil. It is uncertain which species of *Olea* is meant in this text. Today, in Iran and Iraq, the *O. europa* L. is common. The oil is extracted from the olives, and the leaves are used in a decoction for coughs (Hooper 146). *Cf.* al-Kindī (no. 304). Al-Kindī G. (130b) has olive oil used in perfumery. One of the most common uses for olive oil in the Near East is as a stomachic.

286. *Ushna* is fragrant (tree)-moss, *Alectoria usneoides* Ach. In al-Kindī A (93a), this lichen is used with galanga in a treatment for fistula; it is also used in a collyrium for the eyes (al-Kindī A 125a). *Cf.* al-Kindī (no. 293), Maim. (11).

287. *Nammān* is serpolet, wild thyme, especially *Thymus glaber* Mill., *T. Serpyllum* Fries, and others. Maim. (255) gives synonyms as *sīsanbar,* and in Sp. *qālamānta.* Cf. Loew AP (271 ff.). *Tuḥfa* (282, 378) gives a synonym as *ṣandal al-aḥwāḍ,* supposedly a wild species. Renaud and Colin give an account of the confusion in the meaning of *nammān,* still not clarified. The word *nammān,* is derived from the verb *namma,* "to sprinkle perfume far and wide." The Syr. is *sīsambar* (Budge II 721).

288. *Khaḍrā'* "the green" is the spurge laurel, *Daphne Laureola* L. This plant grows in western and southern Asia.

The laurel was probably known in ancient Babylonia as *MA.NU* in Sum., and *eru, enitum, murranu,* and *iznu* in *Akk.* (DAB 299). Laurel was used in medicine as an aromatic, stimulant, for colic and amenorrhoea.

Diosc. (IV 171–172) χαμελαία or θαμελαία and Theoph. (VI 2) have laurel for various ailments as ulcers, for purges, and in a pessary to kill embryos. Maim. (237) gives synonyms for various species as *asad al-arḍ* "lion of the earth," *tābimāk, bāftirag, al-muʿīn,* and in Sp. *alwaru (lauro).* IB (2058) writes that *māziriyūn,* a synonym for *khaḍrā'* is for the abdomen, bile, and other difficulties.

D. Laureola L. is not found in Yunani or Ayurvedic medicine nor in the present day Near Eastern native practise. *CF.* Loew FJ (III 409 ff.).

289. *Narjis* is narcissus, and may be *Narcissus poeticus* L., *N. Tazzetta* L., or other species. The name comes from the Pers. nargi or nargis (Laufer 427). *Cf.* Loew FJ (203–205), Maim. (254), Diosc. (IV 58).

290. Gloss: "That is, blue bdellium."

291. *Sūsan. Cf.* note 80 above.

292. *Samak* is fish. Fresh fish is a simple in Achundow (215) for

jaundice and rectal difficulties. The species in the text is uncertain but is some kind of sardine (Vullers II 541).

293. *Cf.* J. Friedenwald and S. Morrison, "History of the Enema with Some Notes on Related Procedures" *Bull. of the Hist. of Med.* 8 (1940); Wm. Lieberman, "History of the Enema" *Ciba Symposia* 1694 ff. (1944). The enema was probably used in early Hindu medicine. The ancient Egyptians and Mesopotamians describe enemas in their literature. The enema is frequently found in the early Chinese, Greek, and Arabic medical texts.

294. Probably that of an adult.

295. That is, of the cross-section.

296. That is, the end into which the solution enters the tube.

297. Meaning the skin of a bladder or other kind of container of the clyster solution.

298. This is the end which enters the body.

299. That is, the main exit of the clyster duct.

300. Gloss: "*Al-aᶜfāj,* in people and animals, is the condition of food, after [having gone through] the stomach, that makes the intestines heavy."

301. Gloss: "*Tasmīn,*" where the text incorrectly gives *qasmīn.*

302. *Ḥintat* is some kind of semolina. *Cf.* Maim. (270, 284), IB (1255), Serap. (147), al-Razzāq (855). It is a mixture of wheat with other ingredients; the wheat probably contained the by-products of flour milling, the middlings.

303. *Al-ruzz* is rice, *Oryza sativa* L. In Sum., it is *ŠE.LI.A* and in Akk. *kurangu* (R. Campbell Thompson, *Iraq* 180 ff. (1939). The Sum. *ŠE* is corn and *LI.A* is grass. *Pirinj* is rice in Ar. in Mesopotamia and is cognate to Pers. *gurinj* and Akk. *kurangu.* Rice was known in Mesopotamia in the seventh century B.C. (DAB 106).

Theoph. (IV, IV, 10) wrote, ". . . . (the Indians) sow the cereal called rice of which they make their mash. This is like rice-wheat. . . ." Diosc. (II 95) considers rice, ὄρυζα, as binding in the intestines. Sans. is *vrīhi.* The Gr. probably comes from a South Asian word. Afghan is *vrize* (Carnoy 199). No word for rice is in the *Avesta.* Herodotus mentions only wheat as the staple of the Persians (Laufer 372–373). Galen (VIII, XII, 92) agrees with Diosc. that rice is not good for the bowels.

Al-Ghāfiqī (17) gives ibn Māsawaih's opinion that rice strengthens and tones the stomach. Al-Kindī G. (No. 69) uses rice in an ersatz product for camphor. ᶜAyesha claimed that rice has curative powers and has no sickness within it (*Tibb al-nabbī* of al-Suyūṭī (1505), transl. by C. Elgood, *Osiris* 14, 68 1962).

In the eighteenth century in India (Ainslie I 338), rice is used in dysentery as the least aperient grain. There are hundreds of varieties of rice in India. Some synonyms are, Sans. *dhanya, shali;* Hind. and

Beng. *chaval, dhan;* Mar. *tandula;* Tam. *arishi;* Tel. *dhanyamu;* Mal.*ari;* Bom. *bhatta.* Rice gruel is used today for bowel complaints, in diarrhoea, and dysentery. Rice water is demulcent and a nourishing drink in febrile cases. Rice poultices are used like those with linseed meal.

In Syriac medicine (Budge II 164, 363), rice oil and roasted rice are used for injuries to the nerves and for phthisis. Loew AP (358) gives *ōrez* as Mishnaic and Talmudic is Shabb S. 7. *Cf.* Loew FJ (I 730–738) and Freytag.

Rice is not listed in Maim. since it was so common in his day. IB (42) quotes al-Rāzī on the uses of rice for the abdomen, thirst, and to increase the semen.

304. *Bullūṭ,* evergreen oak, *Quercus infectoria* L., or perhaps another species, is known for its acorn. Al-Kindī A (136b) uses this acorn in medicine. Achundow (157) describes this simple as effective for bloody diarrhoea. It is considered mainly as an astringent in the Near East today (Hooper 161). It is also used for wounds and ulcers. *Cf.* al-Kindī (48).

305. *Ṭīn armanī* is Armenian bole. Ducros (15) states that this simple is red ochre sold in the bazaars as a tonic, desiccative, styptic, and for dysentery. *Cf.* Levey M.A.B. (31). For *ṭīn ḥūrī, cf. al-Kindī* (no. 286).

306. *Aqāqiyā* is acacia, *Acacia arabica* Willd. var. *nilotica* Del. Al-*Kindī* A (103a) uses the juice in a prescription for a pustule. Acacia gum is a constituent of inks (Levey M.A.B. 17, 18, 33, 34). In Babylonia, the bark was used for tanning (Levey CCTM 112). The Ar. name comes from the Gr. *ακακία* (Diosc. I 101).

The gum is used in Egypt today for ulcers internally, and in collyria for the eyes externally.

307. *Isfīdāj* is ceruse. Al-Kindī A (99a) uses white lead for swellings, pulsation of the rectum, and for pain of haemorrhoids. For etymology, *cf.* al-Kindī (no. 102).

In Syriac medicine (Budge 86, 87, 89, 90, 91, 94, 97, 98), white lead with other simples is used in ointments for pain in the eyes where rheum attacks are frequent, for eye sores, and the eyesight. Theophrastus gives the production method of ceruse, "Lead is placed in earthen vessels over sharp vinegar, and after it has acquired some thickness of a kind of rust, which it commonly does in about ten days, they open the vessels and scrape it off, as it were in a kind of foulness; they then place the lead over the vinegar again, repeating over and over again the same method of scraping it, till it is wholly dissolved; what has been scraped off, they then beat to a powder, and boil for a long time; and what at last subsides to the bottom of the vessel is the ceruse." (DACG 136).

J. Ruska (*Das Steinbuch des Aristoteles,* Heidelberg, 1912, p. 125) gives white lead as originating from lead and vinegar, good for the whites of the eyes, and for its pains. It is also effective for fire wounds so that the burned part does not become white. Jābir (54a, 111a, 185a) considers ceruse as dry, cold, and lethal since it is a poisonous mineral. It causes much slime in the stomach and affects the intestines.

It is used in the Near East today mainly as an astringent (Hooper 191). For etymology, *cf.* al-Kindī (102).

308. Gloss: "Wrapped here means that it is put into a piece of cloth and cooked."

309. *Kishk* is gruel of a grain or groats saturated with sour milk or yoghurt for many days, then dried in the sun on the terrace of the home (Dozy).

310. Bust is the name of a city between Herat and Sejistan.

311. *Bizr quṭūnā* is fleawort, *Plantago Psyllium* L. It is unknown in ancient Mesopotamian languages although some guesses have been made (DAB 26–27).

Diosc. (IV 69) states that *psyllion*, ψύλλιον, is for arthritis, tumors, headache, ulcers, and running ears. In Indian medicine, psyllium is used for dysentery. It grows in India, Burma, Sudan, and in the Himalayas (Chopra 355). *P. ispaghula* Flem. is used in India for rattlesnake bites; it comes from Japan where it is called *sin-sin-so* (Ainslie II 116–117).

Maim. (52) gives *asfiyūs* as a synonym, and *bsīl* in Sp. The Syr. is *qṭōnā* which gave rise to the Ar. The Syr. and Gr. mean "stinking." *Cf.* Vullers (99). Al-Ghāfiqī (163) uses the term *asfiyūs*. Other synonyms are *barghūthi, hashīshat, al-barghūth, shabīh al-bārghīth; khar-ghūl* in Pers; *pire otu* in Turk. IB (278) states that al-Rāzī uses fleawort for dyspnoea, constipation, and nausea. The *Tuḥfa* (55) gives *bazarqūṭunā* as the Moroccan pronunciation. The *P. psyllium* L. is very abundant there.

Ducros (20) writes that fleawort is employed in Egypt today as a drug for kidney inflammations, urinary difficulties, and for internal haemorrhoids. *P. ovata* Forsk. is well known in Persia and is used for gonorrhoea and as a diuretic (Hooper 154–155). Loew FJ (III 63) gives psyllium as *qṭōn;* also Loew AP (254). *P. major* is known in China as *lieou-lou*, a diuretic and antirheumatic (Soubeiran 160).

312. *Sukkar aḥmar* is red sugar; it is red because of impurities.

313. *Qūlūn*. Gr. χῶλον.

314. Gloss: "*Farzajat* is a piece of cotton or wool dipped into medicines to make pessaries."

315. Gloss: "*Rikhbīn* is a kind of whey. It is the liquid of cooked milk. It is hot and dry in the second degree. If it is administered

with its suppository, it causes the nature to descend, *Minhāj*"; The latter is probably the first word of the title of a book from which the definition was taken. It is probably the *Minhāj al-dukkān* of *al-Kūhūn* (1260 A.D.).

316. Gloss: "Preparation of *nāṭifā*. Dissolved sugar or honey is thickened on a slow fire and beaten so that when it is removed and cooled it will then break. *Minhāj*."

317. The words for "pessaries" and "suppositories" are often confused in this text so that care must be taken in the reading.

318. *Ṣābūn* is soap. For soap in ancient Mesopotamia, *cf.* Levey CCTM (125–129). Most early soaps were cold or semi-boiled soaps (Levey M.A.B. 36). There is a gloss here which reads "*Muqi*," in place of *Raqqi*. This is incorrect (*muqī* is a vomitive) since the soap of Raqqa, a city of Iraq is well known as *al-ṣābūn al-Raqqī* (Maim. 323).

319. *Wark*.

320. *Cf.* Maim. (178) where *māhīzhara* is a fish poison, perhaps the latex plant, *Anamirta paniculata* Colebr.

321. *ᶜAnzarūt* is sarcocol, *Penaea mucronata* L. or *Astragalus Sarcocolla* Dym. Al-Kindī A (98a) has sarcocol in a salve for black spots on the skin. It is still used for the skin in Persia and Egypt (Ducros 11, Hooper 90). In Hind., it is called *anjira*, Bom. *gujar*. The gum is an aperient (Chopra 465).

322. *ᶜArtanīthā* is sow-bread, probably *Cyclamen europaeum* L. Al-Kindī A (130b) has it in a formula to remove writing from notebooks. Diosc. (II 164, 165) has two *Cyclamens*. κυκλάμινος and κυκλάμινος ἑτέρα. The first is used to cause abortion, for the head, jaundice, spleen, and wounds; the second is a diuretic, and good for the spleen.

The *C. persicum* L., in India, is called *bakhur-i-Miryam*. Its action is as an emetic, emmenagogue, purgative, and diuretic. It is used as a fish poison and as an antidote for snake poison (Chopra 481, Nadkarni I 423).

323. *Dhara* is sorghum, *Sorghum vulgare* Pers. *Cf.* Diosc. (II 97). Al-Ghāfiqī (201) discusses common millet, *jāwars*, *Panicum miliaceum* L. IB (996, 1447) quotes ibn al-ᶜAwwām that the particle size is greater than that of barley. *Dhara* is not listed in the *Tuḥfa*. Maim. (70) discusses *jāwars*, common millet.

The Sans. is *javanala;* Bom., Hind., and Beng. *jowar*. In India, it is used as an aphrodisiac. In modern Persia, it is *dahūra;* Kurd. *zuratspi;* Hind. *dari*, usually the giant millet. It is used as a food (Hooper 173).

324. *Dam al-akhawain* is the dragon's blood plant. In the Orient, it is the resin of *Dracaena cinnabari* Balf. and *Calamus Draco*

Willd., and in the Occident *Dracaeno Draco* L. and others. In al-Kindī A (109a, 118b) this resin is in a cure for haemorrhoids.

The first one is known in India as *hiradukhi* in Hind.; Tam. *kandamurgarittan*. It is an astringent (Nadkarni I 464, Chopra 485).

Cf. al-Dīnawarī (170 Ar.). This plant is also called *dam al-tīs* (*Al-Mu*ᶜ*tamad* 158).

325. *Ḥuḍaḍ* is lycium or lycium juice, *Lycium afrum* L. In al-Kindī A (94a, 100a), lycium juice is used for scrofula and a fistula. For a longer description, *cf.* al-Kindī (no. 91) and Levey M.A.B. (35, 36).

Lycium is not used in Egypt today as a drug (Ducros 168).

326. *Kharbaq abyaḍ* is the white hellebore, *Veratrum album* L. For etymology, *cf.* al-Kindī (no. 132). It is used in al-Kindī A (131a) to kill mice. It is still used as an insecticide today but also as a cardiac and respiratory depressant. *Cf. Al-Mu*ᶜ*tamad* (122–123).

327. *Fautanaj jabalī.*

328. *Baṣal* is onion. This is a general term which requires an adjective to determine the species. It is probably the *biṣru* in Akk. (*Vide* lexical list DAB 52) cognate to Heb. *bĕṣĕl* contra DAB (55). The Gr. *skilla* (σκίλλα) is Maim. (60) is equated with *baṣal al-fār* "onion of the rat." A common Ar. synonym is ᶜ*unṣul.*

Theoph. (I 6; VII 12–13) gives descriptions of bulbous plants especially the onion. Diosc. (II 171) describes what is probably the *Scilla maritima* which is considered an excellent remedy for the stomach, retention of urine, cough, asthma, warts, and is good as an alexipharmic.

Pliny (XX V) claims that onion clears the sight and is recommended for pain in the loins, serpent bites, and dropsy. Celsus (II XXIX–XXXI) describes onion as a laxative and diuretic.

In India, onion is used by the native doctors for bleeding piles and to hasten suppuration. It is called *peeaj* in Hind.; *enggayum* in Tam. The common onion, *Allium Cepa* L. grows in Japan; it is called *soo* or *fitomosi.* In Cochin China, it is *cay-hank* (Ainslie I 269–271). The Sans. is *palandu;* Pers. *piyaz.* In India, it is still used as a stimulant, expectorant, and aphrodisiac (Chopra 563). It is also used as a diuretic and purgative in Egypt, Iran, and Iraq (Ducros 22, Hooper 82). For the species of onion used by the Arabs, *cf.* Leclerc in IB (296, 297, 298, 299, 337, 692, 979).

329. *Tinkār* is borax. Al-Rāzī gives six kinds of borax (MASB VII, 347 (1927)) 1. bread borax, 2. natron, 3. goldsmith's, 4. Zarawandī, 5. "of the willow," 6. *tinkār* (which is gold solder). Borax is found near Urmia and Kerman (DACG 15).

IB (381, 431) quotes ibn ᶜImrān that it is good to fuse gold.

Tinkār probably comes from the Sans. term for borax *tankana* (Dutt 81). Maim. (383) gives a synonym as *dinkār*. The Ar. comes from Pers. *tangār* (Vullers I 469). Ducros (30) has borax used today in Egypt as a detersive, desiccative, and antiseptic for caries. It is called *leḥḥam al-ṣagha* when used in metal work.

330. *Ghubaīrā'* is service tree, sorb, *Pirus Sorbus* Gaertn. Al-Kindī A (105b) uses sorb for the gum and for mouth pustules. For etymology, *cf.* al-Kindī (no. 71).

The sorb is used in the Middle East today for medical purposes.

331. *Qanbīl* is kamala, the red glands that form on the fruit of *Mallotus philippinensis* Muell. Arg. or *Rottlera tinctoria* Roxb. Al-Kindī A (99b) uses kamala for an ulcer.

This simple is called *kamela* in Hind. In Persia today, it is used as an anthelmintic (Hooper 138).

332. *Shīḥ* is wormwood, *Artemisia Abrotanum* L. In al-Kindī A (113b), wormwood is used to remove the decaying part of teeth, for bad breath, and to protect the mouth. Leclerc (IB 1372) believes that wormwood is possibly *A. judaica*. The Ar. is from the Akk. *sīḫu* (DAB 362).

333. *Khaukh* is peach, *Amygdalus persica* L. The Akk. is *ḫabḫu* and Sum. *KIB.KUR.RA*. The former is cognate to the Ar. and to Syr. *ḫabḫā* (Loew FJ III 165, DAB 307).

In Hind., it is *aru*. The peach is native in Persia but cultivated in the Deccan for use as a stomachic, demulcent, antiscorbutic, and aperient. The leaves are laxative, anthelmintic, and sedative (Nadkarni I 1036–1037).

Achundow (194) has this simple for swellings, headache, ears, and haemorrhoids. Al-Kindī G. (30) has it as a substitute for bitter almonds. *Cf.* IB (830). Maim. (397) gives synonyms as *al-tuffāḥ al-fārisī* "Persian apple"; *al-durrāqin* in Syria, and *al-zahrī*. *Cf.* *Nabāt* (315), Loew FJ (III 159), Loew AP (148, 420).

334. *Biṭṭīkh* is melon or watermelon, *Citrullus vulgaris* Schrad. This was known to the ancient Egyptians and Hebrews (*abṭiḥ*). In Syr., it is *faṭṭīḥā* and so the Ar. *biṭṭīkha*. Cf. *al-ᶜAlā'* (31).

The *biṭṭīkh akhḍar* or *hindī* (Indian watermelon) corresponds to *dullāᶜ* of the Maghrib and Syria. It is round and green.

Diosc. (II 134–135) discusses σίκος ἥμερος (species referred to is uncertain) as a good drug for the stomach, bladder, and dog bite. This is also called κύκυον. In pre-Greek, *kuku* is a doubled form of *keu* "to be big" (Carnoy 243). Berendes gives *Cucumis Melo* L. for this plant. In fact, this may be a number of various kinds of round, green melons. The home of the melon is probably South Asia. *Cf.* Paulos (700–701).

In India, Ainslie (216–217) gives the melon as *molam pullum* in Tam. and used as an antiseptic in typhus fever by the Vytians. The *Cucumis Melo* seeds are brought to India from Persia. The Hind. name is *khurbūza.* In Syr. medicine (Budge 644), watermelon is not to be eaten at certain times.

IB (303, 780, 1739) quotes Galen that the watermelon is a detersive and diuretic. Al-Rāzī uses it for the bile. *Vide* ibn al-ᶜAwwām (II 215), Loew FJ (I 550 ff.).

To the Chinese, the watermelon is known as *si kwa* "melon of the West." The origin of the plant may be in South Africa, thence to Egypt and Asia. The melon is probably not Persian in origin since Pers. terms as *hindewāne* "Indian fruit" or *battīkh hindī* "Indian melon" contradict this idea (Laufer 438 ff.).

335. *Sarmaq* is orache, *Atriplex hortensis* L. Diosc. (II 119) gives orache, χρυσολαχανον, from which the Ar. *al-baqla al-dhahabiyya* "the golden vegetable" comes (Carnoy 80). It is considered good for icterus.

Achundow (375) describes *sarmaq.* Maim. (331) gives synonyms as *qaṭaf, sarmaj, baqlat al-Rūm,* and the Lat. is *būlash. Sarmaq* is Pers. (Vullers I 98, II 286). IB (1810) gives it as good for the stomach and bile. Loew AP (337) gives *sarmaj,* ἀτράφαξις, Aram. *atrofliki.*

It is not used much in modern Egypt, Iran, and Iraq. In India today, it is cultivated as a garden herb and used as spinach (Nadkarni I 160).

336. *Isfānākh,* probably a species of *Atriplex.* It may be the *išbabtu* in Akk. which is equivalent to the Sum. *ZID.MÁ.LAḪ,* perhaps related to Heb. *mallūaḥ.* Theoph. (IV, xvi, 5) gives it as αλιμον which is *Atriplex Halimus* L.; it grows in the Mediterranean region. Diosc. (I 91) considers it beneficial for convulsions, for the increase of lactation, and for acute pains of colic. *Cf.* Paulos (615) who uses the root with wine for dysentery. Al-Ghāfiqī (62) has it as spinach, *Spinacia oleracea* L. Al-Rāzī is quoted as employing it for the chest and as a laxative for the abdomen. Ibn Sīnā considers *isfānākh* better than *sarmaq* "orache" for it clears, washes, and controls the bile. IB (63) calls it a common vegetable. Ibn al-ᶜAwwām, in his work on agriculture, devotes much space to its cultivation. The earliest mention of spinach, *po-lin* in Chinese is in the seventh century in the *T'aṅ hui yao.* The latter indicates that it was a novelty coming from Nepal (but originally from Persia). Spinach is not known earlier anywhere (Laufer 392 ff.). The Ar. name comes from the Pers. *aspanāh, aspanāj* or *asfināj.* The Pers. name gave rise to the Arm. *spanax* and Turk. *spanāk.* The English introduced spinach into India.

337. *Mulūkhiyā* is cultivated mauve, probably *Corchorus olitorius* L.

Achundow (273) relates this plant to *khūbazī* (*idem* 194). Maim. (229) gives synonyms as *mulūkh, al-khubbāzī al-bustānī,* or the [Jewish] vegetable. *Tuḥfa* (70) gives it as the last. IB (2173) gives it as a light purgative.

Loew AP (250) and Loew FJ (II 246 ff.) give the Gr. as μολόχη, from which the Syr. and Ar. come. This plant grows mainly in the tropics. *Cf. Nabāt* (170).

338. *Lūbiyā aḥmar* is the kidney bean (?), probably *Phaseolus vulgaris* L.

In Iran today, it is the *lubia* or *lubia-kermiz* in Teheran. In Kashmir, it is *rāzmah* (Hooper 149). *Cf.* Nadkarni (I 942).

339. Gloss: "That is, the roots of the melon plant."

340. *Laft* is turnip and others, *Brassica rapa* L., etc. In Akk., it is *laptu,* Aram. *laftā* (DAB 51).

Maim. (273) gives synonyms as *siljam, shiljam,* and *kūshādh.*

Ducros (15) gives the use of *B. napus* α *oleifera L.* in liniments.

341. *Jazariya* is carrot, *Daucus carota* L. *For* etymology, *cf.* al-Kindī (no. 113). In India, it is used as an aphrodisiac (Ainslie I 56). Al-Kindī A (139a) prescribes carrot seed for the stomach and for the results of excessive intercourse.

In Egypt today, the carrot is recommended for kidney colic, as an emmenagogue, and diuretic (Ducros 21). In Iran, the carrot is used as a laxative and emollient (Hooper 112).

342. *Kawāmīkh.*

343. *Khardal,* mustard, *Sinapis* or *Brassica alba* L. For etymology, *cf.* al-Kindī (no. 133). It is used for erysipelas in al-Kindī A (96a). In ancient Babylonia, it was used in venereal diseases, in beer, in baking, and in seasoning (DAB 203 ff.). *Brassica nigra* L. is today very abundant in Iran and Iraq (Levey M.A.B. 28). Mustard is used in the occident much more as a condiment than in the Near East.

344. Gloss: "That is, the strength of the hellebore is obtained."

345. A kind of dish made of meat, onions, butter, cheese, and others, or of bread and milk.

346. Broth or spoon-meat. In Pers. *zīr-bā.* Plural in text is *zīrbājāt.*

347. Gloss: "'*Ṣamgh ḥurshuf*' is gum of artichoke."

348. *Kankarazd,* of Pers. origin.

349. *Kundus* or *kundush,* struthion, various other soapworts, perhaps like *Gypsophilla Struthium* L. In al-Samarqandī (26a), struthion is in a recipe for a plaster. Usually the root is used (*Al-Muᶜtamad* 437); it is used for phlegm and black bile.

350. Gloss: "'*Raqaᶜ*'. It is a fruit which resembles and is as large as the walnut."

351. *Raqᶜ* or *raqaᶜ* is from *Strychnos Nux vomica* L. The nux

vomica, *jauz al-raqa*ᶜ is from this tree. It grows in tropical Africa and meridional Arabia. The seeds which are emetic are known in European commerce as Mafureira seeds which explains the "Mafura of Yemen" in the text (Maim. 82).

This plant is wild and plentiful in tropical India, in the Madras Presidency, Malabar, and Coromandal Coasts, Cochin, Travancore, Orissa, and Ceylon. The stem bark is used as are also the ripe seeds called nux vomica. The leaves are applied as a poultice to sloughing wounds or ulcers when maggots are formed. The seeds are used in aphrodisiacs, in dyspepsia, in diseases of the nervous system, dysentery, constipation, and many more ailments. Strychnine is obtained from the dried ripe seeds of nux vomica (Nadkarni I 1174–1181).

In Persia today, it is called *kuchūlah*. The seed is imported as a valuable tonic from India. It is used by nomadic tribes to poison wolves and dogs.

352. *ᶜAqīr qarḥā* is pellitory, *Anacyclus pyrethrum* D.C. It is used for blemishes in a prescription by al-Kindī A (101b). For etymology, *cf.* al-Kindī (no. 16).

In Diosc. (III 73) as in modern Egypt, pyrethrum is used for paralysis (Ducros 166). In the Near East, pyrethrum is used also for toothache (Hooper 85).

In Sans., it is *akarakarava*; Hind., Bom., and Ben. *akarkara*; Tam. *akkirakaram*. It grows in Bengal and Arabia, and is used as a cordial, stimulant, and sialagogue (Nadkarni I 97). Loew AP (298) discusses the use of this root.

353. Gloss: "Because it is the easiest time for vomiting since the humors are then easy to bring up and the pores are open."

354. Gloss: "Oil of sesame." In Pers., it means decoction, according to IB (251).

355. *Khark* is probably the gigantic swallowwort, *Calotropis gigantea* R. Br.

Synonyms are *arka, alarka, mandara, surya pattra* in Sans.; *madar* in Hind.; *khak* in Pers.; *akado* in Guj.; *ruvi, akda, akra* in Mah.; *mandaramu* in Tel.; *badabadam, erukku* in Tam.; *erikka* in Mal. This shrub having a milky juice grows in many parts of India and South China. The drug acts like digitalis on the heart. Various parts of the plant are used as a stomachic, tonic, and digestive. The root bark is antispasmodic and expectorant. The milky juice is an abortifacient. In Yunani medicine, this plant is used in paralysis, toxic asthma, and other ills (Nadkarni I 237–241). *Cf.* Maim (236) for *Lathyrus sativus* L.

356. General meanings for *luᶜab* are broader than the Eng. "mucilage" since it may mean "saliva," "web" of a spider, "ray"

of the sun, "drool," etc. When referring to a seed, it is its interior.

357. *Farfakh* is purslane, a species of *Portulaca*. The Ar. probably comes from the Pers. *perpehen* through the Syr. *farfaḥīnā* (Loew FJ 70 ff.). The Gr. name *péplion*, πέπλιον, may be related. *Cf.* Maim. (59).

The wild species is sold in Cairo as a vermifuge (Ducros 24).

358. *Karsanah* is bitter vetch, *Vicia ervila* L. Achundow (246) gives this simple as good for granulation of wounds. In al-Kindī A (98a), bitter vetch is used in a salve for black spots on the skin. For etymology, *cf.* al-Kindī (no. 127).

It is employed in Egypt today to increase lactation, for chest ailments, and to ease expectoration (Ducros 75).

359. *Quṭn* is cotton, *Gossypium herbaceum* L. For etymology, *cf.* al-Kindī (no. 212). To open a chronic swelling, al-Kindī A (101a) uses the seed core in a poultice recipe.

For cotton in Mesopotamia in ancient and modern times, *cf.*, Levey CCTM (101, 111), DAB (113), and Hooper (122–123). In India, cotton seed is used for strangury and gravel (Ainslie I 282–284).

360. *ʿUnṣul* is squill, probably *Allium Cepa* L. (Diosc. II 151) believes that this simple is good for incipient cataract, for opening the orifices of blood vessels, for relieving haemorrhoids, and as a diuretic. The Gr. name is σκίλλα. It is also called *baṣal al-fār, al-ishqīl,* in Ber. *uḥkāl* (Maim. 60, Levey M.A.B. 36). Al-Ghāfiqī (134) believes onion to be injurious to the mind but, when cooked, it is an aphrodisiac. When raw, it is effective in checking the harm of bad water.

361. *Qiththa'* may be cucumber, melon, gourd, and various other species. In Egypt, it is *Cucumis Melo* var. *Chate* Naud. Maim (343) gives *al-sawaf,* and the long species as *al-faqqūs*. The Akk. is *gishshu* and Heb. *qishshūt*. The word *qiththa'* means "penis" and is probably the long cucumber (DAB 86). The Sum. is *UKUŠ.ŠAR*.

362. Gloss: "That is, six and a half dirhams."

363. *Ḥabb al-ṣanawbar* is pine cone. The pine may be *Pinus orientalis* Link., *P. Pinea* L., *P. halepensis* Mill. For etymology, *cf.* al-Kindī (no. 271). In al-Kindī A (115a), the seed of pine is employed in an electuary for a cough from catarrh.

The pine was very common in ancient Mesopotamia and had many uses in medicine (Levey CCTM 123, DAB 258). The turpentine from the pine was used for the eyes, feet, anus, lungs, and swellings. In Arabic times, these uses were still known. In addition, pine had its uses in chemical technology as in the manufacture of inks (Levey M.A.B. 15–16).

364. Gloss: "That is, the sieved part of the root of lily."

365. *Mannā* is a sweet exudate observed on certain desert plants. It corresponds to *mann* of the Bible. The Pers. is *tarangubīn*. Maim. (386) gives an Ar. synonym as *rizq* "provisions." *Cf.* Vullers (I 440). The manna in Sinai is supposed to be found on the *Tamarix nilotica* Ehrenb. var. *mannifera*. *Cf.* Achundow (173) and *Tuḥfa* (259); *vide* earlier note on *taranjubīn*.

366. A very brief passage here is illegible.

367. Gloss: "A *qirāṭ* of the physicians is four grains."

368. Gloss: "That is, the seeds and other than that which are sandalwood, rose, and camphor."

369. Gloss: "*Al-faqad* by having the *fā* precede the *qāf* is the *binjinkusht*, and *qafad* with the *qaf* first is the seed of cuscuta." *Cf.* IB (354, 1691). *Faqad* is vitex, *Vitex Agnus-castus* L.

370. From a gloss. Text has *tīn al-akl*.

370a. *Fustuq* is pistachio, probably *Pistacia Terebinthus* L.

371. *Sūbaq* wine is probably one of the best.

372. *Sunbul al-ṭīb* is Indian nard or some species of spikenard, probably *Nardostachys Jatamansi* D.C. For etymology, *cf.* al-Kindī (no. 264). In al-kindī A (92b, 104b), nard is used for mouth pustules and for the gum; wild nard is in a remedy to make one happy. Indian nard (*idem* 138b) is in an original stomachic by al-Kindī.

This herb grows in the Himalayas, Nepal, Bhutan, and Sikkim. It is called in Sans. *jatamansii;* in Hind. and Punj. *jatamashi;* in Tel. *jatamamshi;* in Tam. *jatamashi;* in Mal. *jatamanshi*. In the *Ayurveda,* it is used to give strength and complexion, in cases of blood impurity. In Yunani medicine, it is a tonic for the heart, liver, and brain. It is diuretic, an emmenagogue, and good for jaundice and kidney stone (Nadkarni I 840). *Cf.* Ducros (130) for the use of Indian nard in Egypt for epilepsy, convulsions, and hysteria; in Iran and Iraq, it is for nervous disorders (Hooper 143).

373. *Ward* is rose, in many species. For etymology and references, *cf.* al-Kindī (no. 299). In al-Kindī A (95a), rose oil is employed for haemorrhoids. Rose oil was used in early times as a stomachic as it is used today. In al-Kindī G. (*passim*), rose oil is used in many perfumery products. The ancient Egyptian *wrt* is probably the cognate to the Ar. *warad*. Rose is used in inks (Levey M.A.B. 26, 28).

374. Here spelled *qarabādhīn*.

375. Times of crisis.

376. Gloss: "Because of the phlegm and strange fever."

377. *Ḥummāḍ*.

378. *Pashādhanaj,* probably the same as *shādhanaj* and *sādhanaj,* haematite. For etymology, *cf.* al-Kindī (no. 241).

In Chinese, haematite is *tay-tchou-tche, tieh-chu, fan-hung, tsee-che*. It is used as a tonic, styptic, against hypochondria, haemorrhage (Soubeiran 23).

In India, haematite, or *suvarna* and *gairika* in Sans., and *sitageru* in Hind., is used as an antidote to arsenic poisoning. It is astringent, antibilious, anti-phlegmatic, generative of bile, and good for haemorrhoids (Nadkarni II 42). *Cf.* Ray (156, 173, 227).

379. *Qaraḍ*. Gloss: "An Egyptian tree from which is extracted acacia. It is thus mentioned in ibn Beithar." The ibn Beithar mentioned here is the IB in the bibliography.

380. *Makhtūm* is a clay used for sealing.

381. Gloss: "That is, macerated in water."

382. *Nashā'* is starch. Al-Kindī A (104b) has starch in a prescription for a mouth pustule and for soft gums. Al-Kindī G (*passim*) has starch in many perfumery products. For etymology, *cf.* al-Kindī (no. 189). *Cf.* also *Maim.* (261), *Al-Muᶜtamad* (523), Levey M.A.B. (39, 42). In the latter, starch is used in inks.

383. *Basad* is correct for coral. An earlier gloss states that *bastad* is the same. In al-Kindī A (113a), coral is used for "worm of the teeth." It strengthens loose teeth. For etymology *cf.* al-Kindī (no. 40). It is still used in the Near East for many illnesses (Hooper 194).

384. *Kākanj* is alkekenji, *Physalis Alkekengi* L. This is a Pers. name (Vullers II 779) probably from the Sans. *kakamāchi* (Chopra 595).

The fruit is sold in Indian bazaars. It is diuretic, alterative, anthelmintic, laxative, useful in strangury, kidney stone, and urinary diseases. Linnaeus is said to have cured himself of gout by the use of this fruit. It contains salicylic salts and levulose. It is called the strawberry tomato (Nadkarni I 950).

In modern Iran, the berries are used for syphilis and are supposed to be intoxicating in sufficient quantity (Hooper 151).

385. Gloss: "Know that medical powders act perfectly from the day of preparation to two months later. They should not be used after two months."

386. Gloss: "There is no difference between the powders and dry stomachics. Etymologically, *qamīḥa* is everything small in body and eaten dry. This is why wheat is called *qamḥ*. Therefore, basically al-*qamḥ* is more general than the *safūf* [powder]."

387. *Nabq* is Christ's thorn fruit, of the *Zizyphus Spina Christi* Willd. *Nabq* fruit is good for yellow bile, skin, and hair roots (Achundow 278). The name of the tree is *sidr* (Maim. 269) which is often confused with the *ḍāl* which is the wild jujube (*Zizyphus Lotus* Lam.), in Heb. *ṣāl.*

IB (1165) discusses the *sidr* fruit, *nabq,* as an astringent and to evacuate bile in the stomach and intestines. Loew AP (283 ff.) discusses Aram. and Syr. *kĕnarā, κόναρος,* in relation to Christ's thorn. *Cf. Nabāt* (194 ff.), *Al-Muᶜtamad* (519).

388. Gloss "With its inner rind and not its external."

389. *Kumathrā* is the pear tree, pear. *Pyrus communis* L., and other species.

Maim. (187) gives the synonym in the Maghrib as "the plum." Achundow (246) claims that it strengthens the stomach. Loew FJ (III 235 ff.) and Loew AP (208) gives the Syr. as *kumtĕrā*.

The Akk. for pear is uncertain but Campbell Thompson gives *kameššaru;* he calls it *Sorbus domestica* L. and that the designation of *P. communis* is unlikely (DAB 305). The Chinese pear, *kumathrā ṣīnī,* is probably the *P. chinensis* Roxb. or *P. sinensis* L. (Bailey 2869).

390. *Ṣamgh ʿarabī* is gum arabic. In Egypt, it is gum of *Acacia sperocarpa* Hochst. It is much used for the manufacture of inks (Levey M.A.B. *passim).* In southern Morocco, it is gum of the *A. gummifera* Willd.; in the Orient gum of the *A. vera* Willd.

391. *Qaṣab* is sugar cane. It probably stands here for *qaṣab al-sukkar,* or other cane as *qaṣab al-dharīra,* an odoriferous reed (Maim. 329). Al-Kindī A (110b) has this in a remedy for head and face pustules of children. In Egypt today, it may be the *wajj, Acorus Calamus* L. (Ducros 189).

392. A biscuit without milk or butter in it. Persian.

393. *Raiḥān* is grand basil, *Ocimum Basilicum* L. in Levey M.A.B. (23), it is used in the preparation of ink.

In India, it is called *bisva tulasi, varavara, manjariki* in Sans.; *babui, tulsi, sabzah* in Hind.; *sabajhi* in Sind.; *tirunirupachai* in Tam.; *kala pingain* in Burm. The herb and seeds are used. It is aphrodisiac and diuretic. The root is febrifuge (Nadkarni I 861–863).

Laufer (586 ff.) believes that this plant had its origin in Persia, then was brought to India. The Chinese is *lo-lo* and was first described in the sixth century.

Maim (10, 48) gives synonyms as *bādharūj, al-ḥauk, al-ḥumāḥim, al-ḥabaq al-nabaṭī.* The Gr. is βασιλικόν (Diosc. III 62). In the Maghrib, it is *ṭarṭūr al-ḥājib.*

Ducros (64) states that this simple is considered as a cephalic, diuretic, and nerve drug in modern Cairo. In Persia today, where the seeds of this plant are imported from India, it is used as a cold infusion for influenza (Hooper 145).

394. *Maqalīthā.* Grilled seeds of garden cress *Lepidium sativum* L. and other species of *Lepidium* and *Nasturtium.*

The Akk. is *saḫlē* and Sum. *ZAG.ḪI.LI* for cress. The Akk. is cognate to Syr. *šailūmā* (DAB 56).

IB (653) quotes abū Ḥanīfa that a synonym is *thuffa* in Ar. It is used for dysentery, for the skin, and for scorpion bites.

In Iran today, garden cress is *tukhm-i-shāhī,* and is tonic, aphrodisiac, and diuretic (Hooper 136).

395. Gloss: "The seeds should not be fried too much or their strength will disappear. The pot or earthenware should be heated and removed from the fire. Put in the seeds and stir them until they are roasted. It will be known by its odor."

396. *Laḥlāḥ* is colchicum, especially *Colchicum autumnale* L. The Syr. is *sūrinjān*, in Ar. *sūranjān*. *Vide* note 143.

397. That is, bringing the impurities to the surface.

398. *Bābūnaj, baibūnaj* is camomile, probably *Anthemis nobilis* L. For etymology, *cf.* al-Kindī (no. 28). In al-Kindī A (93a, 93b). camomile is in a strong dressing for the spleen and in an application to relax the liver and stomach. Camomile is used in Egypt today for intercostal neuralgia, as a stimulant, and febrifuge (Hooper 139).

399. *Jāwars* is common millet, *Panicum miliaceum* L. The Ar. comes from the Pers. *gāwers* which corresponds to *κέγχρος* (Diosc. II 97).

In Akk., millet is *ŠE arzik* and *duḫnu* (DAB 108). The latter is cognate to a synonym for *jāwars* given by Maim. (70) as *dukhn* which is actually "small millet," or sorghum. Loew FJ (I 739) says that it is proto-Semitic. The Mishnaic word is *dōḫan*. For diseases of millet and millet for alcoholic beverages in ancient Mesopotamia, *cf.* Levey CCTM (47).

In Sans., common millet is *chīnā*, and in Ben. *chīnā ghās* (Dutt 267). Millet is lacking in Persia although there is a Pers. name, *shushu*. The Chinese is *šu šu*. The Pers. may be a Chinese loanword (Laufer 565). Al-Ghāfiqī (201) quotes Galen (VII, XII, 16) that millet is useful for colic. IB (460) quotes al-Rāzī that it is a good desiccative and laxative.

Today, it is called *arzan* in Pers., *dukhn* in Iraq, *chīna* in Hind. and Sans. Loew FJ (I 738 ff.) gives the Mishnaic synonym as *pĕraggīm*.

400. Liquid elements of the body which may at times seem to conglomerate, for example in the cervical glands.

401. *Asārūn* is wild ginger, root of *Asarum europaeum* L. In al-Kindī A (108a), this simple is used in an oxymel for quartan fever, for the fever of every second day, jaundice, for thirst and pain of the stomach and liver, and to correct skin color. For etymology, *cf.* al-Kindī (no. 22).

Chopra (28) declares that wild ginger is called *upana* in Sans., and *taggar* in Hind. and Bom. Its roots and leaves are emetic and cathartic. It is indigenous to temperate Europe and North Asia.

Cf. Loew FJ (I 223, III 93, 488), Loew AP (369–370), and Paulos (624).

402. *Faufal* is areca nut, *Areca Catechu* L. This word is derived from the Sans. *pūgaphala* (Laufer 548). In India, it is commonly

mixed with betel leaf (*Piper Betle* L.) and some pulverized limestone to be used as a masticatory. Maim. (311) calls it also *al-bunduq al-hindī* and *al-atmūt*.

In modern Egypt (Ducros 109–110), it is used as a collyrium and dentifrice. In Iran today, it is used with sugar and coriander to induce labor (Hooper 86). In India, it is chewed to prevent decay of teeth, for the stomach, and is a vermifuge. In Hind., Guj., and Mah., it is *supari*. In Tam., it is *kamugu* and *pakku*.

403. *Māmīthā* is horned poppy, glaucium, *Glaucium corniculatum* Kurt (?) *Cf.* Achundow (272–273), al-Kindī (no. 163). In al-Kindī A (137b) and Ḥunain (160, 178, 181), it is employed for ophthalmic disorders especially pterygium. Arabic writers have this simple for erysipelas, tumors of the umbilicus, and gout (IB 2059).

404. Gloss: "Like the flour of fenugreek and seed of flax."

405. *Lisān al-ḥamal* is plantain, *Plantago major* L. In Akk., it is *lišan kalbi* "tongue of a dog." In Babylonia, it was used as a stomachic, for urinary troubles, jaundice, menstruation, cough, and eyes (DAB 26).

Diosc. (II 126) gives ἀρνόγλωσσον (*arnóglōsson*) as its name, meaning "tongue of a lamb," also the meaning of *lisān al-ḥamal* (Carnoy 38).

Achundow (265) claims it is for the liver, kidneys, and haemorrhage after tooth extraction. Maim. (213) gives synonyms as *lisān al-kalb* "tongue of the dog," *dhanab al-fār*, "tail of the rat," Sp. *balantāyin* (*plantagine*). In the Maghrib, he says the name is *maṣṣāṣa* "pipe," and in Ar. Pers. *karkūs*. The latter is *khargūsh* "ear of an ass" (Vullers I 680). *Cf.* abū al-ᶜAlā (21). *Cf.* Loew AP (242–244).

In modern Egypt, plantain is used to wash inflammations, it is also prescribed as an astringent and tonic in diarrhoea (Ducros 119). In present day Iran, plantain is called *bārhang* in Teheran, and in Iraq *bizr dinbil*; the seeds are used for affections of the bowels (Hooper 154). In India today, it is called *lahurīya* in Hind., *bartang* in Bom.; it is used in urinary disorders and in dysentery (Nadkarni I 986–987).

406. Gloss: "That is, leaf of cypress."

Sarw is cypress, *Cupressus sempervirens* L. For etymology, *cf.* al-Kindī (no. 236). In al-Kindī A (104a, 123a), the leaf is in remedies to relieve heat in the face, for haemorrhoids, and pulsation in the rectum. *Cf.* also Achundow (219).

407. *Tūtiyā* is tutty. It is the impure oxide of zinc; it may mean other metallic oxides. In al-Kindī A (127b), tutty is used as a cooling agent for the eyes, to sharpen the sight, and to stop tearing. For synonyms, *cf.* al-Kindī (no. 281). In Levey M.A.B. (28), tutty is used in a recipe for a silver *līq*.

408. *Khamīr* is yeast. In al-Kindī G. (225), it is used in a recipe as a substitute for musk. IB (819) quotes Galen and Dioscorides on a yeast mixture for a gargle against throat tumor.

409. *Rāmik* is an electuary composed of gallnut, musk, and other aromatics. In al-Kindī A (113b), this mixture is used for the teeth and mouth. The *Tuḥfa* (360) considers this mixture to contain gallnut, aromatic drugs as mastic, benjamin, and others. In Jābir (83a, 187a), gallnut is also the main constituent. *Cf.* al-Kindī (no. 213).

410. *Karm* (pl. *kurūm*) is vine. The etymology of this name is uncertain. For synonyms, *cf.* al-Kindī (no. 128). It is probably the grape vine.

411. *Ḥabb al-mulūk* is cherry, fruit of *Prunus Cerasia* Br.

The word for cherry in Akk. is uncertain although one writer claims it is *karšu* (DAB 301). (Diosc. I 113) considers the cherry, *κεράσια*, as good for the sight, appetite, and for urinary calculi.

Maim. (330, 371) gives the synonyms as *sarāsiyā* or *jarāsiyā*, and the Pers. as *shāh-dawrān* "seed of the king" which is also the meaning of the Ar. *ḥabb al-mulūk*.

In Hind., it is *alu-balu*; in Punj. *gilas, olchi*. It is a nervine tonic, and contains some hydrocyanic acid (Nadkarni L. 1014). Loew FJ (III 169) gives Syr. *kersiya* and Ar. *karaz*. Sour cherries are Syr. *gīlāzī* and Turk. *chilās* (Loew AP 90, 93). White cherries are Syr. *gilāstā, gilāsā*. Today in Teheran, the cherry is *kastah-i-ālbālū*. The stones are used in an infusion with barley awns and cherry stems for gonorrhoea (Hooper 158).

412. *Turmus* is lupine, *Lupinus* sp. (?). The Sum. *TAR.MUŠ* is related to the Ar. as are Jud.-Aram. *tūrmūsā* and Syr. *turmēsā*. It may be the *L. termis* Forsk. The Akk. is probably *ararianu* which may be compared with the Syr. *ᶜārᶜārīnā* (Loew FJ II 466, DAB 125–126).

The lupine, *θέρμος* (Theoph. VIII 2 ff.; Diosc. II 109), in Greek times was considered valuable for extracting the embryo, for sciatica, swellings, and for the stomach.

Lupine is used by Ḥunain (154) in an aperient to remove obstructions. Maim. (379) claims that the Gr. name is the original but he was not aware of the Sum. term. Maim. states that it is also called *al-basīla* and *al-jarjar*. IB (406) quotes ibn Sīnā that it is difficult to digest, and al-Rāzī that sugar must be taken with it.

The lupine is well known in Syria *Nabāt Sūriyā* (208). *Cf.* also *Al-Muᶜtamad* (49). In Loew FJ (II 453 ff.), the *turmus* is sweetened. Galen also requires that it be cooked in sweet water. *Cf.* also Krauss (I 115).

In Ducros (29), *turmus* is used for cataplasms and vermifuges.

413. *Māzaryūn* is mezereon, *Daphne Mezereum* L. Achundow considers it valuable for yellow gall, cleansing of wounds, for the liver, scabies, impetigo, and fistulas. Maim. (237) has *al-khaḍrā'* as the name in the Maghrib. There is much confusion in regard to the synonyms for this simple.

In India, the *D. oleoides* Schreib. is used. It is *mashur* in Punj., and *pech* in Bom. (Nadkarni I 433). *Cf.* Loew AP (247) which gives the Aram. and Syr. as *mōrīyōn*. The Gr. is χαμελαία.

414. *Māsh* is mung bean, of the *Phaseolus Mungo* L. The Ar. *manāj* originates from the ancient Akk. term *mangu*. In al-Kindī A (98a, 107b), it is used in a prescription for discoloration of skin, and in a remedy for haemorrhoids and scrofula. Ibn Sīnā has *māsh* as an aphrodisiac. Al-Rāzī considers it a refresher (IB 2060). The Sans. is *masha* (B. Meissner, ZA 6, 293; Loew II 468).

415. An eye remedy brought from Dar-band; also an Armenian cataplasm (Dozy 127). IB (374) has *būsh Darbandiyy* as a plant used for gout.

416. *Luffaḥ* is mandrake, *Mandragora officinarum* L. For etymology, *cf.* al-Kindī (no. 158). In al-Kindī A (131b), one is warned that mandrake is not to be used for the eyes.

In Akk., the mandrake is *pillū*; the Ar. is the metathesis, possibly (R. C. Thompson JRAS (1926) 10). The Ar. name "devil's testicles" corresponds to the Babylonian "male *NAM.TAR* plant." The mandrake is discussed by Achundow (266) and DAB (217).

417. *Birwaq* is asphodel. *Vide* note 425. In Levey M.A.B. (42), asphodel is much used in the bookbinding process. The pronunciation may correctly be *birwāq* (IB 88, 277, 826). If it is *bārwaq*, then it is ceruse (IB 242). It is probably the former. Maim. (395) gives *ishrās* and *junthā* as synonyms. The Heb. is *ᶜīrīth* equivalent to the Syr. *ᶜīrōnā* which is asphodel.

418. *Furbiyūn, furfiyūn* is euphorbium, a resin from *Euphorbia resinifera* Berg., and other species. For these other species, *cf.* al-Kindī (no. 66).

In India, the *E. antiquorum* L. resin is used for rheumatic troubles, internally as a purge and for induration of the spleen and liver (Ainslie I 121 ff.). It is also a rubefacient and vesicant (Nadkarni I 522 ff.). Not only is its resin used but also its bark, stem, and root bark.

419. *Zabad al-baḥr*, "ecumen of the sea," is probably the jellyfish. This meaning is uncertain. It is also claimed that it is a brownish liquor formed by cuttle-fish when it is stored underground. It may, under certain conditions, refer to the compressed bone which is still commonly used in jewelry work for casting gold and silver.

Maim. (141), in his description, states that it may be the sponge, a light stone found in Sicily, and others. Meyerhof states that *zabad al-baḥr* is a translation of ἀλκυόνιον of Diosc. (118), a mixture of sponge, seaweed, and polyps thrown up by the sea. In an early Pers. work on medicine, it is considered as meerschaum which cleanses the skin, and is good for alopecia and ophthalmia. It also cleanses the teeth (Achundow 215). IB (1086) states that there are five kinds of *zabad al-baḥr*. The first is dense, spongy and with a strong fishy odor and heavy: the second resembles sponge and is light, spongy, very porous, and with the odor of algae; the third has a green and purple color; the fourth resembles wool and is light and porous; the fifth resembles mushroom with no odor and is rough and like a stone.

Under the name of alcyon, the ancients knew strange substances, animal, plant, and flotsam (IB 1086). The jelly-fish is frequently thrown up on the shore. Diosc. (V 120) has σπόγγος which is probably *isfinj al-baḥr* (Levey M.A.B. 38), sponge. *Al-Muᶜtamad* (195) follows IB in describing the five possibilities. It is used in al-Kindī G. (13, 14, 64) in the manufacture of perfumes.

420. Gloss: "Sea rue," "gum of land rue."

421. *Zarnīkh* is probably the most common yellow arsenic or orpiment. For realgar, *cf.* al-Kindī (No. 309). Levey M.A.B. (22) and Levey CCTM (96, 161) describe orpiment in Babylonian and Arabic times. The red and yellow were the only sulphides known to the Arabs as types of *zarnīkh*.

422. *Naft* is a kind of flammable petroleum substance. In Achundow (280), the pure oil is used for facial paralysis and rheumatic pain. Internally, it drives off the placenta and foetus. It causes headache, however.

422a. *Qunābarā is some kind of pot herb or moss* (?)

Cf. Maim. (344) where. "This is the plant called *barghast* in Pers. and *ghumlūl* in Ar. Some say it is the *usturghāz*." The word is Syr. and comes from the Gr. The gloss reads "sea rue or gum of land rue." Achundow (245) has *qanābarī* as *Plumbago europaea* L., good for the stomach and insect bites.

423. This should perhaps be "pain."

424. *Murr* is myrrh, *Balsamodendron myrrha* Nees. The Ar. comes originally from *murru* in Akk. *Murr makkī* is Meccan myrrh.

In India, it is an important emmenagogue (Ainslie I 244). In Egypt today (Ducros 214), it is used as an antispasmodic, emmenagogue, astringent, and for other purposes. For etymology, *cf.* al-Kindī (no. 179).

425. *Vide* note 417.

426. *Khilāf* is willow or Egyptian willow, *Salix aegyptiaca* or *S.*

Safsaf Forsk. The willow in Sum. is *ḪA.LU.UB,* and in Akk. *ḫaluppu.* In Babylonia, it was used for the feet, as a stomachic, in childbirth, and in poultices in sorcery. The Sum. and Akk, are cognate to the Ar. and Syr. *ḫelāphā.*

Theoph. (III 13) and Diosc. (I 104) mention the willow. The latter claims it is good for gout, the ears, and for various ailments.

Achundow (195) has it for the spleen, heart, and brain since it is good for the blood. It is also helpful for headache and migraine. Maim. (393) gives the synonyms as *al-ṣafṣāf* (*Salix* Safsaf Forsk.), *al-sindar* (from Pers. *sapid-dar, Salix alba* L., Vullers II 216), *al-gharab* (*Salix babylonica* L., from Heb. *ᶜarābāh*), *al-sawḥar* (Frey. II 290, meaning "willow"), and *al-sālij.* The latter is from Lat. *salix. Cf. Tuḥfa* (412, 438). IB (815, 914, 1180, 2069) quotes al-Tamīmī that *khilāf* is a species of *ṣafṣāf. Bīd-khisht* in Pers., *Salix fragilis* L., is used in modern Persia for thrush (Hooper 168).

426a. For a scholarly discussion of "oily substances" see Sami Hamarneh and G. Sonnedecker, *A Pharmaceutical View of Abulcasis Al-Zahrawi in Moorish Spain,* Leiden, 1963, pp. 78–80.

427. *Yāsamīn* is jasmine, *Jasminum officinale* L. The Ar. name comes from the Syr. (Loew FJ III 396; Loew AP 189). Achundow (283) gives it as good for headache, rheumatic pains, for the brain, and for facial paralysis. Maim. (181) gives the synonym *ᶜarīf.*

In India, its oil is used today as a nerve sedative. Its fruits are narcotic. In Sans., it is *mallika;* Hind. *matiya;* Guj. *dojar.* Many other species of *Jasminum* are used in India (Nadkarni I 702–703).

This plant is *ye-si-min* and *su-hing* in China (Soubeiran 174).

Jasmine is native to Kashmir and Persia but now grows almost everywhere. *Cf. Al-Muᶜtamad* (168–169).

428. This should read *marmākhūr,* not *marmaḥūz.* It is the origan of Egypt, *Origanum Maru* L. This is the equivalent of *marw; vide* note 231.

429. *Balasān* is balm of Gilead, *Commiphora Opobalsamum* Engl. For etymology, *cf.* al-Kindī (no. 30). Achundow (165) considers this drug valuable for epilepsy and pain, as an antidote, and as a warming agent for the liver and stomach, good for the eyes and wounds, and also in elephantiasis.

430. Gloss: "Grains."

431. *Bunduq* is filbert, *Corylus Avellana* L. nut. The word *bunduq* comes from the Greek ποντικὸν κάρυον "Pontic nut." *Cf.* Theoph. (I 12) and Diosc. (I 125); in the latter, the plant is κάρυα βασιλικά· The Dioscorides text considers this, also called the hazelnut, as good for chronic coughs and to restore hair fallen as a result of alopecia.

Al-Ghāfiqī (198) calls it *jillauz.* Galen (VII, XII, 4) calls it a cold substance. The Pers. is *funduq*. Loew AP (48–49) derives the Ar. from the Gr. The Ar. comes from Pers. *jilūz* or *gilūz*. *The* Pontic nut is also called in Ar. *lauz jabalī*, and in Turk. *findiq*.

The Hind. is *findak* and is used in India as a tonic, stomachic, and aphrodisiac (Chopra 478). It is an indigenous Indian plant (Nadkarni I 383).

IB (357, 502) quotes ibn Sīnā that this drug is an emmenagogue. Al-Rāzī considers this nut to be a nourishing food. The latter idea is repeated from Galen to Muwaffaq and later on (Achundow 157). The *Tuḥfa* (64) calls this nut *al-jillauz* but there is some confusion as to its identification.

In a Pahlavi text, the filbert is considered as one of the thirty principal fruits (Laufer 193).

In Egypt today, the filbert is regarded as an astringent, diuretic, and good for thoracic difficulties (Ducros 25–26). In Iran, the *C. Colurna* L., growing in the northwestern Himalayas, Kashmir, and Afghanistan, is eaten raw or roasted (Hooper 106).

432. *Nardīn* is nard, *Valeriana Celtica* L. In al-Kindī A (98b, 123b), Celtic nard is used for the bladder and kidneys. For etymology, *cf.* al-Kindī (no. 186). *Vide* note 134.

433. *Rāsin* is elecampane, *Inula Helenium* L. In al-Kindī A (138b), it is in a strengthener for the stomach, for digestion of food, and to drive away the rheums. *Rāsin* is a loanword from the Pers.

In India, it is used in chronic bronchitis and rheumatism (Nadkarni I 683; Chopra 498). In Teheran, elecampane is employed for bronchitis and tuberculosis, and in Egypt as an emmenagogue and stimulant (Ducros 155; Hooper 129–130).

434. *Qardamānā* is bastard cardamom, *Lagoecia cuminoides* L. This name comes from the Gr. Maim. (334) gives it as *al-karāwiyyā al-rūmiyya*. Other species resembling this are known. Achundow (245) has it for epilepsy, asthma, and facial paralysis. *Cf.* Loew FJ (III 439 ff.), IB (1747).

435. *Jauz bawwā* is nutmeg, *Myristica fragrans* Houtt. Al-Kindī A (112a, 135b) uses nutmeg in a tooth medicine and to aid the spirits. For a full description, *cf.* M. Levey, *Journ. Hist. Med.* **16**, 404 (1961). In al-Kindī G., it is used in perfumery operations; especially in 37, 49, 62. Nutmeg is popular for medicinal purposes. In Egypt, it is an astringent (Ducros 37, 68); in India, it is a cardiac remedy (Ainslie I 250); in Iran, it is also well known (Hooper 142).

436. *Maiʿa* is storax, especially from *Boswellia Carterii* Bird. It is described in al-Kindī (nos. 154, 161); al-Kindī A (122a, 136b) has it for rheumatism. Achundow (532) has this storax coming from *Styrax officinalis* L.; it may be dry or liquid. It is used in perfumery in al-Kindī G (no. 65).

437. *Nisrīn* is eglantine, *Rosa canina* L. It is Pers. (Vullers II 1312).

Diosc. (I 94) gives it, *κυνόσβατος*, as good for the belly.

Its oil is good for nervous diseases (Achundow 280). *Al-Muᶜtamad* (522 ff.) claims it is a white rose and that its strength is that of the jasmine. *Cf.* Maim. (253), Loew AP (276) for synonyms *al-ward al-barrī* "wild rose," and *al-ward al-ṣīnī* "Chinese rose."

In China, it is called *kin-yn, tsin-in-tsee;* it is used as a tonic and astringent (Soubeiran 268).

437a. *Aqḥuwān* is feverfew. The identification of this plant is in doubt. IB (121) says that it is the camomile (*bābūnaj*) to the Arabs and known in Egypt as *kirkāsh*. It may also be the *parthénion*, *παρθένιον* in Diosc. (III 138), *Pyrethrum Parthenium*, some kind of large chrysanthemum as *Matricaria parthenoides* Desf. (in Sontheimer). It is a febrifuge, and is used for a balm together with other drugs.

438. Gloss: "Bulging of the eyes." *Shukhūṣ*.

439. *Khīrī* is yellow gillyflower or wallflower, *Cheiranthus Cheiri* L. It is used in the manufacture of inks (Levey M.A.B. 15, 48).

Diosc. (III 123) has it, *λευκόϊον* (Carnoy 160) for amenorrhoea and gout. It is employed in perfumery (al-Kindī G. 28). Achundow (195–196) also has it for amenorrhoea and the head. Maim. (294) states that the Egyptians call it *al-manthūr*. The wild species may be *al-khuzāma* and *al-bābūna*. *Cf.* Loew *AP* (40, 199, 252).

In India, *C. Cheiri* L. is *todrisurkh* in Hind. and *khueri* in Ben. It is used as an emmenagogue (Chopra 474). Today, it is not used medicinally in Egypt, Iran, and Iraq.

439a. *Buṭm* is terebinth, *Pistacia Terebinthus* L. It is native to Asia. Persia has three species, *P. vera, terebinthus,* and *acuminata.*

Achundow (162) gives *buṭm* as *ḥabbat al-khaḍrā'* "the green seed," but it is a different species, possibly. Levey M.A.B. (19) has terebinth in an instant ink. In Babylonia, it was used as a detersive substance (Levey CCTM 124). The Akk. is *buṭuttu;* Syr. *beṭmĕtha;* Heb. *bōṭem*. In early Arabic times, the oil was used for facial paralysis, spleen, and phlegm.

Twan Ch'en-shi, in his *Yu yang tsa tsu* (*ca.* 860 A.D.), wrote that there is a tree which bears the hazel-nut one year and the next year *a-yüe* (pistachio ?) (Laufer 247).

The terebinth is still used in Persia today as an astringent and for dyeing. It grows freely near Banni and in the hills of Sherag (Hooper 153).

440. *ᶜAṣā al-rāᶜī* is knotweed, *Polygonum aviculare* L. or *P. equisetiforme* Sibth & Sm.

Diosc. (IV 4) gives knotweed, *πολύγονον ἄρρεν*, as an herb good for the spitting of blood, strangury, ulcers, for the stomach, inflammations, and wounds.

Achundow (234) gives *ᶜasa'l-rāᶜī* as good for nosebleed, stomach, wounds, spitting of blood, and for the ears. Maim. (298) gives the synonyms as *al-baṭbāṭ, shabaṭbāṭ,* and in Pers. *barsiyāndārū. Cf.* Loew AP (368), Loew (I 4).

In Egypt today, knotweed is known as an astringent, for diarrhoea and haemorrhage (Ducros 92). In modern India, *P.aviculare L.* is known as *miromati, nisomali* in Sans.; *endraru* in Sind.; *kuwar* in Hind. and Punj.; *hozar, bandak* in Pers. It is used in malaria, chronic diarrhoea, lithiasis, leucorrhoea, and for ulcers (Nadkarni I 999).

441. Gloss: *"Baqla al-ḥamqā'."*

442. *Shabath* is dill, *Anethum graveolens* L. For etymology, *cf.* al-Kindī (no. 238). In al-Kindī A (95a), dill is used in a plaster to be applied to frozen limbs, and is used as a diuretic. It is also employed for the kidneys and bladder (*Idem* 98b).

Dill is today a condiment and carminative in Iran and Iraq (Hooper 148–149).

443. *Tīn al-ḥanṭ* is red fig. *Ḥanṭ* is redness in Pers. Vide red fig in *Al-Muᶜtamad* (56). The ordinary fig is *Ficus Carica* L. in the Near East. It is used in al-Kindī A (103b) to eradicate freckles.

444. Gloss: "A kind of swelling."

445. This is the instrument for application of collyria.

446. Gloss: "That is, the part which is the thinnest of the white."

447. *Jashmīzaj* is from the Pers. *chashmīzak,* "a black, shining grain resembling a pippin, with which, when pulverized, they anoint the eyes (Steingass). It is the *Cassia Absus* L. which is *khasamīzaja* in Ar.; *chohsha-makn* and *chasauma* in Pers.; *chakur* in Hind. and Duk.; *chaksoo* in Punj.; *chowan* in Sind. It grows from the Himalayas to Ceylon. Some Arabic writers claim that the seeds strengthen the sight when used as a collyrium.

In India, it is used as an application for sores of the penis. In purulent ophthalmia and conjunctivitis, a grain of the powdered seeds after being baked is introduced beneath the eyelids. The receptacle of the seeds possesses diuretic and stimulant properties (Nadkarni I 282). In modern Iran, it is called *chasm,* in Iraq *ḥab al-sudan, chaksu* seed. *Chaksu* is "eye" in Sans. It is used as a plaster for wounds and sores (Hooper 96).

448. Gloss: "A kind of simple."

449. *Jarab* may also mean "granular conjunctivitis."

450. Gloss: *"Mūm raughan."* A kind of wax and oil mixture.

451. *Bayāḍ.*

452. *Baᶜar al-ḍibb.*

453. *Lū'lū'* is pearl. In al-Kindī A (112a, 130a), unpierced pearl is in a remedy for the gum, tonsils, uvula, and throat. Al-Akfānī (39a) has pearl for the eyes and wounds.

In India today, it is often used as an aphrodisiac. *Cf.* al-Kindī (no. 159).

454. Gloss: "Something resembling a sea-shell."

455. *Qalīmiyā al-dhahab, qalīmiyā al-fiḍa* are scoria of gold, scoria of silver. Ruska *Aristoteles* (138) relates the preparation of gold scoria. *Cf.* also Levey M.A.B. (36). Sometimes, it is spelled *iqlīmiyā*. In al-Kindī A (94a), scoria of gold is in a recipe for scrofula. Cf. al-Kindī (no. 101).

456. *Abār* is lead. It is cognate to the term for lead *abaru* in Akk. The Sum. is *A.BÁR* or *A.GÚG*. *Anaku* in *Akk.* and *AN.NA* were most often tin but sometimes lead. Diosc. (V 96) describes the preparation of burned lead, "One puts it in a crucible or in a large deflagrating spoon. Over it is flung a little sulphur. It is placed in the smith's or jeweller's furnace and one blasts underneath until it is burned (as a sulphide of lead). It is cold in the second degree and desiccating. When used in laving, it desiccates ulcers of the eye and cicatrizes fissures. . . ."

The other burned lead is probably the oxide, the oxidation being carried out in the open air without the addition of any other chemicals.

457. *Sulāq*.

458. Perhaps, "cataract."

459. Gloss: "That is, its drugs should be dry *kuḥl* powders. That means neither drops nor dressings."

Some consider *kuḥl* to be an antimony powder for the eyes. This majority opinion is probably incorrect. *Kuḥl* is most likely simply a dry powder for the eyes; the constituents are uncertain.

460. The word for collyrium in old Arabic does not have the same meaning it is given today. For the ancient physicians, *collyrium* designated a medicament, liquid or solid, to be introduced into natural or accidental openings in the body. Today, the meaning is confined to designate certain remedies for the eyes. *Cf.* P. De Koning, *Traité sur le Calcul dans les Reins et dans la Vessie*, Leyde, 1896, p. 49, note 3; Ḥunain (200–201).

461. *Ithmid* is stibnite, Sb_2S_3. *LIŠ.A.BÁR*. in Sum. is antimony sulphide used in collyria. It is also found in prescriptions for the ears and penis (DAB 116).

The hieroglyphic Egyptian name is *s.d.m.y*. In Coptic, it is *CTHM, stim,* and is found frequently in Egyptian tombs well preserved.

Diosc. (V 94) gives *στίβι* and Galen (XII 236) *στίμμι* as good to cicatrize ulcers in the eyes. It is roasted in coal, removed, and then quenched with the milk of a woman who bore a male child. It is washed as is cadmia, then used.

In India, stibnite in the eighteenth century was brought from Hamadan, Persia. In fact, the Persians call it *surmah ḥāmādānī*. Native Indian practitioners use it as an emetic in intermittent fever, and in collyria with ripe pomegranate (Ainslie I 496 ff.). *Cf.* Ray (137, 151).

Jābir (65) mentions stibnite as an important simple. Al-Ghāfiqī (106) gives the synonym as *kuḥl*. Maim. (27) gives synonyms as *kuḥl al-zurqa* "dark dry collyrium," and *kuḥl isbahānī* "collyrium of Isfahan." The former is found in the Maghrib and the latter in the East.

For use in Syriac medicine (Budge 87, 90), it was prepared for the eyes, for eyelashes which penetrate the eyes, and for eye pain. In Syr., it is *sṭokhōs*, showing a Gr. origin in the Syr. medicine, at least in this case.

IB (18) quotes Galen (XII 236) that stibnite is desiccative and astringent. It is good for the eyes. Aristotle described it as good for this purpose. Ruska's *Alaune* (no. 51) claims that the best *ithmid* comes from Eastern mines; it is more useful for the eyes when mixed with musk. Arabic synonyms are *kuḥl aswad, kuḥl isfahānī, kuḥl kirmānī,* and *sukra*. The Turk. is *surma*.

In Egypt, it is still sold in the bazaars as *kuḥl al-ḥajar, kuḥl sulīmānī,* and *kuḥl jilā* (Ducros 197).

462. *Marqashīthā* is pyrite, especially crystallized marcasite. For etymology, *cf.* al-Kindī (no. 166). Al-Kindī A (126b) has this simple in a remedy for the eyesight. In Levey M.A.B. (24), marcasite is used in an ink recipe.

463. *Rūsakhtaj* is burned copper. It is Pers. for *nuḥās maḥrūq* (IB 1071, 2216, 2217). There are many methods of preparation of this product in the alchemical and technological literature. The Babylonian literature has copper scale (DAB 97). Diosc. (V 76) has burned copper χαλκὸς κεκαυμένος, as being mainly a sulphide. It is used for cicatrizing ulcers, for the eyes, and for vomiting. Dioscorides also discusses the preparation of flowers of copper and copper scales for whose preparation brass is supposed to be used. He distinguished between the two oxides, the red and black. *Cf.* Achundow (325).

464. *Saraṭān baḥrī* is 'sea crab." It is a stone brought from India (IB 1172), or from China coming from the petrified member of a particular species of crab (?). This calcareous petrification from the East is probably not the *ᶜayūn al-saraṭān* used in Egypt today (Maim. 286; Ducros 97). The "sea crab" may also be the burned ash of a crab.

465. *Milḥ Andāranī* is Andāranī or *Dāranī* salt. Cf. Levey M.A.B.

(32), al-Rāzī (MASB 375). The latter gives this salt as a hard salt of two types, one white and one red. In India, it is called *namak Lāhūrī* "Lahore salt." In Iraq, *Andāranī* is called *Tabarzad* (MASB 347). The latter is transparent. In Akk., the *Andāranī* is probably *ṭābat amāni* (DAB 6).

466. *ᶜUrūq ṣufr* is Chelidonium or celandine, *Chelidonium majus* L. Maim. (205) has this confused with *kurkum*. Achundow (235) has *ᶜurūq-i-ṣufr* as a yellow root which has a cleansing effect. It is good for toothache, scabies, and eczema. Loew AP (219) also confuses this simple with *Curcuma longa* L. as does Ducros (90, 91).

467. *Lāzward* is lapis lazuli. This stone was known to the Sumerians (BA 383–385) and Egyptians (*ḫsbd* in Middle Egyptian). In India, in the *Rasakalpa,* it is *rajavarta* (Ray 156). *Lāzward* is described in many Arabic works (Levey M.A.B. 15). It is not found in al-Kindī A.

468. Gloss: "Egyptian ink." For *midad* "ink", *cf* Levey M.A.B. (46).

469. *Kurrāth* is leek, *Allium porrum* L. For etymology, *cf.* al-Kindī (no. 149). In al-Kindī A (97a, 124a), leek is effective for headache and for venereal disease.

In Iran, a few species are used as demulcents and stimulants (Hooper 82).

470. *Zinjār* is most often verdigris. *Cf.* Ḥunain (214–215).

471. *Dahnaj* is malachite. In al-Kindī A (101a), malachite is employed for sores. Achundow (318) has it for boils. IB (966) considers it an antidote. In ancient Babylonia, it was much used for the eyes just as it is today in the Near East.

472. *Zinjarf* is sulphide of mercury or its oxide. *Zinjarf* is related *to zanjafr* which is usually cinnabar.

In Maim. (134), Meyerhof gives a Diosc. (V 94) reference to κιννάβαρι. However, in *Tuḥfa* (147) *zanjafūr* is believed to be the oxide. Under Diosc. (V 99), *psoricum* is considered to be a compound made from vitriol and calamine.

Zinjarf comes from Pers. *shangarf* (Vullers II 471) which is the sulphide of mercury. Cf. Levey M.A.B. (21) for *zanjafr*. In the lapidary of Aristotle (71), it is made from vinegar and copper. Then it is used for sores, leprosy, burns, and fistulas.

473. Gloss: "Which is copper."

474. *Yabruḥ* is mandrake, *Mandragora officinarum* L. *Vide* note 121.

475. Gloss: "That is, pulverized, and two cloths are made of it. The cloths are for the wounds."

476. Gloss: "That is, pulverized fine and cooked until it becomes a porridge."

477. Groats mixed with sour milk and dried in the sun. Also a dough of bulgur and sour milk, cut into small pieces, dried, and used for the preparation of other dishes. There are various methods of preparation.

478. *Rūsakhtaj.*

479. *Dam^ca* is epiphora, weeping discharge. Ḥunain (182–183).

480. Gloss: "We know that the strength of salves remains for six months."

481. *Mardāsanj* is litharge. Litharge was known in ancient Babylonia (DACG 137) and ancient Egypt.

Diosc. (V 87) considers it, λιθάργυρος, good for cicatrization of wounds and for the eyes.

Achundow (275) uses it for perspiration odor, as an astringent, and for cicatrization. Maim. (239) gives the synonym as *martak.* In Pers., *mardāsang* is "impure stone" (Vullers II 1157). The Syr. is *mardĕkā. Martak* is conserved in Sp. as *almartaga. Tuḥfa* (256) gives the synonym as *murtaq.*

Litharge is much used in India today for ulcers, baldness, and the skin (Nadkarni II 86). *Cf.* also Hooper (191) for *murda sang* "death stone," and *Al-Mu^ctamad* (492).

482. *Rātinaj* is the resin of pine, mostly from *Pinus orientalis* Link. A gloss here reads, "Gum of pines." This simple is used for ulcers in al-Kindī A (99b). A resin from the terebinth is prescribed in Egypt today for the chest (Ducros 190).

483. *Qinnah* is galbanum, resin of many species of *Ferula,* especially *F. galbaniflua* Boiss. and Buhse. Achundow (244) has it to drive away the black gall. Galbanum is used by al-Kindī A (91b) for black gall, nerves, and rheumatism.

In Iran and Iraq today, it is used externally for sores and wounds. Internally, it is a stomachic (Hooper 118–119). In Sans., it is called *gaoshira* and *javashira,* used in vaginal and uterine catarrh, in paralytic affections, hysteria, chronic bronchitis, and asthma (Nadkarni I 541).

484. *Qalqaṭār* is perhaps the brownish peroxide of iron, sometimes a product of calcination of impure blue vitriol. *Cf.* Ḥunain (220–221), Levey M.A.B. (16). Although this is not really a vitriol, it is discussed with the vitriols in the latter reference.

485. *Nuḥās maḥrūq.*

486. *Rūsakhtaj.* IB (1071) states that these two are synonyms (I.e., the terms in notes 485 and 486.). "The best is red but the black has little value (IB 2217)." The latter statement is from Diosc. (V 76). According to Dioscorides, burned brass is red and appears like cinnabar. Burned copper is made of ship nails with sulphur or salt, then burned in a pot for days. Alum may be used instead of sulphur

or salt. Other methods of preparation are given by Dioscorides. The difference, if any, betwen the two burned coppers is not known. Al-Muᶜtamad (520) also states that the best is *nuḥās maḥrūq* which is red and equivalent to *rūsakhtaj*.

487. *Nūrah* is quicklime. It is also *naura*. *Tuḥfa* (290) gives this term as a mixture of lime and orpiment for depilation. Levey M.A.B. (10, 39) has this used in bookbinding processes.

488. *Duhn ḥill* is pure, old oil, probably oil of sesame (Ḥunain 214–215).

489. *Sanām al-jamal.*

490. *Bārzad* is galbanum. *Vide* note 483. *Bārzad* is the Pers. name of the resin sold in Cairo bazaars as *qanna-washaq* for fumigation in epilepsy, for asthma, and for applications as unguents for tumors (Ducros 191). In Persia today, *bārījah, bariz, rish-shar,* or *gavshira* (from *gāv* "cow" and *shīr* "milk" alluding to the milky juice of galbanum) is taken as a stomachic. Externally, it is used as a plaster on sores and wounds (Hooper 118–119).

491. *Sandarūs* is sandarach, resin of *Thuya orientalis* L. or *T. articulata* L. *Cf.* Achundow (222). In al-Kindī (no. 232) there are other references.

In India, the Arabs use it for diarrhoea and menorrhagia (Ainslie I 380). It is used for the same purpose in modern Morocco and Egypt. Sandarach is used by al-Kindī G. (13, 14, 64) for perfumery. Sandarach is used in Nafuran ink (Levey M.A.B. 17).

492. *Ḥijr al-Khwārizmī* is an unidentified stone. Khwarizm is a geographic entity in Persia.

493. *Shajarat al-baqq* is the elm tree, *Ulmus campestris* L.

Diosc. (I 84) discusses the elm as good for leprosy, and the bark as a swathing band.

Maim. (91) gives *dirdār,* and the Sp. as *fresno* (ash). The Pers. is *dardār.*

In India, the leaves are used in medicines (Nadkarni I 1254).

In IB (861, 1305), Leclerc states that the tree is called *shajarat al-baqq* "tree of the gnats" because of the tiny flies which develop on it.

494. *Shaqāyiq* or *shaqāyiq al-Nuᶜmān* is anemone, probably *Anemone coronaria* L. Red anemone is used in al-Kindī A (93b) for scrofula and moist ulcers. It is also used in ink manufacture (Levey M.A.B. 17).

Diosc. (II 176) considers it good for the eyes, purging of the head, and leprosy.

In Maim. (359), Meyerhof explains that some scholars believe the name to be of Ar. origin. *Cf.* Loew AP (380), Loew FJ (III 118).

In modern Egypt, anemone is a detersive, good for the eyes, for cicatrization of ulcers, and for leprosy (Ducros 77).

495. *Nūshādir* is sal ammoniac. Al-Kindī A (106b) has this salt in a contracting drug to aid childbirth. It is much used in India today by Tamil practitioners and others as a diuretic and emetic, for female obstructions and enlargements (Ainslie I 365 ff.).

The etymology of *nūshādir* is uncertain.

496. *Qalī* is soda. Levey M.A.B. (9, 10, 24, 43, 44) has it for dyeing of paper, in the preparation of ink, and in the dyeing of leather. *Salicornia fruticosa* L. was most often the plant in ancient and mediaeval times to obtain this ash which was mainly a mixture of sodium and potassium carbonates.

497. *Ushnān* is a soda mixture from the ash of plants. It is made from many species of plants. In al-Kindī A (95b), *ushnān* is in a prescription for haemorrhoids when they appear as papillae. The difference between *qalī* and *ushnān* is undetermined. It is probable that these different ash products come from different plants.

In the Chinese materia medica, soda is *keen, kan,* or *kien,* mined in Mongolia, and used as a purgative and deobstruent. Sometimes, it replaces alum to purify water (Soubeiran 14). Soda is mentioned for glass by Livy (Bailey 191). *Cf.* al-Dīnawarī (41 Ar.).

498. "Killed" because the properties of the mercury are changed according to an ancient Indian process to make the element less reactive. It is no longer mercury, of course, but one of its compounds. *Zībaq* or *zaibaq* is mercury. Al-Kindī A (124a) has mercury introduced into the penis for the dripping of urine, and for calculi.

To kill mercury, it is rubbed with ingredients of the *vida* and roasted in a closed crucible. The ingredients may include vegetable matter, sulphur, and other matter (Al-Rāzī 102–104; Aristotle's lapidary 61; Ray 134). Mercury has many uses in Levey M.A.B. (21, 36, 47).

499. *Shabb* is alum. The Ar. name comes from the root *sh.b.b* "to burn" or "to disinfect." In al-Kindī A (108a), alum of the Yemenite variety is used for toothache. For discussion of alum and its synonyms, *cf.* al-Kindī (no. 240).

In India, alum is used as an astringent by native practitioners for obstinate diarrhoea and diabetes (Ainslie I 13). Alum is used for its detersive properties in the Near East (Ghasānī 257).

500. *Tūbāl al-ḥadid* is scales of iron. Diosc (V 78) states that it, λεπὶς στομώματος, is for washing and for purging. Ḥunain (168, 163, 159) uses iron scales in eye remedies. Scales of iron are drying and useful in cases of malignant ulcers.

Tuḥfa (402) gives *tūbāl* as that which falls from copper, iron and other metals when one forges them. *Tūbāl* is Pers. (Vullers I 476).

IB (438, 1795) quotes ibn Sarāfyūn (ninth century) on the use of copper scales of Cyprus. The scales of metals seem to be of very ancient usage in medicine.

501. Gloss: "It is a stone which is used to rub the foot." *Qisūr* or *qishūr* is *probably* meerschaum (Maim. 141). IB (1721, 1865) gives its equivalent as *fīnak*. It is burned and put in aromatic wine; this is done twice more and then used.

502. *Khushkurīsha* is from Pers. *khushk-resha*.

503. *ᶜAfṣ* is gallnut. Gallnut is used in al-Kindi A (100a) in a remedy for an external fistula. It is used, as it is used today, in inks (Levey M.A.B. 16). Gallnut is to be found used in very early Mesopotamia mainly for tanning (Levey CCTM 79, 162).

504. Gloss: "Yellow of the teeth." This also means "caries."

505. *Qalḥ* Gloss: "Solidified moisture between the teeth."

506. *Masḥūqūniyā* is dross of glass. IB (2129) states that it is for prurigo and itch.

507. *Fīnak.* Vide note 501.

508. *Kazmāzaj* is tamarisk gall. The gall of *thamar al-ṭarfā'* is the gall of *Tamarix gallica* or *T. nilotica* Bge. For etymology, *cf.* al-Kindī (no. 275). In al-Kindī A (113a), tamarisk gall is used for the teeth.

In Egypt today, the tamarisk is used for haemorrhage, dysentery, in ophthalmology, and in dentifrices (Ducros 56).

509. *Ṭarāthīth* or *ṭarāshīt* is the mushroom of Malta, *Cynomorium coccineum* L. This is a plant parasite of the Mediterranean region. Achundow (231, 330) gives this plant as a stomachic, and for palpitation of the heart, and chronic liver difficulties. Maim. (174) gives synonyms as *liḥyat al-taïs* "beard of the male goat," *zubb rubbāḥ* "penis of a monkey," Sp. *fushāla* (*husillo*). IB (1459) quotes al-Rāzī that it is for nasal, uterine, and anal haemorrhage.

510. *Vide* note 465.

511. *Mūbarij* is barberry, *Berberis vulgaris* L. This is a Pers. name, probably equivalent to *amīrbārīs* (Maim. 17). Another Pers. name is *zarashk*. Achundow (142) has it to strengthen the liver and stomach.

Al-Ghāfiqī (15) has Ar. *ᶜud al-rīḥ* and *ambarbārīs* as synonyms. Turk is *qadīn tuzlughy*. The Ber. name for the bark of the root is *ārghīs* (IB 4). *Cf.* Issa (30).

The fruit is an astringent in Egypt for dysentery and inflammatory and bilious fevers (Ducros 32–33). In Persia today, it is used as a decoction for the general health and to sweeten the breath (Hooper 91). The plant grows in India and Iran. In Punj., it is called *zirishk, kashmal*. It is used in present day India for disorders of the bile and urinary passages, for scarlet fever, brain affections, stomach, and leprosy (Chopra 468).

512. *Murrī*. Gloss: "It is made with numerous simples so that its properties are multiple."

513. *Kharnūb* is the Syrian carob or St. John's bread, *Ceratonia siliqua* L. It was originally *kharubu* in Akk.; *ḥarrūb* in Heb.; *ḥarrūbā* in Aram. The tree is native to Palestine (Levey M.A.B. 20). Theoph. (I, 11–13; IV, 2, 4) knew it as κερωνία, and Diosc. (I 114) as κεράτια. *Cf.* also al-Muᶜtamad (119) and Achundow (193). The last two references consider this simple as a strong astringent and good for a prolapsed uterus; it also suppresses mentruation and strengthens the weak stomach. *Nabāt* (307) describes the C. *siliqua* L.

514. *Ḥabb al-rashād* is garden cress, *Lepidium sativum* L.

In Akk., it is probably *saḫlê*, and in Sum *ZAG.ḪI.LI*, neither of which is cognate to *rashād*.

Disoc. (II 155) describes cress, κάρδαμον, as good for the spleen, as an antidote for serpent's poison, falling hair, to suppurate carbuncles, sciatica, and to dissolve oedemata and inflammations.

Maim. (163) gives the synonyms as *ḥurf, al-tufā* (probably *thuffā'*), *ḥabb al-rashād, al-maqalīthā* (from Syr.). Other species are *ḥurf abyaḍ, ḥurf bābilī, ḥurf madanī*. IB (578, 653) gives the Syr. as *muqlayāthā*, quoting abū Ḥanīfa. It is used for the stomach, especially in dysentery, and for scorpion bites. The modern Maghribi is *ḥabb al-rshād,* according to *Tuḥfa* (167). The word *ḥurf* is in the Iraqi dialect (*Tāj al-ᶜarūs* 1/49). *Cf.* abū Ḥanīfa (276).

In India, it is called *chandrasaura* and *ahaleeva* in Sans.; *chansaur, hurf, akalam* in Hind.; *asaliya* in Guj. and Bom.; *ahera* in Sind.; *aditalyu* in Tel.; *alivirai* in Tam. It is grown all over Asia and in much of Europe. The seeds are aperient, diuretic, demulcent, aphrodisiac, galactagogue, and emmenagogue (Nadkarni I 736–738).

In Egypt today, it is used as a diuretic, and externally for ulcerous scrofula (Ducros 72; Loew AP 178, 396, 419; Loew FJ 506 ff.). In Iran, *L. sativum* L. is called *tukhm-i-shāhī* today, and is used as a tonic, aphrodisiac, and diuretic (Hooper 136).

515. As it is, it means "yeast." A gloss reads, however, "*Al-kamīr* meaning sycamore fig."

516. *Maībakhtaj* is concentrated musk. In al-Kindī A (106a), this juice is in a prescription for paroxysmal fever. This simple is prepared by boiling the juice of the grape until only one quarter of it remains (Maim. 84; IB 513). The word is from Pers. *maī-pukhta* "boiled must."

517. Gloss: "That is, *al-madabbar* with jujube and sebesten."

518. The table of contents in the introduction of al-Samarqandī gives the subject of chapter sixteen as sniffing medicines. The latter are included as part of the chapter following.

519. *Shaqāqul* is secacul and others, *Pastinaca Schekakul* Russ.,

Malabaita Secacul Russ., and others. In al-Kindī A (139a), secacul is believed effective as a stomachic, and to increase one's effectiveness in intercourse. For synonyms, *cf.* al-Kindī (no. 246). This simple is noted as good for intercourse in *Al-Muctamad* (268). In the latter, it is listed also as good for the stomach, constriction of the uterus, and for rabies.

520. Gloss: "That is, the top covered."

521. Gloss: "It is said that it is dew which falls on cane, and it is said that it is the sugar taken from cane."

522. Gloss: "That is, sweeten it."

523. Text has *falāfal*. Dozy has *falāfalī*.

524. *Cf.* IB (1519) for *cadas murr*, probably *Sparganium ramosum* L. Al-Ghāfiqī has it as a constituent of a theriac and an antidote. It comes from the Gr. *sparganion*, σπαργάνιον, in Diosc. (IV 21). No etymology is given in Carnoy (249–250). *Sparganium* is a genus of marsh or aquatic herbs.

525. *Tafthia*, is thapsia, *Thapsia garganica* L. Theoph. (IX 9) has thapsia, θαψία, as good for wounds, and when the root is steeped in vinegar good for erysipelas. Diosc. (IV 153) describes thapsia as good for asthma, expectoration, alopecia, leprosy, and other ailments. Carnoy (261) believes that the Gr. word comes from Thapsos, the name of a town in West Sicily; it may, however, be an allusion to the yellow root. IB (440, 2321) has *thāfsiyā* for the Ar., and *adriyās* as the Ber.; it is effective for paralyzed nerves; Galen has it for alopecia. Leclerc has it employed for a plaster used today. According to the *Tuḥfa*, "It is the wild rue, *al-sudhāb al-barrī* which is also mountain rue, *al-sudhāb al-jabalī*." Vide gloss in note 420 above. It is to be found growing in Morocco. The thapsia is not mentioned in *Al-Muctamad*.

526. Gloss: "That is, to be put in a tube and blown."

527. *Al-ḥabba al-sawdā'* is black cumin, *Nigella sativa* L. Maim. (365) gives synonyms as *shūnīz* (Pers., Vullers II 482), *al-shamīth, al-shaibarṭar, al-shashmar, al-kammūn al-aswad*. In Gr., it is μελάνθιον (Diosc. III 79) and in Heb. *qeṣah*. *Cf.* Carnoy (174).

In modern Egypt, it is used as a carminative, emmenagogue, diuretic, and anthelmintic (Ducros 116); in modern Teheran, it is called *tukhm-i-siyāh, siyāh-tukhmah*. In Hind., it is *kala jira, mugrila*. In Iran, it is indigenous. According to the Ar. proverb, "In the black seed is the medicine for everything except death" (Hooper 144).

528. That is, the white and black peppers.

529. *Vide* note 326 above.

530. *Baqla* is Jewish mauve, probably *Corchorus olitorius* L. Maim. (229) has *mulūkhiyā* and *mulūkh* as synonyms. It is "culti-

vated mauve" *al-khubbāzī al-bustānī* or the Jewish legume. The Jewish species was so common that the adjective was often omitted. Serapion (377) and IB (2173) consider *Corchorus* an important drug. It is a mild purgative and better than mauve for gout. The *baqla* plant usually is specified as to the species as in Ḥunain (210–211). The *baqla yamāniyya*, or blite, is also called in Ar. *al-ṣadaḥ*, and in Sp. *blīṭu* (blito). The Syr. is *yarbūzā* giving rise to the names *al-yarbū* and *jarmūz* (Loew FJ I 352 ff.). The blite is the *Albersia Blitum* Kunth. In Gr., it is βλῆτον or βλίτον. *Cf.* Theoph. (VII 1–3) and Diosc. (II 117); the latter claims that the blite has no medicinal virtues. The Berendes edition (216), however, states that it is good for the abdomen even though it is not a drug. IB (318, 2306) quotes Galen and al-Rāzī that it is an edible plant. The *Tuḥfa* (67) and al-Razzāq (145) also give *yarbūz* as a synonym. In the latter, it is given for epilepsy, and for use in fevers and ophthalmia. It also stops thirst (Achundow 160).

531. *Ḥayy al-ᶜalam* is sempervivum, *Sempervivum arboreum* L. Theoph. (VII 15) and Diosc. (IV 88–92) discuss this simple. Diosc. considers houseleek as good for the eyes, dysentery, erysipelas, herpes, and headache.

Maim. (162) says the Gr. is ἀείζωον; Sp. *ubīla rashtaqa*. The Pers. is *hamīsaqūs* (Vullers II 1475). IB (732) quotes Dioscorides and Galen (Bk. VIII). The *Tuḥfa* (187, 277) states that it is *ṣaḥīfat al-mulūk* which is well known in Morocco. It is mentioned in Loew FJ (467). *Cf.* Maim. *Gifte* (102); Loew AP (160, 162). Originally, Pers. is *hamīsha bihār*.

532. *Bāqila* or *bāqilla* is a bean of uncertain species. In al-Kindī A (102a, 117a), the bean is used in a nasal ointment and in a remedy for coughing.

The bean is one of the most staple articles of food in the entire Middle East and North Africa. The medicinal uses of the bean usually follow Galen's ideas in the *De Simpl. Med.* . . . (Kühn 704–775), as for pain of the ear, dysentery, and as a stomachic.

533. *Kibrīt* is sulphur. The Heb. *gophrīth,* Akk. *kibrit* [ilu]*nāri aruqtum* "yellow bank of the river" are cognates. In al-Kindī A (95b) yellow sulphur is used for scabby itch. Ruska (161–162) has it for itch, boils, sores, and chronic fever.

It is still used in Egypt, Iran, and Iraq for skin ailments (Ducros 196; Hooper 193). It was an antidote in early Persia.

534. *Nāranj* is coconut, fruit of *Cocos mucifera* L. Maim. (257) gives the Eastern meaning. It is the *nārijīl* and *rānaj*. In *Tuḥfa* (279), it is the orange from the *Citrus* genus. IB (2203) states that *atwāq* is the milky juice of the nut. Ibn Sīnā calls it *jauz hindī*. *Cf.* Loew AP (118).

In Egypt today, the nut is believed to be an excellent vermifuge and aphrodisiac (Ducros 132).

The Sans. is *tranaraj, sadaphala, narikela*; Hind. *nariyal*; Ben. *narikel*; Guj. *naliar*; Tam. *tengu*; Mal. *ten*. The flower, root, fruit, oil, and ash are used. Coconut milk is aperient, diuretic, and anthelmintic. The oil is used in consumption (Nadkarni I 363 ff.).

In Chinese, it is *ye-chou, tsi-kie, ye-tsü,* and *ye-tsze*. The nut is a styptic. Other products of the tree are used in medicine (Soubeiran 130).

535. Gloss: "That is, composed of grasses and medicines."

535a. *Al nuṭūlāt* are medical fomentations for skin anointing.

536. That is, the more volatile fractions.

537. *Mukhaddirāt* are anaesthetics, drugs, tranquillizers, narcotics.

538. Gloss: "That is, from the oils and milks."

539. *Thūm* is garlic, *Allium sativum* L. For etymology, cf. al-Kindī (no. 276). In al-Kindī A (118a), garlic is used for ear pains, and for its suppuration, pulsation, fistulas. A common synonym is given by Maim. (282) as *saqardiyūn*.

In Iran and Iraq today, garlic is used as a gastric stimulant and to aid digestion (Ducros 60). It is cultivated all over India; there it is used as an antirheumatic, anthelmintic, alterative, and emmenagogue. In Sans., it is *lasuna* or *ugragandha;* Tam. *vellapundu*; Sind. *thum* (Nadkarni I 65).

540. *Lādhan* is ladanum, resin of *Cistus creticus* L., *C. ladaniferus* L, etc.

The Akk. is *ladunu* (DAB 344), and the Heb. *lōṭem*. Diosc. (I 97) has λάδανον. Cf. Achundow (228), Maim. (208), Loew FJ (I 362 ff.), Loew AP (127, 195). According to Maim., it is used as an astringent, antidysenteric, and in the preparation of collyria.

541. Gloss: "That is, the leaf."

Azād-dirakht is azedarach, probably *Melia Azedarach* L. This name is Pers. meaning "free tree" or "noble tree." IB (60) gives a synonym as *ḥar-al-shajar*. Al-Rāzī thought it to be bad for the stomach and nauseating, sometimes fatal. This tree is called the China tree. It is also called "China-berry" and "pride of India." Native to Asia, this tree is common in India and Burma. The tree bears numerous lilac-colored flowers in April and these are succeeded by an abundant crop of yellowish berries.

In India today, the leaves are used as an anthelmintic, antilithic, diuretic, and emmenagogue. Their decoction is astringent and stomachic. In Sans., it is called *mahanimba, himadruma, vraksha,* and *parvatanimba*; Punj. *drek*; Hind. *bakayan*; Tel. *konda-vepa*; Tam. *malaivembu* (Nadkarni I 784).

In China, the fruit is used as a vermifuge, febrifuge, and for urinary troubles. Its nineteenth century synonyms are *tchuen-lien-*

tse, chuen-lien-tsee, xun-lien, ch'uen-lien-tsze, ku-lien-tsze, king-ling-tsze, and *chuen-lien-tszee* (Soubeiran 225).

The bark gives a bitter alkaloid, margosine (Chopra 340 ff.).

542. There seems to be a lacuna following this statement.

543. *Bān* is ben tree or East Indian horseradish tree, probably *Moringa pterygosperma* Gaertn., and *M. aptera* Gaertn. The oil of the nut is frequently found in medical texts. In al-Kindī A (123a), ben nut is used in a recipe to make the hair of the head and beard grow.

In Sans., it is *murungi* with cognates in Tam., Tel., and Sinh. It grows in India and Burma. In Yunani medicine, it is a laxative and antispasmodic, and in the *Ayurveda*, an emmenagogue and aphrodisiac (Nadkarni I 811 ff.).

544. *Khaṭr* is indigo leaf, probably of *Indigofera tinctoria* L. or *Isatis tinctoria* L. It is used much in dyeing as in the manufacture of inks (Levey M.A.B. *passim*).

Under *wasma,* Maim. (126) gives *al-khaṭr* as the leaves of indigo, *al-nīlaj.* "It is *ᶜizlum.* The people of Egypt call it *al-nīl. . . .*"

It was known in ancient Babylonia (DAB 171–172) and to the Greeks (Diosc. II 184). It is common in India. The *I. tinctoria* L. is known in Sans. as *neela* and *nilika.* It grows in northern and southern India. In Ayurvedic medicine, its root is used as an antidote, in colic, and gonorrhoea; the leaves are for jaundice, gout, and fever. In Yunani medicine, it is a haemostatic, sedative, and used for ulcers (Nadkarni I 680–682).

Isatis tinctoria L. was used for a time as a dye substitute for indigo. It grows in Asia, Europe, and North Africa. In China, it is *lan-ts'ai,* and is considered to be very nourishing but used mainly as a dye (Soubeiran 219) Woad is given by Dioscorides and not indigo. The two plants are discussed here together since they were so often indistinguishable to pharmacists.

Gloss: "*Khaṭr* and *wasma* both are "indigo leaf."

545. Gloss: "Two *raṭls.*"

546. *Zāj aḥmar* is "red vitriol" an oxide of iron. In Akk., red vitriol, sesquioxide of iron is *urisḫu,iaraḫu,* and Sum. *ZA.SUḪ.-DIR.TU.* It is colcothar (DAB 97–98), a reddish brown substance left as a residue when ferrous sulphate is highly heated. *Cf.* Levey M.A.B. (16). It may also be a mixture of oxides of iron.

547. The vocalization is uncertain.

Gloss: "*Al-barghand* is the fruit of the pistachio tree. One year it bears pistachio and another year something other than pistachio."

548. In the Leiden MS, the final sentence reads," *The Book of the Principles of Compounding* was completed at the beginning of the month of *Rabiᶜ al-Akhīr* of the year 716 in the city of Sandwar which He guarded from misfortune and protected from evil.

Arabic-English Glossary

burned lead	ابار محرق
savin, juniper, and others	ابهل
citron	اترج
stibnite	اثمد
plum	اجاص
intestines	احشاء
urinary incontinence	ادرار
boils	ادمال
balms	ادهان
hair medicines	ادوية الشعر
collyria	ادوية العين
diuretics	ادوية مدرة للبول
lemon-grass	اذخر
rice	ارز
China-tree	ازادراخت
myrtle	آس
wild ginger	اسارون
istār	استار

atonicity; atonicity or loosening of gums	استرخاء؛ استرخاء اللثات
dropsy	استسقاء زقي
lavender	اسطوخودوس
spinach	اسفاناخ
sponge	اسفنج
ceruse	اسفيداج
a Persian food mixture	اسفيدبا
diarrhoea	اسهال
asphodel [root]	اشراس
gum ammoniac	اشق
soda	اشنان
lichen	اشنة
myrobalan confections	اطريفلات
embrocations	اطلية
dodder	افتيمون
wormwood	افسنتين
opium	افيون
acacia	اقاقيا
feverfew	اقحوان
medical formularies	اقراباذينات
lozenges	اقراص
melilot	اكليل الملك
emblic myrobalan	املج
barberry	انبرباريس
swollen conditions	انتفاخ
anise	انيسون
fīqrā aperient	ايارج
lūghāzīyā aperient	ايارج لوغاذيا
iris	ايرسا
camomile	بابونج
mountain-balm	بادرنجبوية
galbanum	بارزد
bean	باقلى
pustules	بثور

decoction (?)	بختج
fumigants	بخورات
mountain-balm	بدرنجبوية
barghand (?), probably a mythical fruit	برغند
coolants	برودات
asphodel	بروق
fleawort	بزر قطونا
mace	بسباس
common polypody	بسبايج
coral	بسد
clay vessel	بستوقة
dates about to ripen	بسر
onion	بصل
terebinth	بطم
abdomen	بطن
watermelon	بطيخ
Indian watermelon	بطيخ هندى
lizard dung	بعر الضبّ
broad bean	بقلة
blite	بقلة يمانية
balsam	بلسان
phlegm	بلغم
acorn	بلّوط
belleric myrobalan	بليلج
henbane	بنج
filbert	بندق
violet	بنفسج
Isfahan violet	بنفسج اصفهانى
haemorrhoids	بواسير
bauraq, a borate or carbonate mixture	بورق
orchis	بوزيدان
an eye remedy from Dar-band, Persia	بوش
leucoma	بياض
egg white	بياض البيض

maiden hair	برسياوشان
"wild onion"	بيازعصل
thapsia	تافشيا
dissolution [of a tumor]	تحليل
earth, emetic earth	تراب
turpeth	تربد
lupine	ترمس
balm-mint	ترنجان
manna	ترنجبين
filtration	تصفية
apple	تفّاح
tamarind	تمر الهندى
smoothing [of the chest]	تمليس
borax	تنكار
scales of iron	توبال الحديد
tutty	توتيا
fig	تين
red fig	تين الحنط
foeces	ثقل
heaviness of eyelids	ثقل الجفان
gallnut	ثمرة الطرفاء
garlic	ثوم
common millet	جاورس
pig skin	جرادة الاديم
scab, mange	جرب
to peel	جرش
carrot	جزرية
a Persian grain which resembles a pippin	جشميزج
clearing [of the chest]	جلاء
rose water	جلاب
sesame	جلجلان
pomegranate flower	جلنار
castoreum	جند بيدستر
Greek gentian	جنطيان الرومى

stomachic confections	جوارشنات
opopanax	جواشير
nutmeg	جوز بوّا
thyme	حاشا
seed	حبّ
garden cress	حبّ الرشاد
pine cone	حبّ الصنوبر
cherry	حبّ الملوك
to coagulate	حبس
black cumin	حبّة سوداء
pills	حبوبات
"stone of Khwarizm"	حجر الخوارزمي
harmel	حرمل
water-caltrop	حسك
verjuice	حصرم
lycium	حضض
cavity	حفرة
clysters	حقن
fenugreek	حلبة
sorrel	حمّاض
compound fevers	حميات مركبة
henna	حنّاء
semolina	حنطة
colocynth	حنظل
sempervivum	حيّ العالم
mallow	خبّازي
scoria of iron	خبث الحديد
abscesses	خراجات
white hellebore	خربق الابيض
mustard	خردل
gigantic swallowwort	خرك
tamarisk gallnut	خرمانج
carob, St. John's bread	خرنوب
Nabataean carob	خرنوب نبطي

bat excrement	خرو الخطاطيف
mouse excrement	خرو الفار
castor oil plant	خروع
green polishing clay	خزف الجرار الخضر
lettuce	خسّ
poppy	خشخاش
dry scab	خشكريشة
testicle	خصية
spurge laurel	خضراء
indigo leaf	خطر
marshmallow	خطمى
palpitation	خفقان
vinegar	خلّ
cure	خلاص
Egyptian willow	خلاف
dislocation	خلع
wine	خمر
yeast	خمير
peach	خوخ
galingale	خولنجان
purging cassia	خيار شنبر
cucumber and musk melon mixture	خيارين
lesser cardamom	خير بوّا
yellow gillyflower	خيرى
falling out of the hair	داء الثعلب
Chinese cinnamon	دار صينى
long pepper	دار فلفل
hospital	دار مرضى
Darānī salt	ملح درانى
dragon's blood plant	دم الاخوين
menstruum	دم الطمث
brains	دماغ
epiphora	دمعة
ben nut oil	دهن البان

oil of *bakhtaj* [perhaps a kind of decoction] دهن البختج
pure oil دهن حلّ
olive oil دهن الزيت
malachite دهنج
wild carrot دوقو
sorghum ذرة
aromatic powders ذرورات
pine resin راتينج
fennel رازيانج
elecampane راسن
a musk perfume with other aromatics رامك
licorice rob رب السوس
asthma ربو
robs ربوبات
wombs رحام
spoiling, deterioration رحيلة
a sourmilk recipe, a kind of whey رخبين
burned lead رصاص محرق
Mafura of Yemen, nux vomica رقع
ashes رماد
pomegranate رمّان
ophthalmia رمد
gravel and stones [in the kidneys and bladder] رمل والحجارة
burned copper روسختج
Ribes ريباس
grand basil ريحان
lung رئة
rhubarb ريوند
red vitriol زاج احمر
jelly-fish, and others زبد البحر
raisins زبيب
dysentery زحير
long Aristolochia زراوند طويل
arsenic زرنيخ

red arsenic	زرنيخ احمر
azarole	زعرور
saffron	زعفران
pitch	زفت
jasmine	زنبق
verdigris	زنجار
ginger	زنجبيل
red lead, vermilion	زنجفر
hyssop	زوفا
mercury	زيبق
broth meat	زيربا
malabathrum	سادج
Indian malabathrum	سادج هندى
haematite	ساذنج
sebesten	سبستان
irritation of the intestines	سحج
to pulverize	سحق
rue	سداب
Christ's thorn	سدر
sardārūj	سرداروج
vertigo	سرسام
cancer	سرطان
"sea crab" [probably a stone]	سرطان بحرى
orache	سرمق
cypress	سرو
thyme, origan, and others	سعتر
sweet cyperus	سعد
sniffing remedies	سعوطات
quince	سفرجل
drug powders	سفوفات
scammony	سقمونيا
sukk	سك
sagapenum	سكبينج
apoplexy	سكتة

sugar	سكر
red sugar	سكر احمر
crystalline sugar	سكر طبرزد
oxymel	سكنجبين
malabathrum oxymel	سكنجبين ساذج
lippitudo of eyelids	سلاق
beet	سلق
cinnamon	سليخة
sumach	سمّاق
fish	سمك
ṭarīkh fish	سمك طريخ
butter	سمن
senna	سنا
camel's hump [fat]	سنام الجمل
nard	سنبل
Indian nard	سنبل الطيب
sandarac	سندروس
dentifrices	سنونات
a kind of wine made from pomegranate seed	سويق
black bile	سوداء
colchicum	سورنجان
lily	سوسن
blue lily	سوسن آسمانجونى
flowing of blood	سيلان الدم
mandrake fruit	شابيزج
haematite	شاذنج
fumitory	شاهترج
hemp	شهدانج
bush basil	شاهسفرم
bush basil	شاهسفرغم
alum	شبّ
aneth	شبث
elm tree	شجرة البقّ
fat, pulp	شحم

duck fat	شحم البطّ
chicken fat	شحم الدجاج
glazed eyes, bulging eyes	شخوص
belleric myrobalan soaked in milk	شراملج
syrup, dose	شربة
siracost	شرخست
barley	شعير
secacul	شقاقل
anemone	شقايق
red anemone	شقايق النعمان
wax	شمع
odorants	شمومات
shell for glazing	شنج
black cumin	شونيز
suppositories, collyria	شيافات
wormwood	شيح
siracost	شير خشت
belleric myrobalan soaked in milk	شيراملج
shīramaraj(?), perhaps *shīramalaj*	شيرمرج
leadwort	شيطرج
soap	صابون
aloe	صبر
headaches, hemicrany	صداع
chest	صدر
shell	صدف
pus	صديد
migraine	صرع
yellow bile	صفراء
yolk of an egg	صفرة البيض
to filter	صفى
gum arabic	صمغ
gum arabic	صمغ عربي
practise [of medicine]	صناعة
sandalwood	صندل

pine	صنوبر
chinaware	صينيات
dressing	ضمادة
tabasheer	طباشير
decoctions	طبوخات
spleen	طحال
cynomorium	طراثيث
cynomorium	طراثيث
tarragon	طرخون
1/24 of a dirham	طسوج
pterygium, perhaps cataract	ظفرة
embrocation	طلاء
menstruation	طمث
Armenian bole	طين ارمني
Isfahan clay	طين الاكل
potter's clay	طين حرّ
sealing clay	طين مختوم
pips of raisins	عجم الزبيب
electuaries	عجونات
lentil	عدس
Sparganium	عدس مرّ
sow bread, cyclamen	عرطنيثا
chelidonium	عروق صفر
honey	عسل
knotweed	عصا الراعي
extract	عصارة
to squeeze out juice	عصر
nervous organs	عضاء العصبية
sternutative	عطوس
gallnut	عفص
pellitory	عقار قرحا
jujube	عنّاب
black nightshade	عنب الثعلب
ambergris	عنبر

sarcocol	عنزروت
squill	عنصل
Indian aloeswood	عود هندى
cūdnī, an aloe or aloe mixture(?)	عودنى
laurel	غار
agaric	غاريقون
agrimony	غافت
service tree	غبيراء
gargles	غراغر
viscous	غرى
epilepsy	فالج
sugar candy	فانيد
pods	فاوس
radish	فجلية
pessaries	فرازج
euphorbium	فربيون
white mulberry	فرصاد
purslane	فرفخ
euphorbium	فرفيون
Barāniyye pistachio	فستق برانى
parsley	فطراساليون
agnus castus	فقد
pepper	فلفل
white pepper	فلفل ابيض
black pepper	فلفل اسود
basil	فلنجمشك
fanjinosh	فنجنوش
mint	فوتنج
mountain mint	فوتنج جبلى
areca nut	فوفل
madder	فوّة
meerschaum	فهنك
cardamom	قاقلة
constipation	قبضة

cucumber	قثّاء
medical formulary	قراباذين
carat	قراط
medical formulary	قرباذين
ulcer	قرحة
bastard cumin	قردمان
paper	قرطاس
carthamus	قرطم
Egyptian mimosa	قرظ
pumpkin	قرع
pustules	قرع
cinnamon	قرفة
clove	قرنفل
wounds	قروح
costus	قسط
currant	قشمش
[sugar] cane	قصب
trachea	قصبة
tar	قطران
cotton	قطن
heart	قلب
tartar	قلح
yellow vitriol	قلقطار
soda	قلى
scoria of gold	قليميا الذهب
scoria of silver	قليميا الفضة
stomachic powders	قمايح
a legume resembling spinach (?)	قنّابرى
kamala	قنبيل
centaury	قنطوريون
galbanum	قنّة
binders, constipators	قوابض
colic	قولنج
colon	قولون

a cerate or salve	قيروطي
meerschaum (?), a sandstone	قيسور
southernwood	قيصوم
camphor	كافور
alkekenji	كاكنج
cubeb	كبابة
liver	كبد
caper	كبر
sulfur	كبريت
flax	كتان
gum tragacanth	كثيراء
antimony powders	كحال
leek	كراث
bitter vetch	كرسنة
celery	كرفس
cabbage	كرنب
vines	كروم
caraway	كرويا
coriander	كزبرة
tamarisk gall	كزمازج
fracture	كسر
gruel mixture	كشك
dodder	كشوث
biscuit made without milk or butter	كعك
cataplasms	كمادات
pear	كمثرى
Chinese pear	كمثرى صينى
cumin	كمون
sycamore fig (?)	كميز
frankincense	كندر
struthion	كندس
struthion	كندش
emetic resin	كنكرزد
yellow amber	كهربا

vinegar infusion	كوامخ
chyme	كيموس
ladanum	لاذن
lapis lazuli	لازورد
ivy	لبلاب
milk	لبن
storax	لبنى
colchicum	لحلاح
to cicatrize	لحم
borage	لسان الثور
plaintain	لسان الحمل
salivas	لعابات
lohochs	لعقوت
mandrake	لفّاح
turnip	لفت
distortion of the mouth	لقوة
to vomit	لقى
lukk	لكّ
kidney bean	لوبيا احمر
almond	لوز
pearl	لؤلؤ
lemon	ليمو
loose bowels	لين الطبع
cheese water	ماء الجبن
rose water	ماء ورد
humor	مادة
mezereon	مازريون
mung bean	ماش
softeners	ملينة
horned poppy	ماميثا
celandine	ماميران
cocculus	ماهيزهرج
file	مبرد
bladder	مثانة

mithqāl	مثقال
sealing [clay]	مختوم
narcotics	مخدّرات
ink	مداد
diuresis	مدرّة
myrrh	مرّ
Meccan myrrh	مرّ مكي
gall of a cow	مرارة البقر
gall of birds	مرارة الطيور
poultices	مراهم
confections	مربيات
litharge	مرداسنج
marjoram	مرزنجوش
marcasite	مرقشيثا
Egyptian origan	مرماحوز
Egyptian origan	مرو
garum	مرّي
sour-sweet	مزّ
smoothers	مزلقات
dross of glass	مسحقونيا
musk	مسك
dittany	مشكطرا مشير
apricot	مشمش
mastix	مصطكي
filter	مصفاة
ingredients	مصلحات
decoction	مطبوخ
stomach	معدة
electuaries	معاجين
joints	مفاصل
heart strengtheners	مفرحات
simples	مفردات
rectum, anus	مقرّ
false bdellium	مقل

garden cress	مقليتا
vomitive	مقى
dough salt	ملح العجين
Andarānī salt, Darānī salt	ملح اندرنى
nafṭī salt	ملح نفطى
Indian salt	ملح هندى
gentlers	ملطفات
cultivated mauve	ملوخيا
manna	منّا
sieve	منخل
barberry	موزج
concentrated must	ميبختج
mīzumiraj	ميزمرج
storax	ميعة
nard	ناردين
azarole	نارسنجد
ironwood tree	نارمشك
coconut	نارنج
treacle	ناطف
a kind of whey (?)	ناطفا
royal cumin	نانخواة
Christ's thorn	نبق
sweet wine	نبيذ حلو
copper	نحاس
bran	نخالة
narcissus	نرجس
rheums	نزلات
a cold, catarrh	نزلة
sciatic nerve	نسا
prescription, recipe	نسخ
eglantine	نسرين
starch	نشا
natron	نطرون
bath aromatics	نطولات

breathing	نفس
nafṭ	نفط
diminution of semen	نقصان الباه
infusions	نقوعات
medlar	نلك
serpolet, wild thyme	نمّام
fistulas	نواصير
quicklime	نورة
sal ammoniac	نوشادر
indigo	نيل
nenuphar	نيلوفر
chebulic myrobalan	هليلج كابلى
endive	هندباء
diarrhoea	هيضة
small cardamom	هيل
to bruise	وثى
sweet flag	وج
rose	ورد
chemosis, swelling	وردينج
hip	ورك
indigo leaf	وسمة
jasmine	ياسمين
mandrake	يبرح

Abbreviations and Selected Bibliography

Abdāl. Māsarjawaih's *Fī abdāl al-adwiya wamā yaqūm maqam ghairihā minhā.* MS Aya Sofya 4838.

Achundow. Achundow, A. C., *Die pharmakologischen Grundsaetze (Liber fundamentorum pharmacologiae) des Abu Mansur Muwaffak bin Ali Harawi. Hist. Stud. aus dem pharmak. Inst. d. Kais. Univ. Dorpat,* vol. 3, Halle, 1893.

Ainslie. Ainslie, W., *Indian Materia Medica,* London, 1826, 2 vols.

ᶜAjil. M. Sadr al-Din, *Risālat shifā' ᶜājil.* MS Yale Z105 Ar./3.

al-Akfānī. Al-Akfānī's (d. 1348) *Kashf al-rain fī aḥwāl al-ᶜain* MS Ahmet III 1968.

ᶜAbd al-Salām b. M. al-ᶜAlamī. *Ḏiyā al-nibrās fī hall mufradat al-Anṭākī bi lughat Fās,* Fés, 1318 H.

Anawati, G. C. *Tarīkh al-saidalah wa'l-ᶜaqāqīr,* Cairo, 1959.

Anonymous. *Ḥudud al-ᶜalam,* translated by V. Minorsky, London, 1937.

al-Anṭākī. Dā'ūd al-Anṭākī, *Tadhkirat uli al-albāb wa'l-jāmi*ᶜ *li'l-*ᶜ*ajab al-*ᶜ*ujāb,* Le Caire, 1281 H.

Aristotle or Aristotle's lapidary, Ruska J., ed. *Das Steinbuch des Aristoteles.* Heidelberg, 1912 (A mediaeval work attributed to Aristotle).

Asher ben Jehiel (1250?–1328). *Orḥot ḥayyim,* Fürth, 1791.

ᶜAwwām. Abū Zakarīyā Yaḥyā ibn al-ᶜAwwām al-Ishbīlī (end of 12th century) *Kitāb al-filaḥa.* Clement-Mullet, J.-J., translator, Paris, 1864–1867.

Ibr. b. ᶜAr. b. a. Bakr al-Azraqī (after 1412), *Tashīl al-manafi*ᶜ *fī al-ṭibb wa'l-ḥikam,* Cairo, 1947.

BA. Meissner, B., *Babylonien und Assyrien.* Heidelberg, 1925, vol. 2.

ibn Bādīs. Ibn Bādīs, ᶜ*Umdat al-kuttāb wa*ᶜ*uddat* dhawi'l-albāb. MS Univ. of Chicago A 12060.

Bailey, L. H., *The Standard Cyclopedia of Horticulture,* 3 vols., New York, 1950.

Bartholomae, C., *Altiranisches Wörterbuch,* Berlin, 1961.

Bayān. Abu'l-Faḍl Dā'ūd b. a. al-Bayān al-Isrā'īlī, *Al-dustūr al-bīmāristānī* (*fi'l-adwiyah al-murakkabah*). MS Sbath, text published in Cairo, 1933.

Berendes, J., trans., *Des Pedanios Dioskurides aus Anazarbos Arzneimittellehre in fuenf Buechern.* Stuttgart, 1902.

Bik. Yunus b. Isḥāq b. Biklārish al-Isrā'īlī, *Al-musta*ᶜ*īnī fī al-muqradāt al-ṭibbiyah.* MS Lugduno-Batava, Cod. Or. 15.

al-Bīrūnī. Abū al-Raiḥān al-Bīrūnī, *Kitāb al-saidana.* MS Brussa 149.

al-Biṭrīq. Al-Biṭrīq b. Yuḥannā b. al-Biṭrīq, *Kitāb al-sumūm.* MS Aya Sofya 3724.

Boissier, B., *Flora orientalis.* Paris, 1882.

Boerhaave, H., *Historia plantarum*. Rom, 1727.

Boerhaave, H., *Tractatus de viribus medicamentorum*. Paris, 1726.

Bretschneider, B. V., Botanicon sinicum. Notes on Chinese botany from native and western sources. *Journ. Asiat. Soc. of Great Brit. and Ireland, North China Branch,* 1882, vol. 16, pt. 1, 18–230; 1891, vol. 25, parts 1 and 2, 1–1468; vol. 29, pt. 3, 1–623.

Brockelmann, C., *Lexicon Syriacum*. Halis Saxonum, 1928.

Bryson. *Der OIKONOMIKOC des Neupythagoreers 'Bryson' und sein Einflusz auf die islamische Wissenschaft,* ed., transl. by Martin Plessner, Heidelberg, 1928.

Budge. Budge, E. A. W., *The Syriac Book of Medicine,* London, 1913.

Carnoy. Carnoy, A. *Dictionnaire étymologique des noms grecs de plantes.* Louvain, 1959.

Celsus, A. C., *Traité de medecine* de A. C. Celse, Paris, 1876; *De re medica libr. VIII*. Basel, 1905.

Colin, C., *Abderrezzāq el-Jezāiri un medecin arabe du XIIe S. Heg.* Montpellier, 1905.

Colin, G., *Avenzoar sa vie et ses oeuvres.* Paris, 1911.

DAB. Thompson, R. C., *A dictionary of Assyrian botany*. London, 1949.

DACG. Thompson, R. C., A dictionary of Assyrian chemistry. Oxford, 1936.

al-Damīrī. Kamāl al-Dīn al-Damīrī, *Kitāb ḥayāt al-hayawān al-kubra.* Le Caire, 1309 H.

de Candolle, Al. P., *Distribution géographique des plantes alimentaires.* Genf, 1936.

Idem. Géographie botanique raisonnée. Paris, 1855.

Idem. Origine des plantes cultivées. Paris, 1883.

Idem. Essai sur les propriétés médicales des plantes comparées avec leur forme extérieure et leur classification naturelle. Paris, 1804.

Dickson, J. H., *The fibre plants of India, Africa, and our colonies.* Dublin, 1865.

Dietrich, A., *Zum Drogenhandel im islamischen Aegypten.* Heidelberg, 1954.

Dillmann, A., *Lexicon linguae aethiopicae cum indice latino.* Lipsiae, 1865.

al-Dīnawarī. Lewin, B., ed. *The book of plants of Abū Ḥanīfa Dīnawarī.* Uppsala, Wiesbaden, 1953 (Alīf to zā only).

Diosc. Wellmann, M., ed. *Pedanii Dioscuridis Anazarbei de materia medica.* Berolini, 1907–1914.

Dozy. Dozy, R., *Supplément aux dictionnaires arabes,* Leyde, 1881.

Dubler, D. E., *La 'Materia Medica' de Dioscórides,* Barcelona, 1953–1959.

Ducros. Ducros, M. A. H., Essai sur le droguier populaire arabe de l'inspectorat des pharmacies du Caire, *Mém. prés. á l'Inst. d'Égypte,* vol. 15, Cairo, 1930.

Dunlop, D. M., Arabic Medicine in England, *Journ. Hist. Med.* 11, 166–182 (1956).

Dymock, Wm., *The vegetable materia medica of western India.* London, 1883.

Ebeling, E., Parfümrezepte und kultische Texte aus Assur, *Orientalia* 17, 129–143, 299–313 (1948); 18, 404–418 (1949); 19, 265–278 (1950).

Ebstein, W., *Die Medizin im alten Testament.* Stuttgart, 1901.

Elgood, C., *A Medical History of Persia and the Eastern Caliphate.* Cambridge, 1951.

Idem,Tibb-ul-Nabbi [*of al-Suyuti*] *or Medicine of the Prophet, Osiris* 14, 33 ff. (1962).

Engler, A., *Die pflanzenwelt Afrikas.* . . . Leipzig, 1908–1925.

Idem, Die natürlichen Pflanzenfamilien nebst ihren Gattungen. . . . Leipzig, 1924.

Farès, B., *Le livre de la thériaque,* Le Caire, 1953.

al-Fāriqī, Aḥmad b. Yūsuf, *Tārīkh al-Fāriqī.* Cairo, 1959.

al-Fasi, M., *Al-ṭibb al-aṭbā' bi'l-maghrib,* Rabat, 1959.

Fihrist. Ibn al-Nadim's *Fihrist,* G. Flügel, ed., Leipzig, 1871–1872.

Fonahn, A., *Janus* **14**, 347–353 (1909).

Forskal, P., *Flora Aegyptiaco-Arabica sine descriptiones plantarum.* Hauniae, 1775.

Freytag. Freytag, G. W., *Lexicon arabico-latinum.* Halle, 1830–1837.

GAL. Brockelmann, C., *Gesch. d. arab. Literatur.* Leiden, 1943, 1949; Supplement [S], 1937, 1938, 1942.

Galdston, I., *Bull New York Acad. Med.* **13**, 512–538 (1937).

Galen. Kühn, W., ed. *Claudii Galeni opera omnia.* Leipzig, 1821–1833.

Gesner, K., *Thesaurus de remediis secretis liber physicus, medicus, et partim chymicus.* Tigur, 1552.

al-Ghāfiqī. Meyerhof, M. and G. P. Sobhy, eds. *The abridged version of "The Book of Simple Drugs" of . . . al-Ghāfiqī.* Cairo, 1932–1938 (incomplete).

Ghasānī, Y. (694H.), *Al-muᶜtamad fī al-adwiyah al-mufradah.* Cairo, 1951.

Grapow. Grapow, H. *et al, Grund. d. Med. d. alten Aegypter.* Berlin, 1954 ff.

Grohman, A., *Arabic Papyri in the Egyptian Library.* Cairo, 1934–1962.

Gstirner. Gstirner, F., *Handbuch d. Galenischen Pharmazie.* Berlin, 1936.

Gunther, R. T., *The Greek Herbal of Dioscorides.* New York, 1959.

Ḥāfiz . . . al-Dhahabī, *Al ṭibb al-nabawī.* Cairo, 1961.

Hamarneh, S. K., *Some pharmaceutical aspects of al-*

Zahrawi's al-Tasreef (ca. 1000). Univ. of Wisconsin thesis, Madison, 1959.

al-Hamdānī, Kitab al-iklīl. vol. 8, Baghdad, 1931.

Hance, H. F., *Adversaria in stirpes imprimis Asiae orientalis criticas minusve notas, interjectis novarum plurimarum diagnosibus.* Paris, 1866.

Hessler, A. F., *Susruta. . . .* Erlangen, 1852–1855.

Heyd, W., *Histoire du Commerce du Levant au Moyen-Age.* Leipzig, 1885–1886.

Hippocrates. Fuchs, R. German translation, *Hippocrates, sämmtliche Werke.* München, 1895–1900.

Hoernle, A. F. R., *Susruta. . . .* Calcutta, 1897.

Holmyard, E. J., *Kitāb al-kanz al-afkhar wa-al-sirr al-aᶜẕam fī tasrīf al-mukarram.* Paris, 1923.

Idem. The Arabic Works of Jābir ibn Ḥayyān. Paris, 1928.

Idem and D. C. Mandeville, *Avicenna's de congelatione et conglutinatione lapidum. Sections of the Kitāb al-shifā'.* Paris, 1927.

Hooper, D., *Introduction to materia medica for India.* London, 1901.

Hooper. Hooper, D. and H. Field, *Useful plants and drugs of Iran and Iraq.* Chicago, 1937.

Hort, A., *Theophrastus' enquiry into plants.* London, 1916.

ibn Hubal al-Baghdādī, *Kitāb al-mukhtārāt fī al-ṭibb.* Hyderabad, 1362–4 H.

Ḥunain. Meyerhof, Max, *The book of the ten treatises on the eye ascribed to Hunain ibn Ishaq* (809–877 A.D.). Cairo, 1928.

Ḥunain A. Hunain ibn Ishaq, transl (author unknown). *Fī abdāl* al-adwiyah al-mufradah. MS Aya Sofya 4838.

Hyrtl, J., *Das Arabische und Hebräische in der Anatomie*. Wien, 1879.

IB. *Vide* Leclerc.

al-Idrīsī. M. al-Idrīsī, *Kitāb al-jāmi^{c} li-ṣifāt ashtāt al-nabāt*. MS Fatih 3610.

Muḥammad al-Idrīsī, *Maghrib, sūdān, miṣr, wa-al-andalus*. Dozy, R. and M. J. de Goeje, eds., Leyde, 1866.

Ishbīlī, *Kitāb al-falāḥa*. Hyderabad, 1926, 1932.

Isḥāq b. S. al-Isrā'īlī (fl. 905 A.D.). *Kitāb al-Ḥummayāt*. MS Leiden, 1305.

Issa. Ahmed Issa Bey, *Dictionnaire des noms des plantes en latin, francais, anglais, et arabe*. Le Caire, 1930.

IAU. Ibn abī Uṣaibi^{c}a, *^{c}Uyūn al-anbā' fī ṭabaqāt al-aṭibbā'*. ed. A. Mueller, Le Caire, 1882.

Jahier, H. and A. Noureddine, *Kitāb khalq al-janīn wa-tadbīr al-h'abālā wa'l-mawlūdīn*. Alger, 1956.

Jābir. Siggel, A., ed., *Das Buch der Gifte des Gābir ibn Ḥayyān*. Wiesbaden, 1958.

^{c}Abd al-Raḥīm b. ^{c}Umar al-Dimashqī al-Jaubarī, *Kitāb al mukhtār fī kashf al-asrār wa-hatk al-astār*. Cairo, 1908.

ibn Jazla. Yaḥyā ibn ^{c}Isā, *Taqwīm al-abdān* (in Pers.) MS Yale z105 Ar./6.

al-Jazzār, abū Ja^{c}far . . . , *Kitāb ṭibb al-fuqarā' wa'l-masākīn*. MS Gotha 2054.

Idem. Kitāb i^{c}timad al-adwiya al-mufrada, MS Aya Sofya 3564.

al-Jildakī. Aidamir b. ^{c}Alī al-Jildakī, *Nihāyat al-ṭalab fī sharḥ al-muktasab fī zirā^{c}at al-dhahab*. MS Berlin 4184.

Joret, C., *La flore de l'Inde*. . . . Paris, 1901.

Idem. Les plantes dans l'antiquité et au moyen âge. . . . Paris, 1897, 1904.

JRAS. *Journ. of the Royal Asiatic Society*.

Kahle, P., *Opera Minora*, Leiden, 1956.

de Karabacek, J. *et al, De codicis Dioscuridei Aniciae*

Iulianae, nunc Vindobonensis Med. Gr. I, Lugduni Batavorum, 1906.

Katzenellenbogen, L., *Ein altfranzösische Abhandlung über Fieber.* Würzburg, 1933.

Kaviratna, K. A. C. *Charaka samhita.* Calcutta (1890) 1925.

ibn Khaldūn, *The Muqaddimah,* translated by F. Rosenthal, New York, 1958. Ar. text used, Beirut, 1900.

ibn Khallikān, *Kitāb wafayāt al-a^cyān ilkh.* Cairo, 1299 H.

al-Kindī. *The 'Aqrābādhīn' or Medical Formulary of al-Kindī with a Study of its Materia Medica* by Martin Levey, Madison, 1966.

al-Kindī A. *Aqrābādhīn* of al-Kindī. MS in Aya Sofya 3603.

al-Kindī G. al-Kindī's *Kitāb kīmiyā' al-^ciṭr wat-taṣ^cīdāt,* ed. and transl. by K. Garbers. Leipzig, 1948.

de Koning, R., *Traité sur la calcul dans les reins et dans la vessie* par . . . al-Rāzī. Leyde. 1896.

Idem. Trois traités d'anatomie arabes par . . . al-Rāzī, . . . ibn al-^cAbbās, ibn Sīnā. Leide, 1903.

Kraus, P., Jābir ibn Ḥayyān. *Mém. prés. á l'Inst. d'Égypte,* vols. 44, 45, Le Caire, 1943.

Krauss, S., *Talmudische Archäologie.* Leipzig, 1910–1912.

Langkavel, B., *Botanik der späteren Griechen von III bis XIII* Jahrh. Berlin, 1866.

Laufer. Laufer, B., "Sino-Iranica." *Field Museum of Natural History, Anthrop. ser.* **15**, 185–630 (1919).

Leclerc, L., *Histoire de la médecine arabe.* Paris, 1876.

Leclerc, L., *Kachef er-romouz d'Abd er-Rezzaq ed-Djezairy. . . .* Paris, 1874. This may be abbreviated to al-Razzāq.

Leicester, H., *The historical background of chemistry.* New York, 1956.

Levey CCTM. Levey, M., *Chemistry and chemical technology in ancient Mesopotamia.* Amsterdam, 1959.

Levey M.A.B. Levey, M., *Mediaeval Arabic Bookmaking and its Relation to Early Chemistry and Pharmacology.* Philodelphia, 1962.

Levey, M., *Journ. Hist. Med.* **17** (1962).

Levy, J., *Neuhebraisches und chaldaisches Wörterbuch über die Talmudim* und Midrashim. Leipzig, 1876–1889.

Linnaeus, K., *Materia medica.* Stockholm, 1749.

Lisān al-ᶜarab. Jamāl al-Dīn ibn Mansūr's *Lisān al-ᶜarab.* Cairo, 1300–04 H.

Lobscheid, W., *English and Chinese Dictionary.* Hongkong, 1866.

Loew AP. Loew, I., *Aramaeische pflanzennamen.* Leipzig, 1881.

Loew FJ. Loew, I., *Die Flora der Juden.* Wien, 1924–1934.

Loret, V., *La flore pharaonique.* Paris, 1892.

Lucas. Lucas, A., *Ancient Egyptian materials and industries.* London, 1945.

Maḥī, T., *Muqaddimat fī tarīkh al-ṭibb al-ᶜarabī.* Khartoum, 1959.

Maim. Meyerhof, M., ed. and trans. *Maimonides' Sharḥ asmā' al-ᶜuqqār. Mém. prés. á l'Inst. d'Égypte* **41**, Le Caire, 1940.

al-Majūsī. ᶜAlī ibn al-ᶜAbbas al-Majūsī. *Kāmil al-ṣināᶜa al-ṭibbiya.* Cairo, 1294 H.

Māsarjawaih. *Vide Abdāl.*

Māsawaih. Abū Zakariyā' Yuḥannā b. Māsawaih, *Jawāhir al-ṭibb al-mufrada.* Text published by P. Sbath, *Bull. de l'Inst. d'Égypte* **19**, 5–27 (1936/7); translation and commentary by Martin Levey, *Journ. Hist. Med.* **16**, 394–410 (1961). Māsawaih died in 857 A.D.

Meyerhof, Max, *Quellen u. Studien z. Gesch. d. Naturw. u. d. Medizin* 3, 88–206 (1941).

Mieli. Mieli, A., *La Science Arabe*. Leiden, 1938.

Minhāj. Abu'l-Munā ibn Abī Naṣr al-Isrā'īlī, Minhāj al-dukkān. Bulaq, 1287 H.

Müller, R. F. G., *Grundsätze altindischer Medizin*. Kopenhagen, 1951.

Muntakhib. ibn Sīnā, *Kitāb muntakhib shifā' al-ṭibb*. MS Aya Sofya 3752.

Muntner, S., ed. Moshe ben Maimon, *Aphorisms of Moses in the Hebrew* translation of R. Nathan Hameathi (1283 A.D.). Jerusalem, 1959.

Idem. ed., Moshe ben Maimon, *Regimen sanitatis in the Hebrew translation of R. Moshe ibn Tibbon*. Jerusalem, 1957.

Mustawfī. *The Geographical Part of the Nuzhat al-Qulūb by Ḥamd-Allāh Mustawfī* (1340 H.) trans. by G. LeStrange, Leiden, 1919.

Al-Muᶜtamad. Vide. al-Ghasānī.

Nabāt. Vide Post.

Nadkarni. Nadkarni. A. K., *Indian Materia Medica*, Bombay, 1954.

M. Hāskim al-Nadwī, ed. Badr al-Dīn a. Al. M. b. Burhān al-Dīn a. Isḥāq Ibr. b. Saᶜdallah b. Jamāᶜah al-Kinānī al-Ḥamawī al-Shāfiᶜī. *Tadhkirat al-sāmiᶜ* ilkh. Hyderabad, 1353 H.

Nansich, Abraham b. Solomon. *'Alêh terûfâh*. London, 1785.

abū al-Naṣr, ᶜAdl, *Tarīkh al-Nabāt*. Beirut, 1962.

ibn abī Naṣr, Dā'ūd, *Minhāj al-dukkān*. Cairo, 1940.

Opitz, K., Translation of a work of "Avicenna . . . das

lehrgedicht über die heilkunde (Canticum de medicina)." *Quellen u. Studien z. Gesch. d. Naturw. u. d. Medizin* 7, 150–220 (1939).

Oribasius. *Commentaria in aphorismos Hippocratis. . . .* Venice, 1533.

Ortolff von Bayerlandt (ca. 1450), *Arzneibuch*. Augsburg, 1479.

Paracelsus von Hohenheim (fl. 1526), *De natura rerum libri septem*. Basil, 1573.

Paulos. Paulus Aegineta (7th cent. A.D.) *Sieben bucher. . . .* Translated into German by J. Berendes. Leipzig, 1914. Abbrev. is Ber.

Peñuela, J. M., *"Die Goldene" des ibn al-Munāṣif*. Rome, 1941.

Post, G. E., *Nabāt sūriah wa-falasṭīn wa'l-qiṭr al-miṣrī wa-bawādīkā*. Beirut, 1884.

Preuss, J., *Biblisch-talmudische medizin. . . .* Berlin, 1923.

ibn al-Qifṭī. *Tarīkh al-ḥukamā'*. J. Lippert ed. Leipzig, 1903.

al-Qumrī, Abū Manṣūr . . . , *Maqālāt fī al-ṭibb*. MS Aya Sofya 3749.

al-Qurba. Levy, R., Ibn al-Ukhuwwa's *Ma*ᶜ*ālim al-Qurba fī aḥkām al-ḥisba*. London, 1938.

ibn Qurra, Thābit, *Al-dhakhīra fī* ᶜ*ilm al-ṭibb*. Cairo, 1928.

al-Qurtubī, ᶜArib ibn Saᶜīd al-Kātib, *Kitāb khalq al-janīn wa-tadbīr al-ḥabālā wa'l-mawlūdūn*. Alger, 1956.

Rabbinowicz, I. M., *Einleitung in die Gesetzgebung und die Medicin des Thalmuds*. Leipzig, 1883.

Ray, J., *Historia plantarum*. London, 1686–1704.

Ray, P., History of chemistry in ancient and medieval India. Calcutta, 1956.

abū Bakr M. ibn Zakariyyā' al-Rāzī, *Kitāb manāfi*ᶜ *al-aghghiya wa-daf*ᶜ *madhārrha*. Le Caire, 1305 H.

al-Rāzī. al-Rāzī's *Kitābu'l hawī fi'ṭ-ṭibb*. Hyderabad, 1955–63.

al-Rāzī's *Kitāb fī abdāl al-adwiya*. MS Aya Sofya 3725.

al-Rāzī A. al Rāzī's *Kitāb al-murshid*. MS Aya Sofya 3724.

al-Rāzī B. al-Razi's *Fī al-adwiya al-maujūda fī kull makān*. MS Yale Z105 Ar./2.

al-Razzāq. *Vide* Leclerc Kachef. . . .

Rechinger, K. H., *Flora aegea*. Vienna, 1943.

Reinaud, M., *Relation des voyages faits par les Arabes et les Persans dans l'Inde et la Chine (Salsalat al-tawārīkh)*. Paris, 1845.

Renaud, H.-P.-J., and G. S. Colin, *Documents Morocains pour servir à* l'histoire du "mal Franc." Paris, 1935.

Ritter, H. and M. Plessner, *"Picatrix" Das Ziel des Weisen von Pseudo-Majrīṭī*. London, 1962.

Ritter, H., *Das biographische Lexicon des Salaḥaddīn Khalīl ibn Aibak aṣ-Safadī*. In *Bibliotheca Islamica* 6a, pt. 1, Wiesbaden, 1962.

ibn Rushd. ibn Rushd's *Kitāb al-adwiyah*. MS Ahmet III 2030.

Ruska, J., "Al-Rāzī's Buch Geheimniss der Geheimnisse." *Quellen u. Studien z. Gesch. d. Naturw. u. d. Medizin* 6 (1937).

Ruska, J., *el al,* Abū al-Qāsim ᶜAbd Allah b. ᶜAlī b. M. b. abī Tāhir al-Qāshanī's *Kitāb jawāhir al-ᶜara'is wa-aṭāyib al-nafā'is*. Istanbul, 1935.

Idem. Das Buch des Alaune und Salze. Berlin, 1935.

Idem. Das Steinbuch des Aristoteles. Heidelberg, 1912.

Idem. Sal ammoniacus, Nūšādir und salmiak. Heidelberg, 1923.

S. is the supplement to GAL.

ibn Sahl, Sābūr (d. 869 A.D.). *Aqrābādhīn*. MS Munich 808.

al-Sahmī, *Tārīkh Jurjān*. Hyderabad, 1950.

al-Samarqandī. His *Aqrābādhīn*. MS Aya Sofya 3555.

al-Samarqandī, Najīb al-dīn, *Uṣūl tarkīb al-adwiya*. MSS Leiden 1352, Aya Sofya 3554.

Sayili, A., "Islam and the rise of seventeenth century science," *Belleten Türk Tarih Kurumu* 22, 353–368 (1958).

Sbath, P. and C. D. Avierinos, *Deux traités medicaux*. Le Caire, 1953.

Schonak, W., *Die Rezeptsammlung des Scribonius Largus*. Jena, 1912.

Schrader, H. A., *Systematische Sammlung kryptogamische Gewächse*. Göttingen, 1796.

Schweinfurth, G., *Arabische Pflanzennamen aus Aegypten, Algerien, und Jemen*. Berlin, 1912.

Serapion. Guiges, P., "Les noms arabes dans Sérapion au liber de simplici medicina. . . ." *Journ. Asiatique* (1905).

Sigerist, H. E., *Studien u. Texte z. frühmittelalterlichen Rezeptliteratur* in vol. 13 of *Studien z. Gesch d. Medizin* (1923).

Siggel, A., ᶜAlī ibn Sahl Rabban al-Ṭaubarī's Gynokologie, Embryologie . . . aus dem "Paradies der Weisheit" über die Medizin. *Quellen* und Studien z. Gesch. d. Naturw. u. d. Medizin 8, 216–272 (1941).

ibn Sīnā. Abū ᶜAlī al-Ḥusain b. ᶜAl. b. Sīnā al-Qānūnī. *Kitab al-saᶜādah wal-iqbāl*. MS Ahmet III 2050.

Idem. Kitāb al-shifā'. Cairo, 1956–1960.

Soubeiran, J. L., *La matière médicale chez les chinois*. Paris, 1874.

Stahl, G. E., *Fundamenta pharmaciae chimiae*. Dresden, 1728.

Steingass, F., *A comprehensive Persian-English dictionary*. London, 1892.

Stromberg, R., *Griechische Pflanzennamen*. Götenburg, 1940.

Siddīqī, M. Z., *Studies in Arabic and Persian medical literature*. Calcutta, 1959.

al-Ṭabarī. ᶜAlī ibn Rabban al-Ṭabarī, *Firdausu'l-ḥikmat*. Siddīqī, M. Z., ed. Berlin, 1928.

al-Ṭabarī A. Abū Jaᶜfar M. b. Jarīr al-Ṭabarī, *Kitāb akhbār al-rusul wa'l-mulūk*. Goeje, M.J. ed. Leiden, 1879–1901.

Tabernaemontanus, J. T. (1520–1590), *Ein newes Artzney Buch*. Frankfurt, 1577.

Tāj. M. Murtaḍā al-Zabīdī al-Ḥanafī, *Tāj al-ᶜarūs min jawāhir al-qāmūs*. Cairo, 1306–1310 H.

Temkin, O., "Medicine and Graeco-Arabic alchemy." *Bull Hist. Med.* **29**, 134–153 (1955).

Theoph., Hort, A., ed. *Theophrastus' inquiry into plants*. London, 1916

Theophrastus, *De causis plantarum*. Hort, A., ed. London, 1948.

Thiebaut, J., "Flore Libano-Syrienne" in *Mém. prés. à l'Inst. d'Égypte* **31**, **40** (1936, 1940).

Tuḥfa. *Tuḥfat al-aḥbāb*, transl, and ed, by Renaud, H.-P.-J. and G. Colin. Paris, 1934.

Uhlenbeck, C. C. *Kurzgefasstes etymologisches Wörterbuch*. Amsterdam, 1899.

von Kremer, A., *Culturgeschichte des Orients unter den Chalifen*. Vienna, 1877.

von Lippmann, E. O., *Gesch. d. Rüben (Beta)*. Leipzig, 1925.

Vullers, J. A., *Lexicon persico-latinum etymologicum*. Bonnae,, 1855–1867.

Walzer, R., *Greek into Arabic, Essays on Islamic Philosophy*. Oxford, 1962.

Wellmann, M., *Vide* Diosc.

Wiedemann, Wiedemann, E., articles in *Beiträge z. Gesch. d. Wissen. Sitz. d. Physikalisch-medizinischen Soz. in Erlangen.*

Wiedemann, E., "Über arabische Parfüms," *Archiv. f. Gesch. d. Med.* 8, 83–88 (1915).

Willdenow, K. L., *Linnei species plantarum.* Berlin, 1797.

Williams, M., *A Sanskrit-English dictionary.* Oxford, 1872.

Williams, S. W., *An English and Chinese vocabulary.* Macao, 1844.

Wüstenfeld, F., *Jacut's geographisches Wörterbuch.* Leipzig, 1866–1870.

al-Yaᶜqūbī, Aḥmad b.a. Yaᶜqūb b. Jaᶜfar, *Tarīkh al-Yaᶜqūbī.* Beirut, 1960.

al-Zahrāwī. Vide Hamarneh.

al-Zirkilī. *Iᶜlām* . . . [Biog. dict.]. Cairo, 1954–1959.

Arabic Text in Photocopy

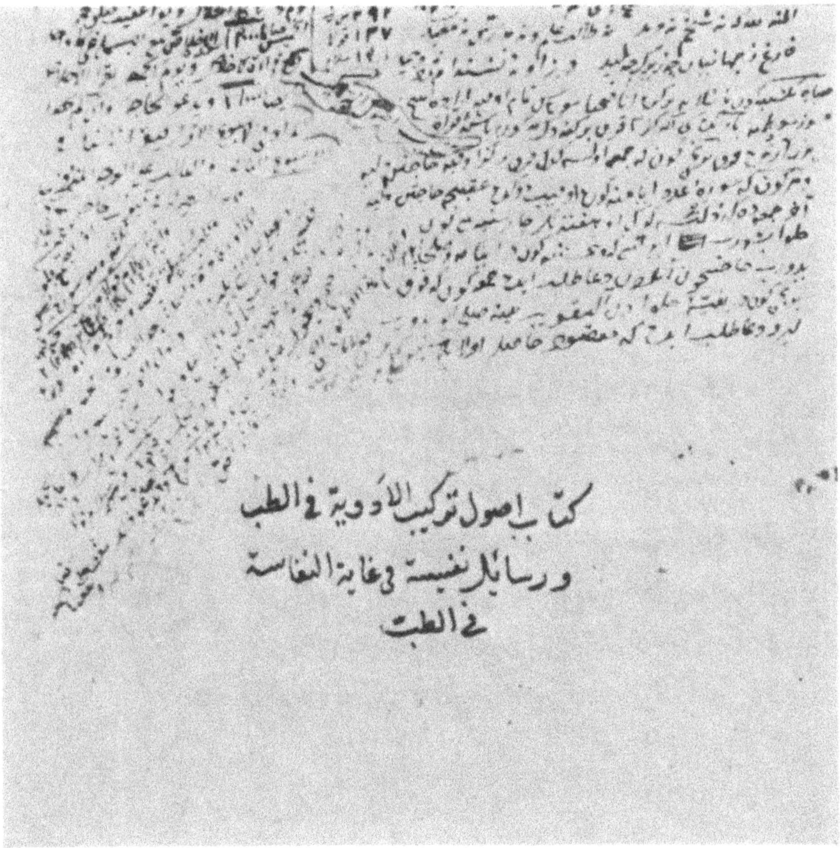
كتاب اصول تركيب الادوية في الطب
ورسائل نفيسة في غاية النفاسة
في الطب

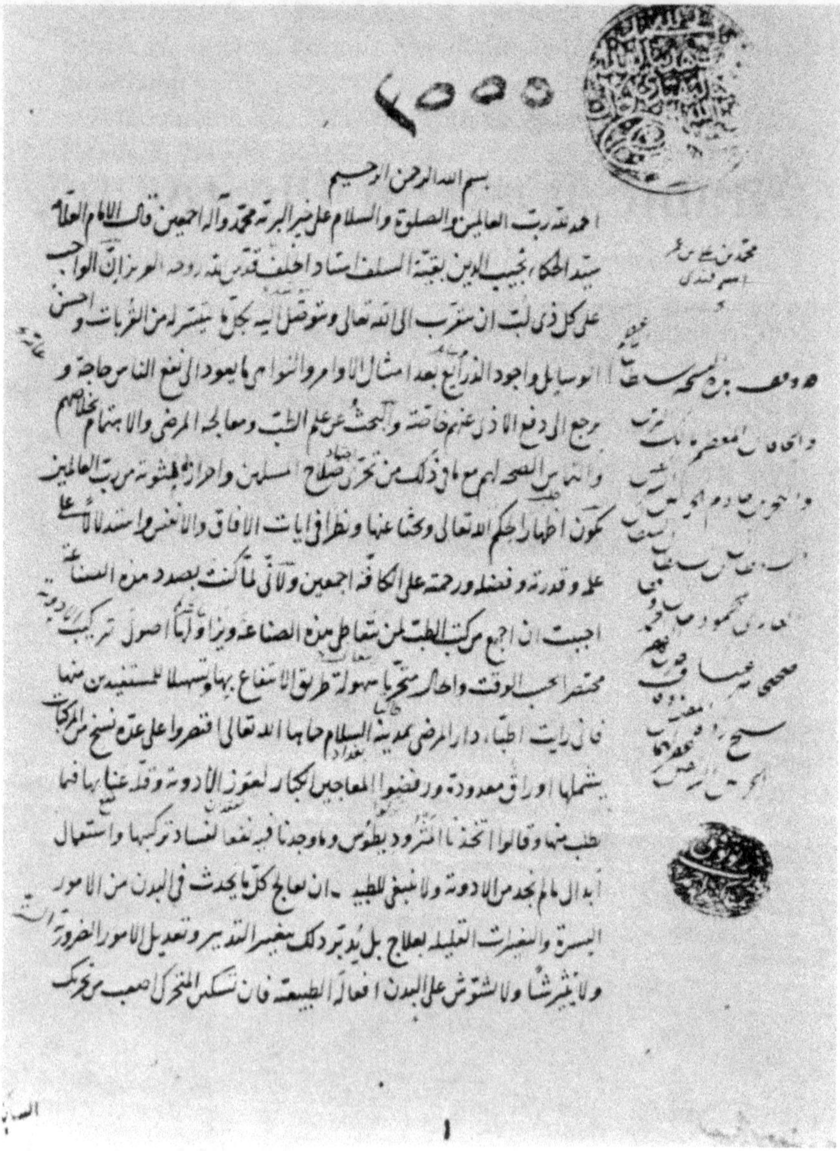

بسم الله الرحمن الرحيم

الحمد لله رب العالمين والصلوة والسلام على خير البرية محمد وآله اجمعين قال الامام العلامة
سيد الحكماء نجيب الدين بقية السلف استاد الخلف قدس الله روحه العزيز ان الواجب
على كل ذي لب ان يتقرب الى الله تعالى ويتوصل اليه بكل ما يتيسر له من القربات واحسن
الوسايل واجود الذرايع بعد امتثال الاوامر والنواهي ما يعود الى نفع الناس حاجة و
يرجع الى دفع الاذى عنهم خاصة والبحث عن علم الطب ومعالجة المرضى والاهتمام بخلاصهم
والتماس الصحة لهم مع ما في ذلك من تحري صلاح المسلمين واحراز المثوبة من رب العالمين
لكون اظهار حكم الله تعالى وبحثا عنها ونظرا في ايات الافاق والانفس واسند لالة على
علمه وقدرته وفضله ورحمته على الكافة اجمعين ولاني لما كنت بصدد من الصناعة
احببت ان اجمع مركبات الطب لمن يتعاطى من الصناعة وزنا وكما اصول تركيب
مختصرا بحسب الوقت واحال متحريا سهولة طريق الانتفاع بها وتسهيلا للمستفيدين منها
فاني رايت اطباء دار المرضى بمدينة السلام حماها الله تعالى قد قصروا على عدة نسخ من المركبات
يشتملها اوراق معدودة ورفضوا المعاجين الكبار لعوز الادوية وقد عنيا بها فيما
طلب منها وقالوا اتخذنا الترود يطوس وما وجدنا فيه نفعا لفساد تركيبها واستعمال
ابدال ما لم يجد من الادوية ولا ينبغي للطبيب ان يعالج كل ما يحدث في البدن من الامور
اليسيرة والتغيرات القليلة بعلاج بل يدبر ذلك بتغيير التدبير وتعديل الامور الضرورية
ولا يشوش على البدن افعال الطبيعة فان تسكين المتحرك اصعب من تحريك

١

الساكن ومتى قدر ان يعالج بالاغذية الدوائية لا ينبغي ان يعالج بالادوية وان اضطر
فبالادوية الغذائية وان احتيج الى الادوية الصرفة فلا يتجاوز المفردات منها ما امكن
لان ذلك اخف على الطبيعة وابلغ نفعا في المرض كما قال جالينوس في الادوية المركبة ان
الادوية الموصوفة يمكن ان ينفع لا ينفع ولا في واحد من تلك الخلال نفعا عظيما قويا بل
احرى انها لما ركبت من ادوية شتى ينفع كل واحد منها من عدة من العلل كان ادخل
في الشربة الواحدة من الدواء المركب ينفع علل كثيرة مقدار يسير من الدواء النافع من كل
واحد منها فلا يبلغ ابدا من النفع في العلل التي تستحق ايها ما يبلغ ذلك المقدار من الادوية
المفردة النافعة من تلك العلل وهذا خصوصا قد بلغ الامر في هذا الزمان من دروس
معالم العلوم وكساد بضايع الصناعات الى ان فقدت جل الادوية سيما المفردة فلم يبق
الا اسماؤها وما وجدت وجدت اما مغشوشة واما عتيقة ضعيفة قد بقيت
دهورا طويلة واكثر الادوية لا يبقى قوتها بعد سنتين وحينئذ فترك المركبات
الكثيرة الاخلاط في هذا الزمان اولى وان اقتصرنا على الاقل منها عند ضرورة التركيب
اخرى حتى ترجح منها المنفعة ولا يحقق قول الناس في المثل اكذب من قراباذين
وتركيب الادوية في الحال والوقت على مراعاة قوانين التركيب بحسب احتياجه و
العلل وكيفيات الامزجة اولى من نقل النسخ من القراباذينات التي ملئت اكثرها
حشوا وفضولا وغلطا وتحريفا وتركا وتصحيفا وقد احلها قوم محل كتاب الله تعالى
الذي لا ينبغي ان يغير ويبدل ولا يقدر الجن والانس على ان ياتوا بمثله وهم الذين

دتهم جالينوس وبيخز منهم وقال ان كثيرا منهم ضاعت نسخهم فماتوا غما وآخرون بقوا
حيارى آخر اعمارهم لا يهتدون بشئ منها وضمن لمن احكم معرفة قوى الادوية و
قوانين تركيبها ان يركب متى شاء وحيث شاء ادوية اجود وابلغ منها فيما
اراد والامور الداعية الى التركيب عند تعذر دواء واحد يبلغ الغرض المقصود
بعضها من جهة طبيعة العلل والادواء وبعضها من احوال الاعضاء وبعضها بسبب
الدواء وجميع ذلك بضعة عشر شيئا احدها مقدار سوء المزاج حيث لم يوجد دواء
مقابل له في مقداره فيركب الاقوى منه ويكسر مع الذي دونه فيها فيجتمع منهما مزاج متقاوم
لذلك المزاج الردي والثاني قوة المرض وشدته حيث لم يوجد دواء واحد يقاوم
ه فيركب ليعين بعضها بعضا في مقاومته والثالث اختلاف حال المرض ومقتضى
علاجه فلم يوجد دواء يفعل فعلا متضادة مثل الجلاء والتمليس في امراض الصدر و
التحليل والردع في الاورام فيركب والرابع الاستظهار ليكون عدة لمعاودة سموم
… وامراض شتى وهذا اشرف المركبات لانه يستفيد من التركيب قوة فوق قوى
جميع المفردات لكن الشأن في وجود مفرداته الخامس بعد العضو الآلم عن المعدة
فيركب مع الدواء الذي فعله … ويوصله اليه بسرعته كالزعفران مع الكافور
و… مع النشادر والسادس قوة العضو وشرفه وكثرة منافعه فيخلط
بدوائه المحلل للاورام والملطف للاخلاط فيه ما يحفظ عليه قوته من الادوية القابضة
العطرة والسابع بشاعة الدواء وكراهته حتى يطيب وتحتمله الطبيعة والثامن

زيادة قوة الدواء كخلط الزنجبيل بالتربد والتاسع دفع مضرة الدواء ببعض الاعضاء
كالمصلحات مع المسهلات والعاشر نقص قوة الدواء كالصمغ في شياف الزنجار
والحادي عشر كسر عادية الدواء كخلط جندبيدستر بالافيون والثاني عشر حفظ
قوة الدواء المركب زمانا طويلا كخلط الافيون بالمعاجين الكبار والثالث عشر
اختلاف الادوية في اجرامها واستعمالها في الجهة المرادة كخلط الفيروزج بالادوية
المحتضرة في المراهم والرابع عشر عوز الدواء الواحد النافع من العلة كخلط الفيروزج
بالزنجار ليحصل منهما دواء نافع للقروح حيث لم يوجد الادوية التي تصلح للقروح فهذه
هي الاسباب الموجبة للتركيب والمضطر اليها عند عوز دواء مفرد يفي بجميع ما يراد منه
فاما سبب اختلاف اوزانها فهي اسباب سبعة مفردات واسباب مركبة من
المفردات اما السبعة المفردات فاحدها قوتها وضعفها في كيفياتها والثاني كثرة
منافعها وقلتها والثالث شرف منفعتها وخستها والرابع مشاركتها في منفعة
وانفرادها بها والخامس مواضع الاعضاء العليلة بحسب قربها من المعدة وبعدها عنها
والسادس وجود ادوية في المركب تضعف قوتها وعدمها والسابع وجود مضرة
فيها لبعض الاعضاء او لبعض الادوية وعدمها اما اختلاف اوزانها بحسب قوتها و
ضعفها فان شدة قوة الدواء في التسخين والتبريد توجب التقليل منه في المركب وضعف
قوته توجب التكثير ليقوم بكثرته مقام ما يراد منه من قوته واما اختلافها بحسب كثرة
المنفعة وقلتها فكثرة المنافع توجب التكثير وقلتها اعني كون الدواء ذا منفعة واحدة

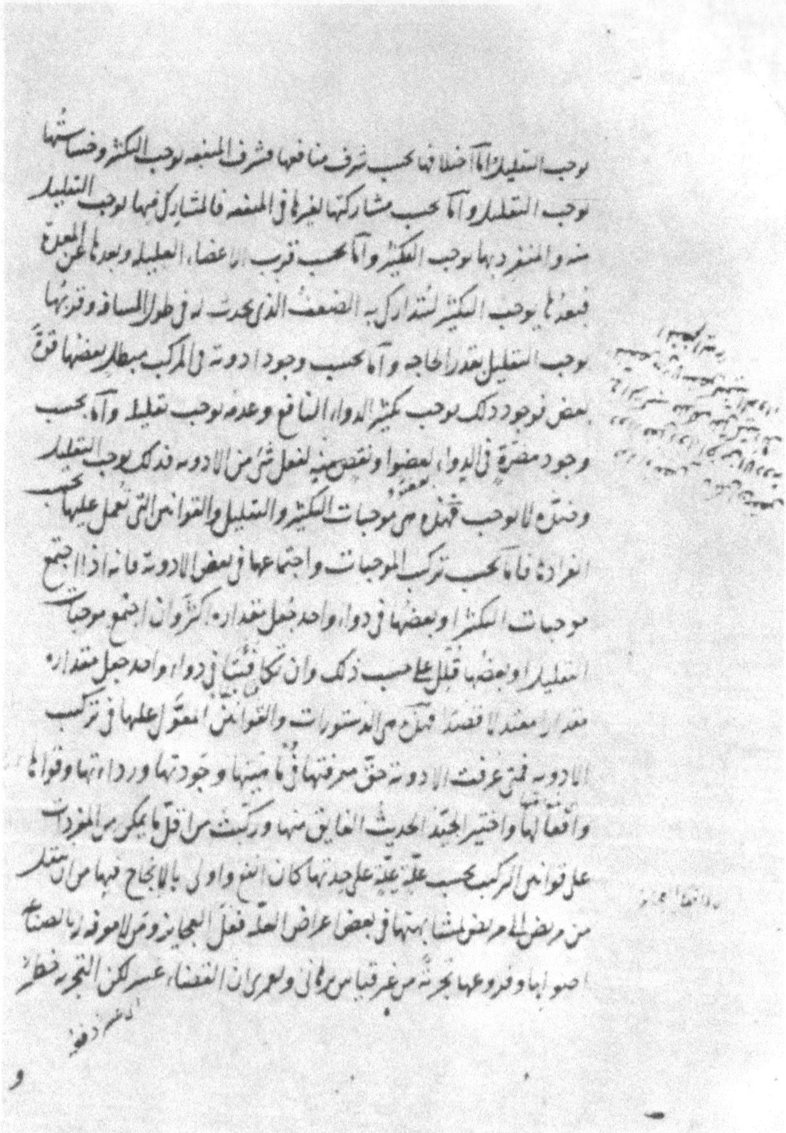
يوجب التقليل واما اختلافها بحسب شرف منافعها وشرف المنفعة يوجب التكثير وخساستها
يوجب التقليل واما بحسب مشاركتها لغيرها في المنفعة فالمشارك منها يوجب التقليل
منه والمنفرد بها يوجب التكثير واما بحسب قرب الاعضاء العليلة وبعدها عن المعدة
فبعدها يوجب التكثير ليتدارك به الضعف الذي يحدث له في طول المسافة وقربها
يوجب التقليل بقدر الحاجة واما بحسب وجود ادوية في المركب يبطل بعضها قوة
بعض فوجود ذلك يوجب تكثير الدواء النافع وعدمه يوجب تقليله واما بحسب
وجود مضرة في الدواء لبعض الاعضاء ونقص منه لفعل شيء من الادوية فذلك يوجب التقليل
وضده لما يوجب فهذه هي موجبات التكثير والتقليل والقوانين التي تعمل عليها بحسب
انفرادها فاما بحسب تركيب الموجبات واجتماعها في بعض الادوية فانه اذا اجتمع
موجبات التكثير او بعضها في دواء واحد جعل مقداره اكثر وان اجتمع موجبات
التقليل او بعضها قلل على حسب ذلك وان تكافئتا في دواء واحد جعل مقداره
مقدارا معتدلا فهذه هي الدستورات والقوانين المعول عليها في تركيب
الادوية فمتى عرفت الادوية حق معرفتها في ماهيتها وجودتها ورداءتها وقواها
ومنافعها واختير الجيد الحديث الفائق منها وركبت من اقل ما يمكن من المفردات
على قوانين التركيب بحسب علة علة على حدتها كان انفع واولى بالانجاح فيها من ان يستعمل
من مرض الى مرض لمشابهتها في بعض اعراض العلة فعل العجائز ومن لا معرفة له بالصناعة
اصولها وفروعها بجرأة من غير قياس برهاني ولعمري ان القضاء عسر لكن التجربة خطر

وطريق القياس مأمون مستعمل معتمد عليه في جميع التدابير الطبية وغيرها ولو وجب
تركه فان الاوائل ركبوا جميع ما ركبوا بطريق القياس ثم وجدوه بعد تجربته على غاية
ما املوا منها حتى دعاهم ذلك الى ان دونوه وخلدوه في الكتب فيجب ان يكون
اسوة لنا في اتخاذ المركبات على انحاء التركيب بحسب ضروب الحاجات وكما ان
المصالح الان في مركبات علمنا قوانينها واغراضهم في تركيبها ان اتفق ان سنح لنا
اغراض مثل اغراضهم فنسق الجواهر على الحاجة كما يقع الحافر على الحافر وانا اثبت
من ذلك القبيل بعض ما بدا ولله ايدي التجارب وابرزته عن القوة الى الفعل على طريق
المثال حتى ينتفع به عند الحاجة بموضعه واستعماله في مستحقه وتقاس عليه ابواب في
وهي تسعة عشر بابا آ في الاشربة والربوب ب في الجوارشنات والمعجونات
ج في الحبوبات والايارجات د في المطبوخات والمنقوعات ه في الحقن و
والشيافات والفرازج ز في ادوية القيء ح في المعوقات ط في الاقراص ي
في السفوفات واللعوقات يا في الاضمدة والاطلية والكمادات يب
الادهان يج في ادوية العين يد في المراهم والذرورات يه في السنونات
يو في الغراغر في المرتبات يز في السعوطات والمطوسات والشمومات
والبخورات يح في النطولات يط في ادوية الشعر الباب الاول
الاشربة والربوب اما المفرد من الاشربة الذي هو في غاية البساطة فالماء
القراح وهو انفع شراب للمحموم من حمى حادة لشدة لطافته وسرعة نفوذه

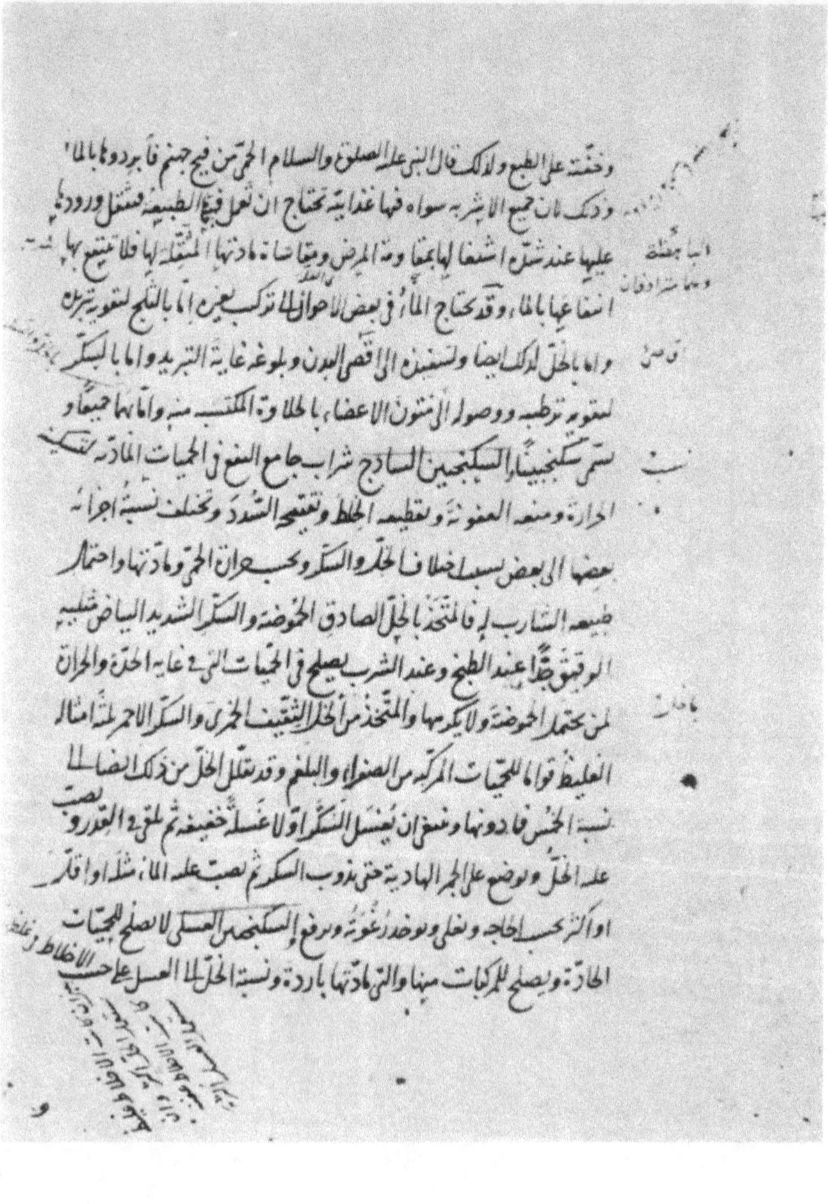
وخفته على الطبع ولذلك قال النبي عليه الصلوة والسلام الحمى من فيح جهنم فابردوها بالماء
وذلك لان جميع الاشربة سواه فيها غذائية تحتاج ان تعمل فيها الطبيعة فتشتغل ورودها
عليها عند شروع اشتغالها بما هو المرض ومقاساته مادتها المشتغلة لها فلا تنتفع بها
انتفاعها بالماء وقد يحتاج الماء في بعض الاحوال الى تركيب بغيره اما بالثلج لتقوية تبريده
واما بالخل لذلك ايضا وليستنفذه الى اقصى البدن وبلوغه غاية التبريد واما بالسكر
لتقوية ترطيبه ووصوله الى متون الاعضاء بالحلاوة المكتسبة منه واما بهما جميعا و
تسمى سكنجبينا السكنجبين الساذج شراب جامع النفع في الحميات المادية لتسكين
الحرارة ومنعه العفونة وتقطيعه الخلط وتفتيحه السدد وتختلف نسبة اجزائه
بعضها الى بعض بسبب اختلاف الخل والسكر وبحسب ان الحمى ومادتها واحتمال
طبيعة الشارب له فالمتخذ بالخل الصادق الحموضة والسكر الشديد البياض شديد
الوثوق جدا عند الطبخ وعند الشرب يصلح في الحميات التي في غاية الحدة والحرارة
لمن يحتمل الحموضة ولا يكرهها والمتخذ من الخل الثقيف الخمري والسكر الاحمر لمثل امثال
الغليظ فاما للحميات المركبة من الصفراء والبلغم وقد يقلل الخل من ذلك النصاب الى
نسبة الخمس فما دونها وينبغي ان يغسل السكر اولا غسلة خفيفة ثم يلقى في القدر ويصب
عليه الخل ويوضع على الجمر الهادية حتى يذوب السكر ثم يصب عليه الماء مثلا او اقل
او اكثر بحسب الحاجة ويغلى ويؤخذ رغوته ويرفع والسكنجبين العسلي لا يصلح للحميات
الحادة ويصلح للمركبات منها والتي مادتها باردة ونسبة الخل الى العسل على حسب الاخلاط وغلظ

ولزوجتها ورقتها وشدة عفونتها فان الخل مبرد مسكن والعسل مسخن ملطف
وقد تتخذ بحل المفصل في العلل الباردة جدا ومنها الخل حار جلاء مقطع
والسكنجبين البزوري قد تركب السكنجبين مع البزور لانه ينفع للسدد اما في
الحميات الحارة فمع البزور الباردة واما في الحميات التي مادتها باردة وغيرها
من الامراض فمع البزور الحارة واما في المركبة فمع الحارة والباردة جميعا مع مراعاة
نسبتها الى الاخلاط والى الاعضاء مثلا ان اتخذ للحميات الحارة والاخلاط الصفراوية
وسدد العروق اتخذ من بزر الهندباء وقشر اصله وبزر الخيارين والبطيخ لانه
من البزور المدرة الباردة مخصوصة بسدد العروق والادرار الصفراء ويجعل
من بزر الخيارين والبطيخ اكثر مقدارا لضعفها وبعد مسلكها ومن قشور اصل
الهندباء اقل لوجود مشاركتها في المعنى معها وقصور منفعتها عن بزرها ومن
بزر الهندباء اكثر من قشور اصله لزيادة المنفعة وعظمتها ولانه كالعمدة المعول
عليه في تفتيح سدد العروق عند الحميات الحارة واقل من بزر الخيارين والبطيخ
لقوته فيجعل من بزر الخيارين والبطيخ من كل واحد خمسة دراهم ومن قشور اصل
الهندباء درهمان ومن بزر الهندباء ثلثة دراهم واما في الحميات التي مادتها باردة
فيتخذ من بزر الكرفس والانيسون وبزر الهندباء لانه مركب الاجزاء معتدل النفع
ومن بزر الرازيانج واصول واصول الكرفس والغافث والكشوث والريوند
ويجعل من البزور مثلا من كل واحد ثلثة دراهم ومن الاصول خمسة دراهم لتقوى البزور

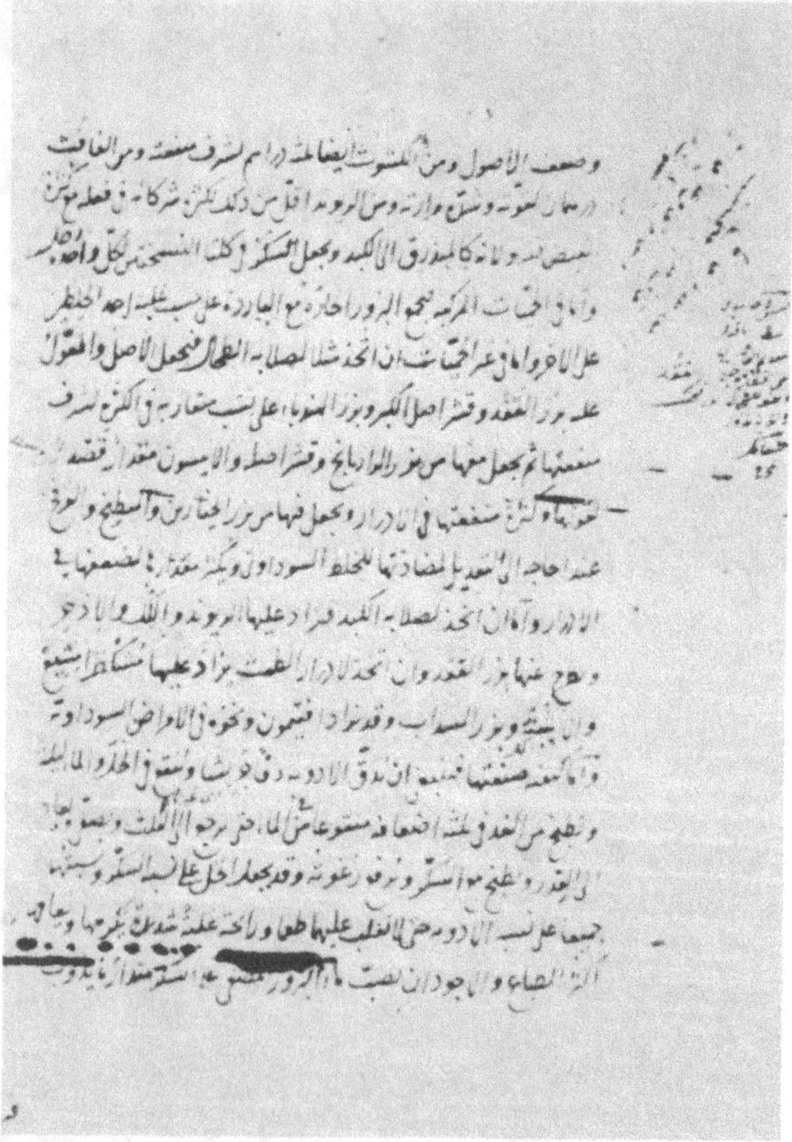

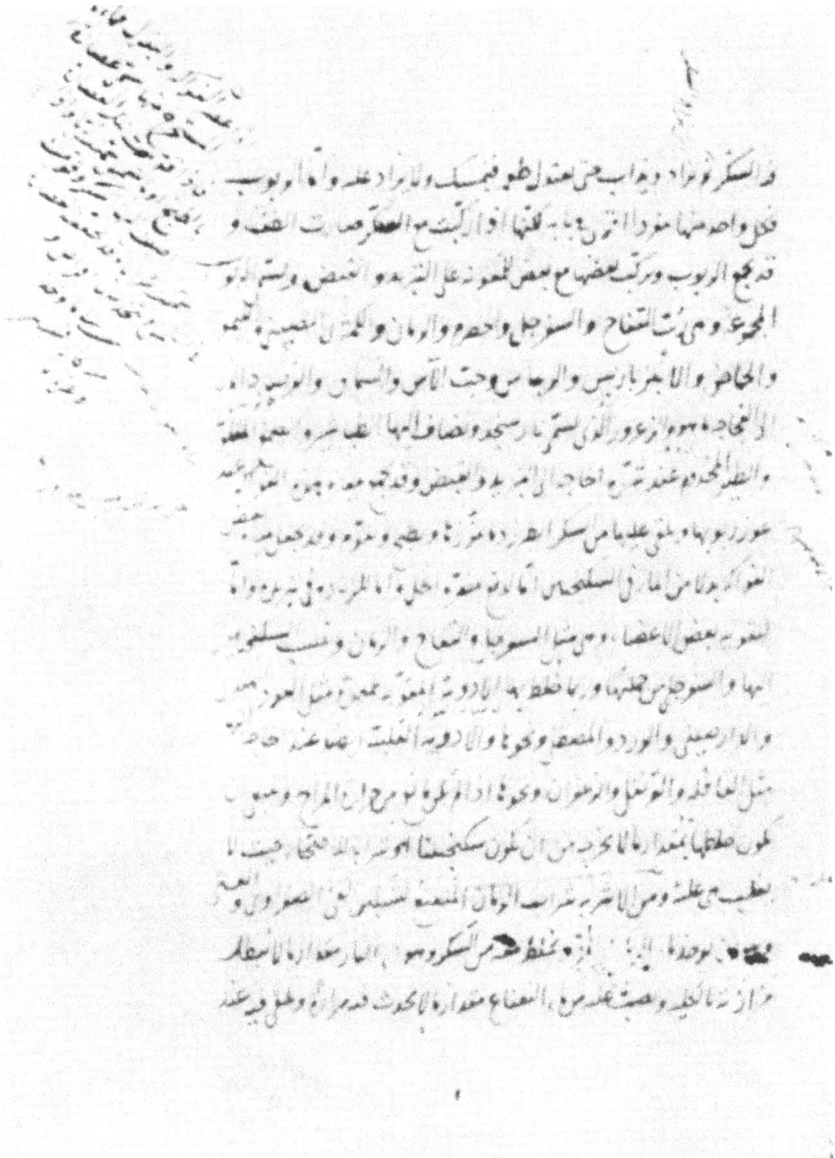

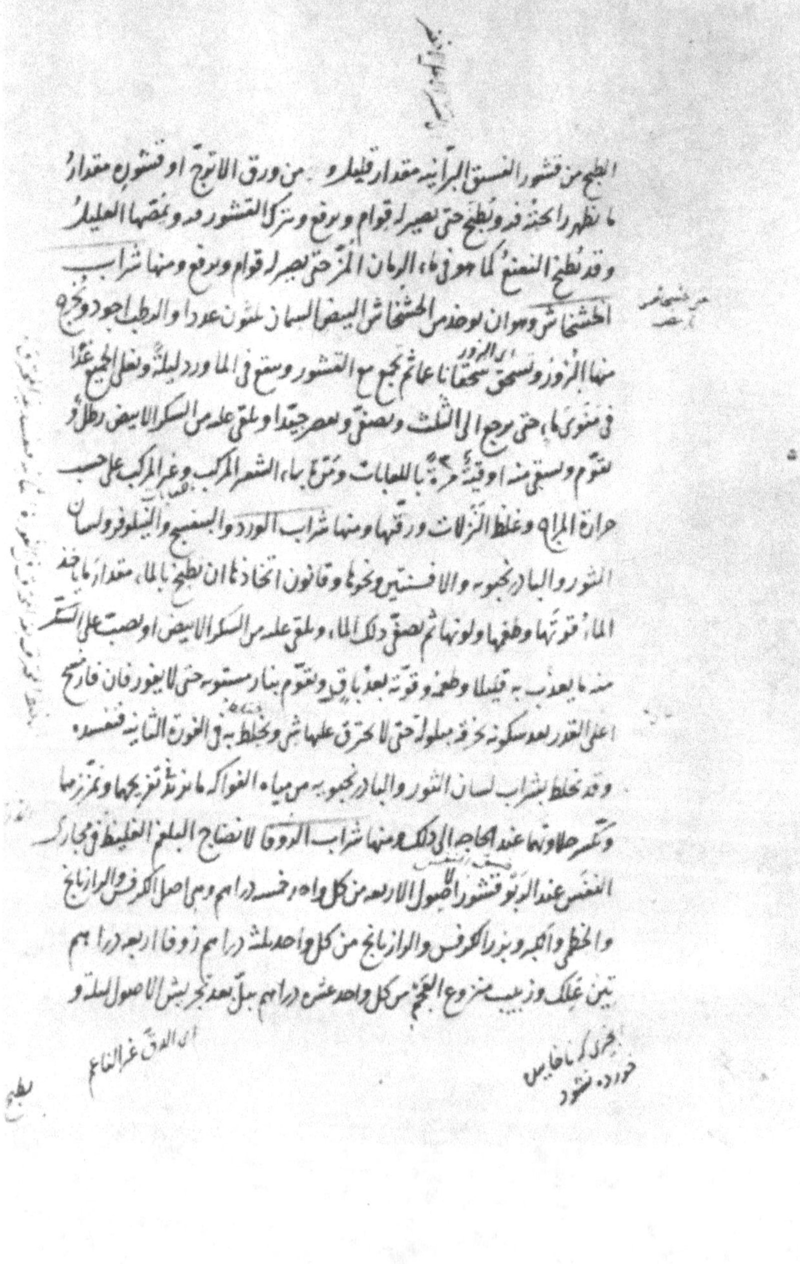
الطبخ من قشور الفستق البرانية مقدار قليل و ... من ورق الاترج او قشوره مقدار
ما تظهر الحموضة و يطبخ حتى يصير له قوام و يرفع و يترك القشور منه و بعضها العليل
وقد يطبخ النعنع كما هو في ماء الرمان المز حتى يصير له قوام ويرفع ومنها شراب
الخشخاش وهو ان يوخذ من الخشخاش الابيض السمان ستون عددا والرطب اجود ويخرج
منها البزور وتسحق سحقا ناعما ثم يجمع مع القشور وينقع في الماء ورد ليلة ويغلى الجميع غليا
في مثل ماء حتى يرجع الى الثلث ويصفى ويعصر جيدا ويلقى عليه من السكر الابيض رطل و
يقوم ويسقى منه اوقية ... باللعابات ... الشعر المركب وغير المركب على حسب
حرارة المزاج وغلظ النزلات ورقتها ومنها شراب الورد والبنفسج والنيلوفر ولسان
الثور والبادرنجبويه والافسنتين ونحوها وقانون اتخاذها ان يطبخ بالماء مقدار ما ياخذ
الماء قوتها وطعمها ولونها ثم يصفى ذلك الماء ويلقى عليه من السكر الابيض او يصب على السكر
منه ما يعذب به قليلا وطعمه وقوته بعد باق ويقوم بنار مستوية حتى لا يفور فان فار مسح
اعلى القدر بعد سكونه بخرقة مبلولة حتى لا يحترق عليها شي ويخلط به في الفورة الثانية فيفسده
وقد يخلط بشراب لسان الثور والبادرنجبويه من مياه الفواكه ما يزيد تفريحهما و...
ويكسر حلاوتهما عند الحاجة الى ذلك ومنها شراب الزوفا لانضاج البلغم الغليظ في مجاري
النفس عند الربو قشور الاصول الاربعة من كل واحد خمسة دراهم وهي اصل الكرفس والرازيانج
والخطمي والاذخر وبزر الكرفس والرازيانج من كل واحد ثلثة دراهم زوفا اربعة دراهم
تين علك وزبيب منزوع العجم من كل واحد عشرة دراهم يبل بعد تجريش الاصول ثلثة و
اى الدق غير الناعم

ويطبخ بثلثة ارطال ماء حتى يرجع الى رطل ونصف ويصفى والشربة خمسة اساتير خمسة عشر درهما سكنجبين
وقد يزاد عند الحاجة الى زيادة القوة اصل السوسن الاسمانجوني واصل سوسن و
البرسياوشان وينقص بعض الادوية الحارة عند حرارة المزاج ويجعل بدلها بنفسج
وبزر الخطمي وبزر السونبل والعناب والبستان [illegible] عند الحاجة الى
تليين الصدور ومنع الازمنة ومنها ماء الجبن يسهل المواد المحترقة تغلى اللبن [illegible]
الماعز مقدار رطلين ويصب عليه بعد غليانه ثلثة مقدار خمسة اساتير من السكنجبين [illegible]
ويرفع ويصفى بخرقة صفيقة والشربة عشرة اساتير بالسكنجبين ويشرب معها مسهل
الصفراء والسوداء بحسب الحاجة شراب الصندل لحرارة القلب يؤخذ الصندل [illegible]
مقدار ثلثين درهما [illegible] بالمدق وينقع في نصف رطل من [illegible] وليلة ويطبخ
من الغد في ثلثة ارطال ماء حتى يرجع الى رطل ونصف ويضاف اليه نصف رطل ماء [illegible]
[illegible] ونصف رطل ماء التمر الهندي وثلثة ارطال سكر طبرزد ويقوم على نار [illegible]
[illegible] ثم يلقى عليه طباشير وصندل مسحوق [illegible] درهمان [illegible] مسحوق
زعفران ثلثة دراهم شراب العناب لتسكين [illegible] الدم [illegible]
عناب جرجاني صحيح رطل زبيب [illegible] خمسة عشر درهما عدس مقشر [illegible] درهم [illegible]
[illegible] فينقع الجميع في خل ثلثة ايام ثم يغلى عليه [illegible] ويصفى ويعمل [illegible] بالسكنجبين
ويسقى منه كل يوم عشرة دراهم [illegible] من نقوع الانبرباريس [illegible] يؤخذ عناب
جرجاني [illegible] النوى رطل انبرباريس [illegible] من حبة رطل [illegible]

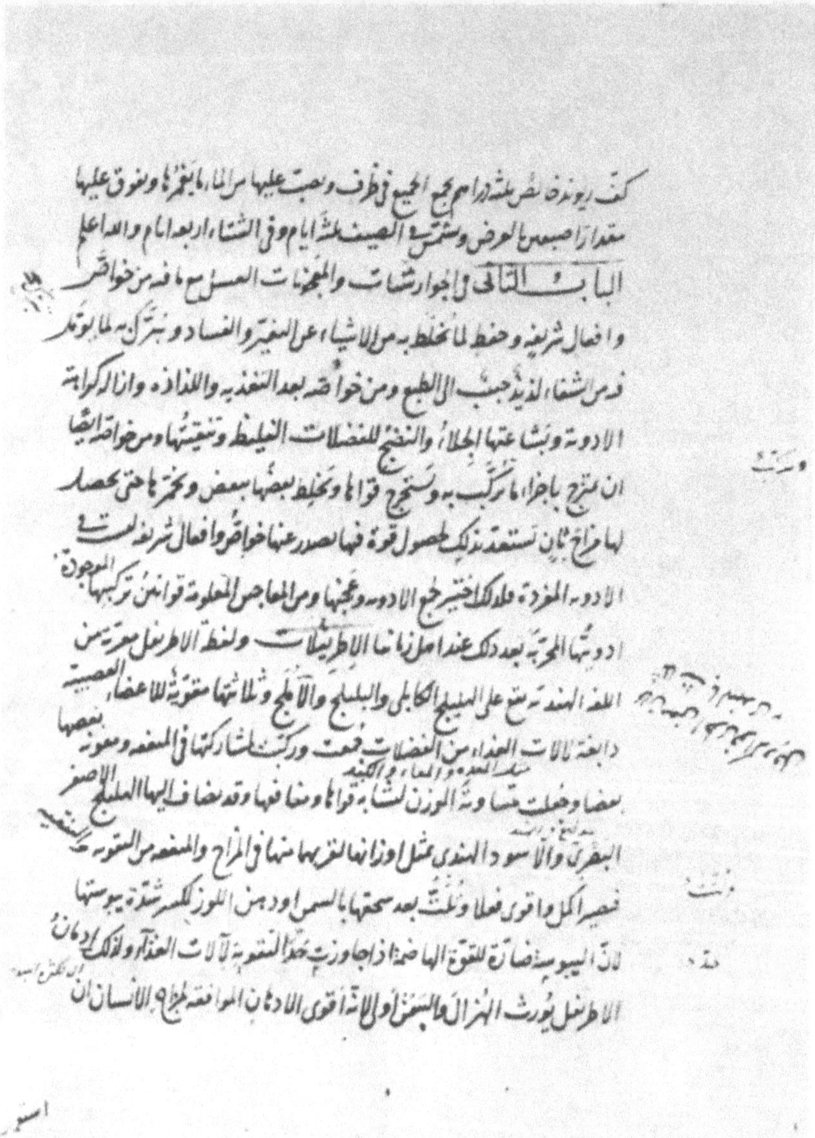

كف ريوند خمسة دراهم ويجمع الجميع في ظرف ويصب عليها من الماء ما يغمرها ويفوق عليها
مقدار اصبع بالعرض ويشمس في الصيف ثلثة ايام وفي الشتاء اربعة ايام والله اعلم
الباب الثاني في الجوارشنات والمعجونات العسل مع ما فيه من خواص
وافعال شريفة وحفظ لما يخلط به من الاشياء عن التغير والفساد ويترك به لما يوثر
فيه من الشفاء الذي يجذب الى الطبع ومن خواصه بعد التغذية واللذاذة وازالة كراهة
الادوية وبشاعتها الجلاء والنضج للفضلات الغليظة وتنقيتها ومن خواصه ايضا
ان يمتزج باجزاء ما يركب به ويستخرج قواها ويخلط بعضها ببعض ويخمرها حتى يحصل
لها مزاج ثان تستعد بذلك لحصول قوة فيها تصدر عنها خواص وافعال شريفة ليست في
الادوية المفردة فلذلك اختير جمع الادوية وعجنها ومن المعاجين المعلومة قوانين تركيبها الموجودة
ادويتها المجربة بعد ذلك عند اهل زماننا الاطريفلات ولفظ الاطريفل معرب من
اللغة الهندية يقع على الهليلج الكابلي والبليلج والاملج وثلاثتها مقوية للاعضاء العصبية
دابغة لآلات الغذاء من الفضلات جمعت وركبت لمشاركتها في المنفعة ومعونة بعضها
بعضا وجعلت متساوية الوزن لتشابه قواها ومنافعها وقد يضاف اليها الهليلج الاصفر
والبطرق والاسود الهندي مثل اوزانها لتقربهما منها في المزاج والمنفعة من التقوية والتنقية
فيصير اكمل واقوى فعلا وتلت بعد سحقها بالسمن او دهن اللوز لكسر شدة يبوستها
لان اليبوسة ضارة للقوة الهاضمة اذا جاوزت حد التقوية لآلات الغذاء ولذلك ادمان
الاطريفل يورث الهزال والسمن اولى لانه اقوى الادهان الموافقة لمزاج الانسان ان

استعمل في الوقت فانه اذا تاخر استعمالها فقد بين الموز اوى ماقت السمن بتمشى ويتغير
رائحته سريعا وقد ينتفع الاملج في اللبس ليزول بخمسه ويستر ثبثر املج وذلك في غير الاحر على
اول وينبغي ان يجعل العسل ضعف الادوية في الاطريفلات حيث يراد تمام نفعها وكا
وقد يجعل مثل اضعافها ليصير احر والطف واقل بشاعة وقد يجعل في المعاجين الاخر
كذلك حيث يراد تحجرها والعسل نيا احر واحد واقرب الى الدوائية ومطبوخ منزوع
الرغوة اسكن حدة وينبغي ان يصب على الماء ويطبخ حتى يعود الى القوام الاول ان
اريد طبخه وقد يتخذ الاطريفل من الهليلجات الثلاث حيث يكون غرض نفعه اهم
من غرض التقوية وقد يقتصر على الثلاث الاول مضاف اليها التربذ والمقل متساوية
للبواسير مع يبوسة الثفل ويغير التربذ اذا لم يكن في الطبع حبس ومع ما دونه انقباض
الحابسة للدم كالكهربا والجلنار وابزمارج والصدف محرق وانس نحوه مدبر
والبسد ونحوها على اوزان دونها اذا كان مع البواسير لين الطبع ويسد ... مدد
وعند ذلك يقلى البليلج والبليلج والاملج بالدهن لتنكسر قوة الاسهالية ويصير
عصرها قبضا وليختلط الدهن قواها الى المسافة البعيدة واسهل ... ان ... ذلك
لما ذكر ويطرح عنها العسل لما فيه من لحق الجلاء والمعونة على الاسهال ويجمع بالمقل
محلولا بماء الكراث لاختصاصه بالبواسير وحبسه الدم ويجب جمع ... نفعا
ليسهل انحلالها ونزولها الى الاسافل ويستر تحت المقل وقد يزاد على الاطريفل
الادوية التي تصلح للمعدة عند سوء مزاجها واجتماع الاخلاط فيها فعند سوء مزاجها البارد

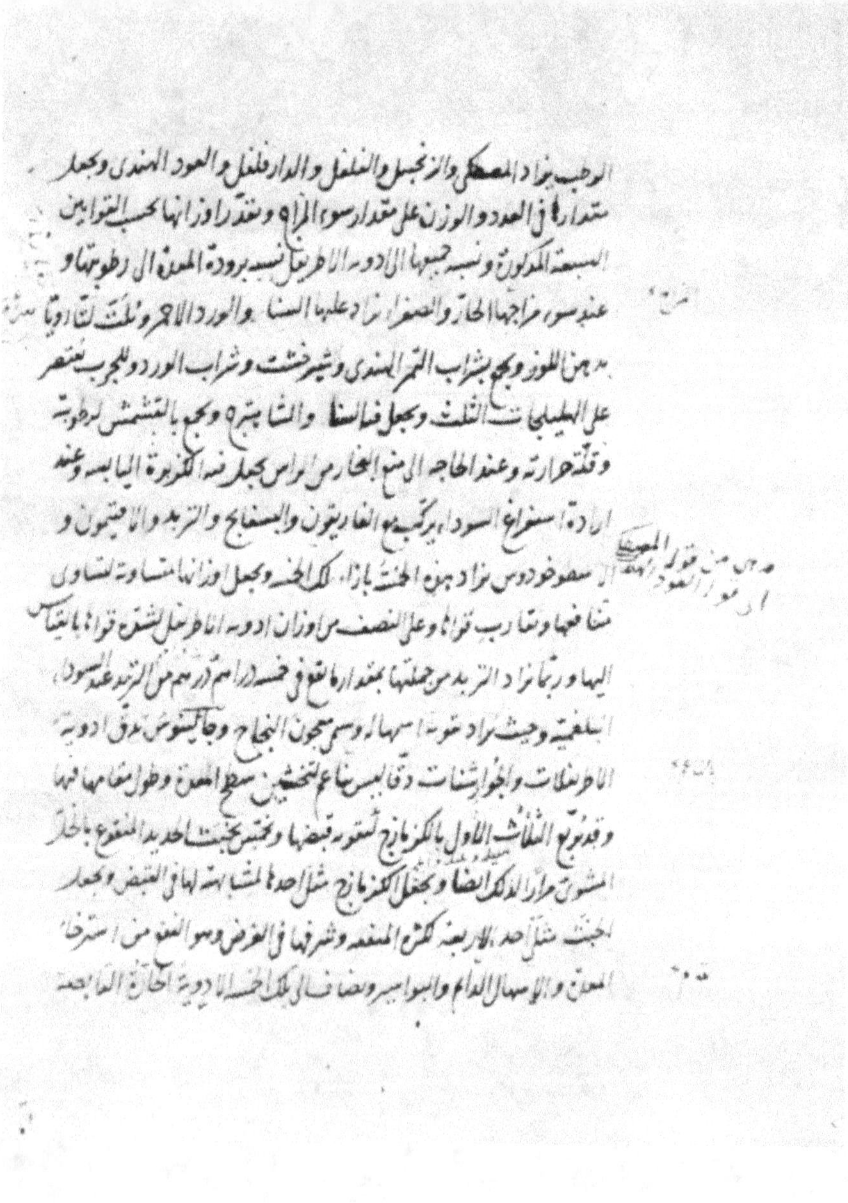

الرطب يزاد المصطكى والزنجبيل والفلفل والدارفلفل والعود الهندي ويجعل
مقدارها في العدد والوزن على مقدار سوء المزاج ويقدر اوزانها بحسب القوابض
السبعة المذكورة ونسبة جميعها الى ادوية الاطريفل نسبة برودة المعدة الى رطوبتها و
عند سوء مزاجها الحار والصفراء يزاد عليها السنا والورد الاحمر [illegible]
بدهن اللوز ويعجن بشراب التمر الهندي وشيرخشت وشراب الورد وللمجرب يقتصر
على الهليلجات الثلث ويجعل فيها السنا والشاهترج ويعجن بالمشمش لرطوبته
وقلة حرارته وعند الحاجة الى منع البخار من الراس يجعل فيه الكزبرة اليابسة وعند
ارادة استفراغ السوداء يركب مع الغاريقون والبسفايج والتربد والافتيمون و
الاسطوخودوس يزاد بوزن الجملة بازاء تلك الخمسة ويجعل اوزانها متساوية لتساوي
منافعها وتقارب قواها وعلى النصف من اوزان ادوية الاطريفل لشدة قواها بالقياس
اليها وربما يزاد التربد من جملتها بمقدار ما يقع في خمسة دراهم درهم من التربد عند السوداء
البلغمية وحيث يراد تقوية اسهالها وسمي معجون النجاح وجالينوس يدق ادوية
الاطريفلات والجوارشنات دقا ليس بناعم لتخشين سطح المعدة وطول مقامها فيها
وقد نوع الثلاث الاول بالكزمازج لتقوية قبضها ويحبس بخبث الحديد المنقوع بالخل
المشوي مرارا لذلك ايضا ويجعل الكزمازج مثل احدها لمشابهته لها في القبض ويجعل
الخبث مثل احد الاربعة لكثرة المنفعة وشرفها في الغرض وهو المنع من استرخاء
المعدة والاسهال الدائم والبواسير ويضاف الى تلك الخمسة الادوية الحارة [illegible]

اما الحارة فلتعديل تلك الخمسة الباردة وتسخن المعدة وتفتح السدد واما القبض فلانه هو المحفظ
الاول وهي مثل قشار الكندر والسعد والسنبل والاذخر والى نحوها المدبر بالخل
على نسبة دونها بمثل كر بعضها بعضا فما براد منها وقد يضاف اليها السكر والورد
لازدياد القبض ولتكون اقرب الى الاعتدال وهو يسمى معجون الخبث والفنجنكشت
معرّبا من الفارسية لمكان تلك الخمسة التي هي كالاصول فيه واما المفرحات فالتي تفعل بخاصيتها
وبما يتبعها من تلطيف الروح الغليظ ونشره وجمع الرقيق وتمتينه وتحيّاتها من تكثير
مادة الروح فينبغي ان تركب بقدر الحاجة اليها واما اذا كان ضعف بلا سوء مزاج فتركب
الحار مع البارد ة لتعتدل الكيفيات فيها وتجتمع الخواص وتكثر فيها عند ذلك ما تفعل
بالخاصية وليست الكيفية تعتد بها كالجواهر ويبالغ في سحقها وتصويلها واستعمال
الادوية المسهلة للسودا في المفرحات غير محمود لانها تثير السودا وتعجز عن اخراجها و
تضر بغوايلها ومزاحمتها لغيرها وقد يركب مع الادوية القلبية ادوية غير قلبية كبزر
الجبارس والفرنج والتوع والخشخش ونحو ذلك عند الحاجة الى كسر يبوسة الادوية القلبية
وتقوية تبريدها وادوية مبدرقة لها من جنسها ان كانت باردة جدا كالزعفران و
العنبر وقد يتخذ من الادوية المسهلات ومصلحاتها معاجين لتكون معدة لعلل و
حاجات تحدث ولا يحتمل الوقت تركيبها منها معجون الخيار شنبر للقولنج الحار والعلل
الصفراوية والبلغمية في الاحشاء يوخذ من البنفسج الاصفهاني والتربد من كل واحد
اربعون درهما ومن الملح الهندي سبعة دراهم ونصف ومن بزر الرازيانج والانيسون و

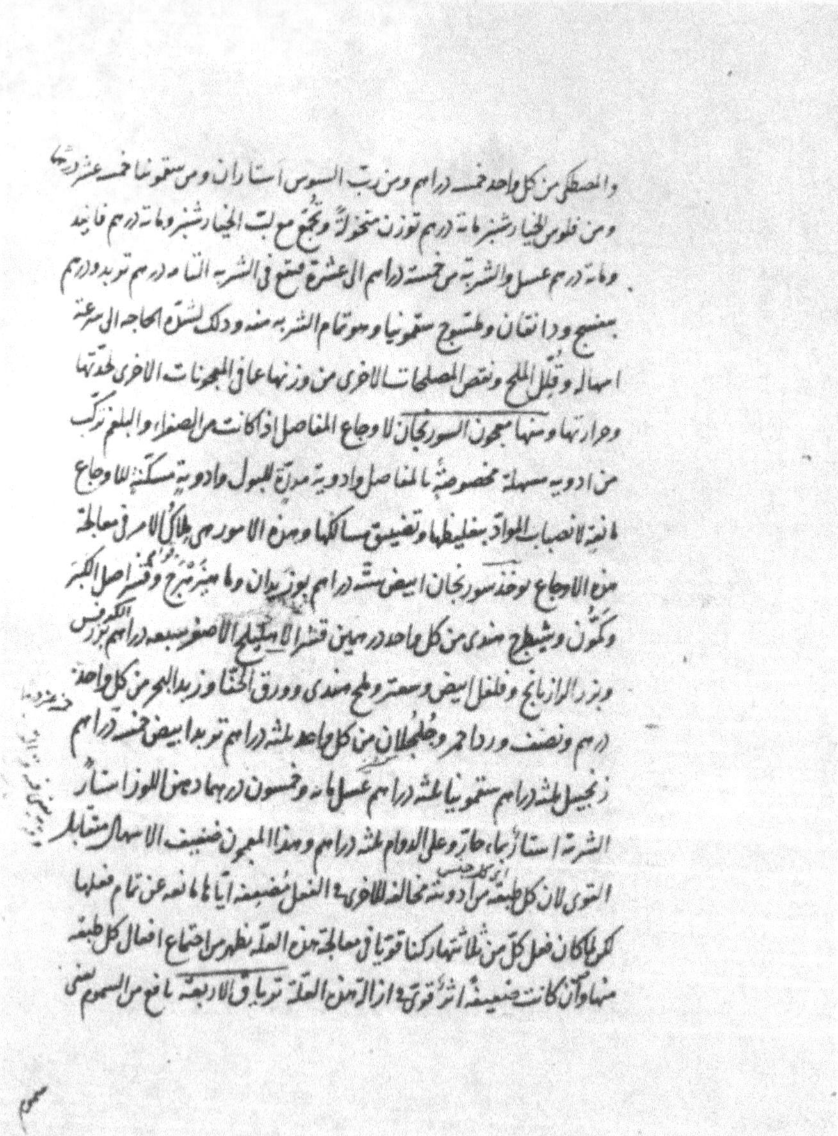

والمصطكى من كل واحد خمسة دراهم ومن رب السوس استاران ومن سقمونيا خمسة عشر درهما
ومن فلوس الخيار شنبر مائة درهم توزن منخولة وتجمع مع لب الخيار شنبر ومائة درهم فانيد
ومائة درهم عسل والشربة من خمسة دراهم الى عشرة ممتع في الشربة التامة درهم تربد ودرهم
بنفسج ودانقان وطبيخ سقمونيا وهو تمام الشربة منه وذلك لشدة الحاجة الى سرعة
اسهاله وقلل الملح ونقص المصلحات الاخرى من وزنها عن المعجونات الاخرى لحدتها
وحرارتها ومنها معجون السورنجان لاوجاع المفاصل اذا كانت من الصفراء والبلغم تركب
من ادوية مسهلة مخصوصة بالمفاصل وادوية مدرة للبول وادوية مسكنة للاوجاع
مانعة لانصباب المواد بتغليظها وتضييق مسالكها وهذه الامور هي ملاك الامر في معالجة
هذه الاوجاع يوخذ سورنجان ابيض ستة دراهم بوزيدان وماهيزهرج وقشر اصل الكبر
وكمون وشيطرج هندي من كل واحد درهمين قشر الاهليلج الاصفر سبعة دراهم بزر الكرفس
وبزر الرازيانج وفلفل ابيض وسعتر وملح هندي وورق الحنا وزبد البحر من كل واحد
درهم ونصف وورد احمر وجلجلان من كل واحد ثلثة دراهم تربد ابيض خمسة دراهم
زنجبيل ثلثة دراهم سقمونيا ثلثة دراهم عسل مائة وخمسون درهما دهن اللوز استار
الشربة استار بماء حار وعلى الدوام ثلثة دراهم وهذا المعجون ضعيف الاسهال متشابه
القوى لان كل طبقة من ادوية مخالفة للاخرى في الفعل مضعفة اياها مانعة عن تمام فعلها
لكن لما كان فعل كل من الاشتهار كنا قويا في معالجة هذه العلة يظهر من اجتماع افعال كل طبقة
منها وان كانت ضعيفة اثر قوي في ازالة هذه العلة ترياق الاربعة نافع من السموم يعني

سموم

سموم الحيوانات القاتلة بلدغها خاصة للعقرب ومن العلل البلغمية جنطيانا رومي
وحب الغار ومر مكي وزراوند طويل من كل واحد جزء يدق ويعجن بالعسل منزوع
الرغوة الشربة مثقال معجون بالخولنجان لتفتيت الحصاة وتنقية آلات البول يدق
الانخواه نا عما ويعجن بعسل الشربة مثقال معجون لتنقية الرئة اصل السوس الاسمانجوني
واصل السوس محكوكان مدقوقان يستعملان كل واحد منهما اما منفردا وللاخر اذا كان غرضا
النضج والتنقية متساويين او زائدا احدهما على الآخر بحسب زيادة احد الغرضين يعجن
بعسل والشربة مثقال او اقل او اكثر بحسب اختلاف وزنيهما واختلاف احوال العليل
في القوة والضعف ونضج اخلاط بالكمال او قصورها عن ذلك معجون لتنقية الامعاء من
البلاغم لب حب القرطم والتين مدقوقين وحليبا بهما متقويين يعجنان متساويين و
الشربة منها اوقية معجون ينفع السعال البلغمي بزر الكتان يقلى قليا خفيفا لتنقص
رطوبته الفضلية ويكتسب غروية وسخونة ازيد ثم يعجن بعسل واما الجوارشنات
فهي مثل المعاجين الا ان المعاجين تكون حلوة ومرة وكريهة وغير كريهة والجوارشنات
لا تكون الا طيبة ولفظ الجوارشن معرب من الفارسي ومعناه الهاضوم واطيب الجوارشنات
والذها جوارشن العود تقوي المعدة ويسخنها تسخينا لطيفا يخلط بالرطل من السكر
درهمان عود هندي مسحوق ويعقد على النار ويزاد عليه الزعفران والقرنفل والقاقلة
ونحوها فرادى ومجموعة بحسب الحاجة اليها وقد يمزج به رب الليمو بقدر ما يرززه فيكون
اطيب وقد يجعل بدله ماء الليمو فيكون اصفى واحسن والافاوية التي تستعمل في الجوارشنات

غرضا

الشربة من عشرة الى خمسة والعسل مقدار الكفاية

١

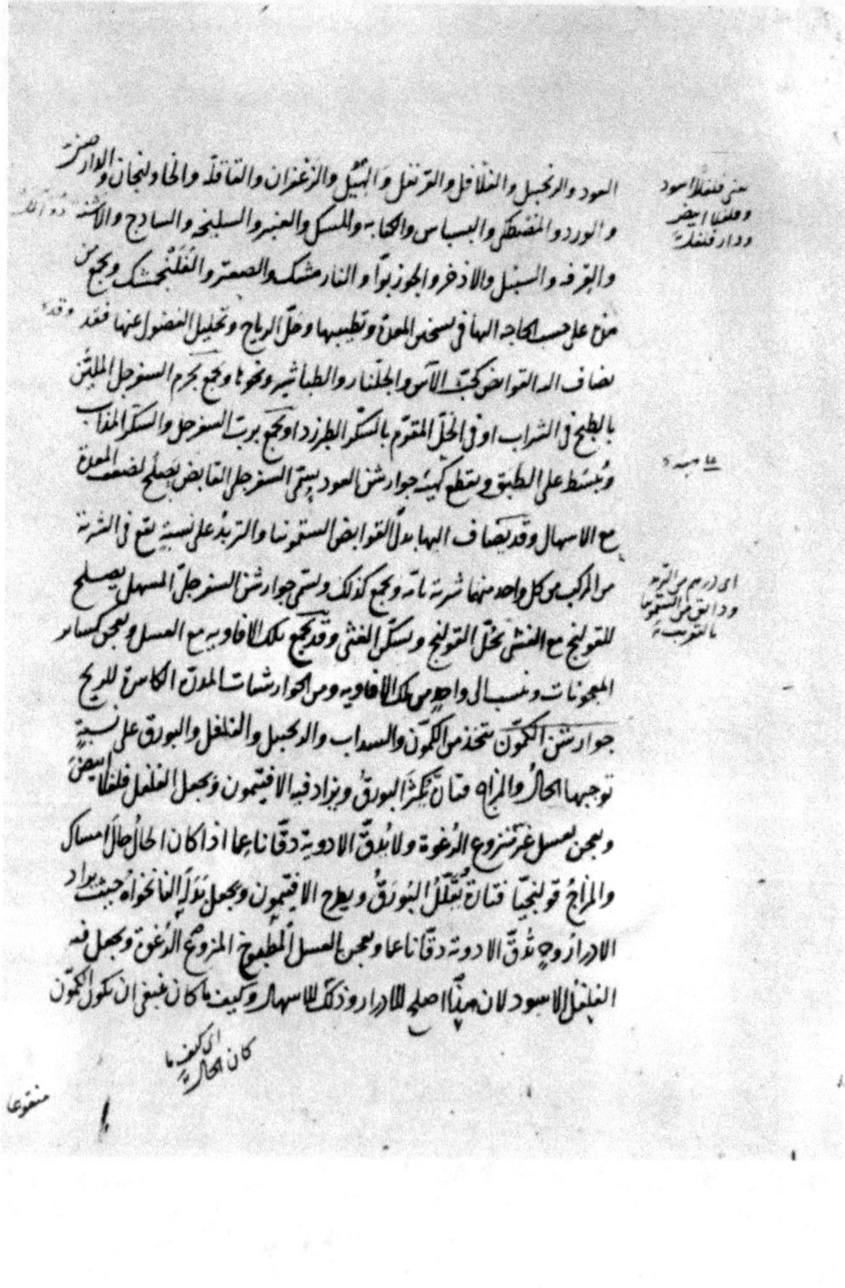

العود والزنجبيل والفلافل والقرنفل والهيل والزعفران والقاقلة والخاولنجان والدارصيني
والورد والمصطكى والبسباسة والكبابة والمسك والعنبر والسليخة والساذج والاشنه
والقرفة والسنبل والاذخر والجوزبوا والنارمشك والصعتر والقلنجمشك ويجمع من
منها على حسب الحاجة اليها في تسخين المعدة وتطييبها وحل الرياح وتحليل الفضول عنها فقد
يضاف اليه القوابض كحب الاس والجلنار والطباشير ونحوها ويجمع بجرم السفرجل الملبق
بالطبخ في الشراب او في الخل المقوم بالسكر الطبرزد او يجمع برب السفرجل والسكر المذاب
ويبسط على الطبق ويقطع كهيئة جوارش العود ويسمى السفرجلي القابض يصلح لضعف المعدة
مع الاسهال وقد يضاف اليها بدل القوابض السقمونيا والتربد على نسبة تقع في الشربة
من المركب من كل واحد منها شربة تامة ويجمع كذلك ويسمى جوارش السفرجلي المسهل يصلح
للقولنج مع الغثي يحل القولنج ويسكن الغثي وقد يجمع تلك الافاويه مع العسل ويعجن كسائر
المعجونات ويسمى باسم واحد من تلك الافاويه ومن الجوارشنات المدق الكامن للريح
جوارشن الكمون يتخذ من الكمون والسذاب والزنجبيل والفلفل والبورق على نسبة
توجبها الحال والمزاج فان كثر البورق ويزاد فيه الافتيمون ويجعل الفلفل فلفلا ابيض
ويعجن بعسل غير منزوع الرغوة ولا يدق الادوية دقا ناعما اذا كان الحال حال امساك
والمزاج قولنجيا فان يقلل البورق ويطرح الافتيمون ويجعل بدل الانخواه حيث يراد
الادرار وحينئذ يدق الادوية دقا ناعما ويعجن بالعسل المطبوخ المنزوع الرغوة ويجعل فيه
الفلفل الاسود لان هذا اصلح للادرار وذلك للاسهال وكيف ما كان ينبغي ان يكون الكمون

يعني فلفلا اسود وفلفلا ابيض ودار فلفل

اي درهم من التربد ودانق من السقمونيا

اي كيف ما كان الحال

منقوعا

منقوعا في الخل يغلو بعد ذلك فان الخل كالمصلح له والمقوي لتلطيفه وقد تتخذ جوارشن
من الادوية الحابسة القابضة ويجعل معها حب الآس ويغلب عليها ويعجن بعسل الطبرزد و
يسمى الخوزي الكبير منسوبا الى الاول من تخذه يصلح للاسهال المعدي مع برودة المزاج والخوزي
الصغير وهو المتخذ من عجم الزبيب المقلو وحب الآس والخرنوب النبطي والجلنار و
الجوارش ودقاق الكندر والنانخواه المدبر بالخل معجونا بعسل الطبرزد او برب السفرجل
يصلح للاسهال المعدي مع حرارة المزاج اذا جعل اكثر اجزائه عجم الزبيب ثم حب الآس
لمناسبتهما لآلات الغذاء بسبب غذائية فيهما ولكثرة منفعتهما ثم الادوية الاخرى
ويجعل دقاق الكندر والنانخواه من اقلها وربما يحتاج ان تكثر اجزاؤه حتى يلحقا الطبقة
التي تليهما في الوزن عند نقصان حرارة المزاج وقد تتخذ معاجين من ادوية كريهة منقية
لامراض شتى مثل التوليج واوجاع المفاصل ونقصان الباه وغير ذلك وتسمى جوارشنات
تطييبا للقلوب المنتان وليناً لها ولايخ ذلك من اثر في بعض النفوس وتجنب عنها واذا اتخذ
المعجون فينبغي ان يودع بستوقة ولا يملأ بل يترك فيها متسع لربوه وبسط فيها اذا غلا
وفار عند التخمر ولا تستوثق من راسها بحيث لا يجد متنفسا يخرج منه الابخرة وتوضع
البستوقة في الشعير ليحصر الحرارة وتعكسها فتتخمر تخمرا جيدا وبعد التخمر ورجوع حجمه الى
الحالة الاولى تخرج من الشعير ويستوثق راسها واولى الظروف بالمعاجين ما لا يوثر فيها ولا
يتاثر منها وهي الصينيات وما يشابهها من الصفائح ويقاربها في الجوهر وهو الزجاجيات
ومن الفلزات الذهب والفضة لانهما لا يصدآن صداء سائر الفلزات وبقاء قوى

المعاجين على قدر بقائها على لينها ولدونتها وطعومها وروائحها وسلامتها من الآفات
العارضة لها والله أعلم. الباب الثالث في الحبوب المسهلة والأيارجات
وهي أدوية مسهلة مجموعة مع مصلحاتها وما يكسر غوائلها ويعين على إسهالها تهيئة للمواد
وتلطيفا لها وإسالة. أيارج والأيارج معناه الشريف وتأويله المسهل المصلح وتفسير
الدواء الإلهي وإنما خصت المسهلات من الأدوية بالأمر الإلهي وإن كان جميع الموجودات
منه تبارك وتعالى لأن خواص المسهلات وقواها ليست من عالم الخلق والطبيعة بل من عالم
الأمر وهي أعني الأيارجات أقدم استعمالا من الحبوب استعملها القدماء وكانوا يقتصرون
عليها آمنين من غوائلها لكثرة المصلحات والفاذزهرات فيها واستفادتها من العسل
نحوا أو مزاجا ثم جسروا بعد ذلك على استعمال الحبوب وهي تصلح للادخار وتزداد جودة
به بخلاف الحبوب فإنها تصلح للوقت والحال قبل الجفاف والقانون المطرد في اتخاذ
الحبوب أن يجمع الأدوية المسهلة التي يحتاج إليها شربات تامة ويجمع مع مصلحاتها ثم يحسب عدد
المسهلات فيقسم الجميع على عددها إن كان اثنين فنصفين أو ثلاثة فأثلاثا أو أربعة فأرباعا
أو خمسة فأخماسا فيكون كل قسم شربة تامة ولكن لما لم تكن حاجتنا إلى جميع الأدوية المسهلة
التي ركبنا منها الحبوب وإلى أعمالها متساوية في جميع الأوقات بل تكون حاجتنا إلى
بعضها أكثر وإلى بعضها أقل واحتجنا كثيرا إلى أن نقع في الشربة منها شربة كاملة من واحد
منها فلو جمعناها شربات متساوية وقسمناها على أعدادها ما حصل لنا في شربة واحدة منها
من ذلك الواحد المطلوب فعله أكثر إلا شيء قليل قاصر عن بلوغ مرادنا ويجتمع عندنا شربات

ضعيفة لا يبلغ الواحد منها غرضنا وجعل الباقي ونضعف ونجمع في جل ذلك نصف
ذلك القانون وتركناه وصيرنا النسخة بدوا هو العاد والمعول عليه في غرضنا وتمنا
وزن الشربة منه على حسب ما توجب الحال والقوة ثم نتلو ذلك بالمسهلات الاخرى
المحتاج اليها على مراتبها بحسب الحاجة الى كثرتها وقلتها ثم بحسب اوزانها ونقتصر في
اقل الشربة على ثلثة دراهم ولا نتجاوز في اكثرها من اربعة دراهم ثم نكتب مصلح كل منها بأن
على الربع منه او على الثلث ان اردنا توهين قوته ثم نجمع الجميع بالمثل والكثير ان وقع فيه
ويجب حبوبا كبارا ان اتخذناها للدماغ والمعدة ليبطؤ نزولها او صغارا ان اتخذناها
للاسافل والاطراف حتى لا يطول وقوفها في المعدة فيحصل لنا شربة وافية تفي بغرضنا
وتسهل على مقدار حاجتنا وسأكتب من الحبوب نسخا على سبيل المثال والدستور ليحتذى
فيما يراد تركيبها منها حب لتنقية البدن من الاخلاط المختلفة تربد مثقال قشر
الاهليلج الاصفر نصف درهم افتيمون دانق ونصف غاريقون نصف درهم انطاكي
دانق ونصف ملح هندي دانق ونصف شحم الحنظل دانق ونصف زنجبيل دانق مصطكي
دانق انيسون دانق مقل دانقين كثيرا طسوج ورد احمر دانق آخر يسهل
السوداء والبلغم وينقي الدماغ تربد مثقال ايارج فيقرا درهم اسطوخودوس دانقان
غاريقون نصف درهم انطاكي دانق ونصف زنجبيل دانق ورد احمر دانق مقل دانقان
وايارج فيقرا مصلح للسقمونيا لما فيه من الافاويه فمتى اجتمعا كفاه مصلحا له آخر
يسهل الصفراء صالح للصدور وهو حب البنفسج بنفسج درهمان تربد مثقال

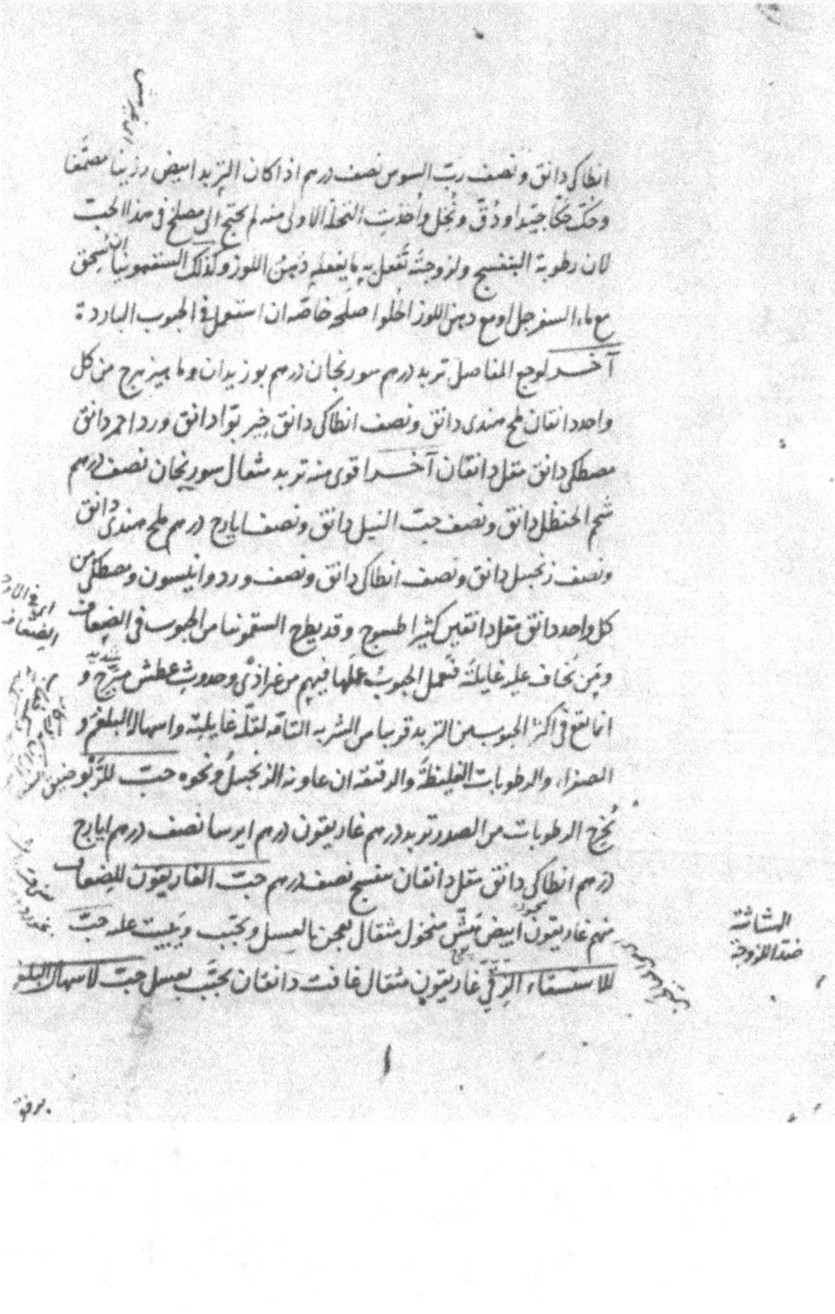

انطاكي دانق ونصف رب السوس نصف درهم اذا كان التربد ابيض رزينا مصمتا
وحك حكا جيدا ودق ونخل واخذت النخالة الاولى منه لم يحتج الى مصلح في هذا الحب
لان رطوبة البنفسج ولزوجته تفعل به ما يفعله دهن اللوز وكذلك السقمونيا ان يسحق
مع ماء السفرجل او مع دهن اللوز الحلو اصلحه خاصة ان استعمل في الحبوب الباردة :
آخر لوجع المفاصل تربد درهم سورنجان درهم بوزيدان وماهيزهرج من كل
واحد دانقان ملح هندي دانق ونصف انطاكي دانق خربق دانق ورد احمر دانق
مصطكي دانق مثقال دانقان آخر اقوى منه تربد مثقال سورنجان نصف درهم
شحم الحنظل دانق ونصف حب النيل دانق ونصف ايارج درهم ملح هندي دانق
ونصف زنجبيل دانق ونصف انطاكي دانق ونصف ورد وانيسون ومصطكي من
كل واحد دانق مثقال دانقين كثيرا الطبيخ وقد يطرح السقمونيا من الحبوب في الضعاف
ومن يخاف عليه غايلته فتعمل الحبوب عليها فيهم من غرادي وحدوث عطش مبرح و
انما نفع في اكثر الحبوب من التربد قريبا من الشربة التامة لقلة غايلته واسهال البلغم و
الصفراء والرطوبات الغليظة والرقيقة ان عاونه الزنجبيل ونحوه حب للتربو ضيق النفس
يخرج الرطوبات من الصدور تربد درهم غاريقون درهم ايرسا نصف درهم ايارج
درهم انطاكي دانق مثقال دانقان سنبج نصف درهم حب الغاريقون للضعاف
منهم غاريقون ابيض هش منخول مثقال يعجن بالعسل ويحبب ويبيت عليه حب
للاستسقاء الزق غاريقون مثقال غافث دانقان يحبب بعسل حب لاسهال البلغم

المشاشة ضد اللزوجة

برفق وهو دواء التربد توبد مثقالان زنجبيل نصف درهم يحبب بعسل حب لاسهال الصفراء
والبلغم برفق منضج درهمان تربد مثقال يحبب بشراب الورد حب يحط الثفل والنفخ
ويهضم ويبعث الشهوة وهو حب الأمير مصطكي ودارصيني وزنجبيل وقرنفل و
فلنجة ودار فلفل ونار مشك وسقمونيا وسكر من كل واحد عشرة دراهم تتخذ حبوبا كالحمص
من دانق الى دانقين ويؤخذ منها واحد فيستعمل مجلسا او اثنان فيستعملان مجلسين حب
لطيب النكهة يؤخذ منه في الفم غدوة وعشية ويبلع ماؤه سك وقرنفل قرفة زنجبيل
جوزبوا سعد سنبل قشور الاترج عود ني بالسوية يجمع برب المشمش وتتخذ حبوبا
كالحمص حب الملوك لمن يعاف المسهل وتعبيته تربد درهم وثلث درهم غاريقون
ثلث درهم هليلج اصفر دانق ونصف هليلج اسود دانق ونصف افتيمون نصف درهم
مصطكي ربع درهم لسان الثور سدس درهم فلنجمشك مثله زعفران مثله ورد احمر
مثله ويعجن بجلاب ويحبب واما الايارجات الكبار المنسوبة الى الاطباء
الاقدمين مثل هرمس وروفس وجالينوس وغيرهم فلتقدمها وكثرة تداول ايدي
الناسخين لها كثرت تخاليطها وهجرت لذلك ولما ترك لها اكثر المركبات وهم
وان كانوا مهتمين بتركيبها ومتدبرين لتآليفها وهي كالمعجزات الباقية عنهم زمانا طويلا
فالآن قد اندرست بتمامها وانطمس رسمها وما بقي الا اسمها للمتنبي شعر
تخلف الآثار عن اربابها حينا فيدركها الفناء فيتبع فسبيل المنتفع بها والمستمر
اياما ان يعرضها على قوانين المركب ويتصرف فيها بحسبها حتى يستقيم عليها ثم يجربها

بعد ذلك ولعل الله سدده لها ووفقه للصواب فيها وجدد تلك الموهبة لعباده
فالله تعالى هو المرشد والهادي اولا واخرا وقد اتخذت ايارج لوغاذيا على النسخة
المكتوبة والادوية الموجودة رايت ممن استعمل امرا عجيبا وذلك انه كان يجلس كل مجلس
بالاخلاط الثلثة متمايزا بعضها من بعض وقانون سقي ايارجات الكبار ان يسقى الشربة
منها معجونا مع درهم ملح النفط محلولا في مطبوخ من صفته افتيمون اربعة دراهم زبيب
منزوع العجم عشرة دراهم اهليلج اسود سبعة دراهم اسطوخودوس ثلثة دراهم يطبخ برطل
ونصف من الماء حتى يبقى نصف رطل ويصفى ويحل الايارج فيه ويسقى ويتجرع شيئا من
خلال الاسهال ماء العسل وماء السكر ويسقى بعد الاسهال بزر الخطمي والخبازي بجلاب
ودهن اللوز واما الايارج الفيقرا ومعناه المر فهو الصبر مع مصلحاته ولما كان الصبر
في نفسه بطيء الاسهال وكثر مصلحاته صار اسهاله ابطأ فيتاخر الى يوم او يومين ان سقي
مفردا ولم يتقو بمسهلات اخرى سريعة الاسهال والصبر وان كان اكثر اسهاله للصفراء فهو
ايضا يسهل البلغم فاذا ركب مع الافاويه والادوية الحارة الكثيرة صار اسهاله للبلغم اكثر
فهو اذن نافع من الامراض البلغمية المعدية والدماغية وادويته نسخة حب البلسان
وعوده وسنبل وسليخة واسارون ومصطكي ودارصيني وزعفران ثم الصبر
ضعف مثل الجميع وقد تصرف فيه المتاخرون وزادوا فيه ادوية واستبدلوا بعضا
ببعض بحسب اغراضهم ولم ذلك اذا ارادوا سقيه مفردا فاما اذا وقع في الحبوب المسهلة
واضيف اليها بحسب العلة وحال العليل فعند ذلك عن غيره نفسه غني واجود تصرفاتهم

فان ابدلوا الزعفران بالورد الاحمر جدا ان في بعض الاحوال عن حديد [illegible] وان

زادوا فيه المقل على وزن احد مصلحات الصبر شيئا مفترقة على اسهل وان عسوا الصبر

بماء الهندباء وجففوه لذوى الامراض الحارة والمتروك منه [illegible] عن قرب والمعجون

بالعسل اقوى اسهالا واسخن وتبقى قوته من سنة شهر الى اربعة [illegible] مثل سم

من الغايلة والشربة التامة منفردا [illegible] دراهم الباب [illegible] في المطبوخات و[illegible]

المطبوخات في المطلقات للمواد واما مسهلات [illegible] المطلقات [illegible]

الادوية الحارة وهي اما اصول مثل اصل الكرفس والرازيانج و[illegible]

والسوس والوج والعاقرقرحا والزنجبيل و[illegible]

الزراوند والبوزيدان واما بزور مثل بزر الرازيانج والكرفس والهندباء [illegible]

السداب والدوقو والشونيز والكروايا [illegible]

وبزر الكتان والمرز والحلبة والكمون واما حشايش [illegible]

والاذخر والقنطوريون والبرسياوشان والسنبل [illegible]

النور والفلنجمشك واما ثمار كالتين والزبيب والتمر والعناب والسبستان

وما يقرب منها كالعسل والفانيد والسكر فتركب منها المطبوخات لانضاج المواد

بحسب انواعها واصنافها وعلى مقدار برودتها وغلظها ولزوجتها واما المسهلات

من المطبوخات فقانون تركيبها مثل قانون تركيب الحبوب والامارجات على تفاوت

مقادير الشربة منها ومن المطبوخات وهي الطف منها والين واخف على الطباع

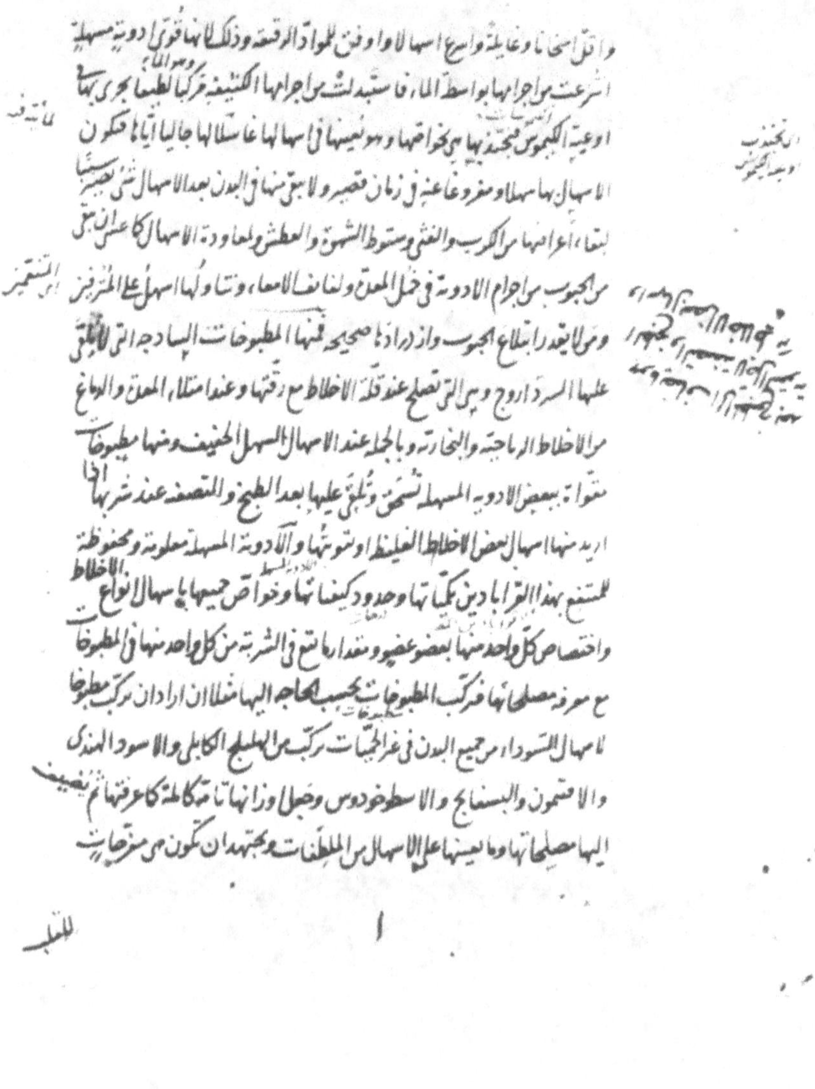

وأقل إسهالا وغايلة وأسرع إسهالا وأوفق للمواد الرقيقة وذلك لأنها قوى أدوية مسهلة
أسرعت من أجرامها بواسطة الماء فاستبدلت من أجرامها الكثيفة فركبا لطيفا يجري بها
أوعية الكيموس فيجذب بها من خواصها وهو نفسها في إسهالها غاسلا لها جاليا إياها فيكون
الإسهال بها سهلا ومفرغا في زمان قصير ولا يبقى منها في البدن بعد الإسهال شيء يصير سببا
لبقاء أعراضها من الكرب والغثي وسقوط الشهوة والعطش ولمعاودة الإسهال كما عسى أن يبقى
من الحبوب من أجرام الأدوية في خمل المعدة ولفائف الأمعاء وتناولها أسهل على المترفين
ومن لا يقدر ابتلاع الحبوب وإذا أراد ما صحيحة فمنها المطبوخات الساذجة التي لا يلقى
عليها السكر والأدوية وهي التي تصلح عند قلة الأخلاط مع رقتها وعند امتلاء المعدة والدماغ
من الأخلاط الزجاجية والبخارية وبالجملة عند الإسهال السهل الخفيف ومنها مطبوخات
مقواة ببعض الأدوية المسهلة تسحق وتلقى عليها بعد الطبخ والتصفية عند شربها إذا
أريد منها إسهال بعض الأخلاط الغليظة أو تقويتها والأدوية المسهلة معلومة ومحفوظة
للمتنفع بهذا القراباذين بكمياتها وحدود كيفياتها وخواص جميعها بإسهال أنواع الأخلاط
واختصاص كل واحد منها بعضو عضو ومقدار ما يقع في الشربة من كل واحد منها في المطبوخات
مع معرفة مصلحاتها فتركب المطبوخات بحسب الحاجة إليها فإذا أراد أن يركب مطبوخا
لإسهال السوداء من جميع البدن في غير الحميات تركب من الهليلج الكابلي والأسود الهندي
والأفتيمون والبسفايج والأسطوخودوس وحبل وزنها تامة كاملة كما عرفتها ثم يضيف
إليها مصلحاتها وما يعينها على الإسهال من الملطفات ويجتهد أن تكون من مزاجات

للقلب ايضا مقويات للروح نكاية السوداء فربما خاصة عند حركته و... منه من معارة
فيجعلها مثل الباذرنجبويه ولسان الثور والورد والدرونج والفلنجمشك وجعل ...
من مفتحات السدد ومفتحات المجاري مثل الانيسون والغافت والكشوث وبزر الكرفس
والرازيانج والمضعفات مثل التين والزبيب واصل السوس وما يقوي ... الرئة
وحفظ قواها مثل الراوند وبزر الهندبا للكبد والادوية الطيبة العطرة مثل التي تقدم ذكرها
للقلب والدماغ ثم يدق ما صلب منها دقا جريشا ويبل جميعه خلا الافتيمون ويترك ليلة
ثم يصب عليه من الغد ثلثة ارطال ماء ويطبخ الى ان يرجع الى رطل ثم يصفيه و... ويمرس
الافتيمون باليد وقد انقع في الماء الشديد السخونة ليلة مرسا جيدا ويصفيه بخرقة ويجمع
بينهما ويترك حتى يصفو ثم ياخذ الصافي منه ويحل فيه بعضه من الفلوس الخيار شنبر وزن اوقية
ويصفيه بمصفاة او يحل في بعضه من الشيرخشت والترنجبين ثلث اواق ويصفيه من الشوك
والتراب ويجمع بينهما ويشرب بكرة ان كان الزمان حارا او ضحوة النهار ان كان الزمان
باردا ليكون الاسهال في اعدل اوقات النهار والطفه ويمنع الغثيان ان حدث بمص سفرجل
والتفاح وشمهما وشم الماورد والخل المرشوشين على الطين المحرق في الشمس ومضغ الطرخون
والنعناع وبشد العضدين بعصابة كل ذلك لتسكين النفس وتقويه الروح الطبيعي وجمعه
ومنعه من الحركة الى فوق ومضغ السفرجل ومصه بعد المطبوخات جيدا ان ابطا شيء
عليها وكذلك بعد الجوارشنات ابطات في الانحدار بعد انحلالها لتقوية فم المعدة وعصره عليه حتى
تدفع الدواء الى قعر المعدة فاما تجرع الماء الحار على المطبوخات فمما يومن قوتها بغسلها بخلاف

مجوب فانه برقعها ويتنزل بها من ناحيه في العمل هذا هو المطبوخ السانج وما من اراد
موته وان يسهل السوداء الغليظ ايضا فيلق عند عند الشرب بهذه العلاوة غاريقون
منخول بغرمه قوق درهم ملح نفط دانق ونصف تربد ثلثا درهم سقمونيا دانق مصطكي دانق
والاجود ان يعجنها بشي من المطبوخ ثم يحل فيه وقد يتخذ منه العدوة حب ويسقى قبل سقي
المطبوخ بساعتين تليث فان كانت السوداء متولدة عن احتراق صفراء زيد في المطبوخ الاهليلج
الاصفر والسنا والشاهترج والافسنتين وان كانت متولدة من احتراق البلغم زيد فيه
التربد والبليلج والاملج وفي السوداء وج الزنجبيل والايارج وكذلك اذا كانت العلة مركبة من
خلطين او اكثر كان المطبوخ مركبا بحسب ذلك واذا كانت المادة راسخة في عضو بعينه جعل
في المطبوخ ما يخص ذلك العضو بعد الادوية المشتركة النافعة لجميع البدن مثل اذا اتخذ لوجع المفاصل
جعل فيه من السورنجان والبوزيدان والماهيزهرج وفي علاوته من شحم الحنظل وحب النيل و
متى اتخذ لتنقية الصدر جعل فيه برسياوشان وبزر الخطمي واصله والزوفى والعناب و
السبستان واصل السوس والزبيب وطرح عنه الهليلجات وجعل بدلها البنفسج وكذلك
اذا اتخذ للحميات تطرح الهليلجات ايضا لتجفيفها وايراثها بعد الاسهال يبوسة في
المجاري بسبب تضييقها وسددها وملاك الامر في علاج الحميات تفتيح السدد التي هي سبب
عفونة الاخلاط ويزاد في الحميات ما يسهل بالارخاء مثل البنفسج والفواكه كالاجاص
والتمر الهندي والمشمش والعناب والسبستان وما يفتح السدد مثل اصل الهندباء وبزره و
والريوند والغافت والكشوث وكذلك ان اتخذ لتنقية الدماغ سقي مع شراب الورد

وجعل في العلاوة الايارج وكذلك للمعدة مثل الافسنتين وللطحال مثل ...
مثل ورق عنب الثعلب ونحوه وهكذا الافسنتين للامعاء ...
... والزجاجية او للجلد وتنقيته من مادة الجرب ...
والحجارة ... لكل واحد منها ما يختص بذلك العضو وتلك المادة وكلما ... حاجة
ونقصت اخرى يزاد وينقص بحسبها واما المنقوعات فهي اضعف من المطبوخات
الساذجة ونسبتها الى المطبوخات الساذجة نسبة المطبوخات الساذجة الى المطبوخات
المقواة بالسرداروج لان الغليان والطبخ يعين على الادوية في استخراج قواها وتحلل
بعض اجرامها بالماء ويحلل ما لطف منها خاصة ما كان من الادوية مزاجه رخوا سريع التحلل
الطبخ قواه كالافتيمون وكثير من الحشايش واذا كانت لطائف اجزاء الادوية وحارة
التركيب يبلغ مبلغا يسلب الغسل قوتها كالهندبا ونحوه فكم بالحري ان يحلل حرارة القوية
الشديدة والطبخ الطويل قواها والمنقوع اخف من المطبوخ وابرد ايضا فانه لا يكتسب من
حرارة النار ما يكتسب المطبوخ فلذلك هي اوفق في الحميات والامراض الحارة والمترفين
المستبشعين للادوية الكريهة الطعوم والروائح واكثر ما يراد من المنقوعات في الحميات
تليين البطن مع تسكين الحرارة وفي غير الحميات اخراج المواد بالرفق قليلا قليلا ومن
المنقوعات المستعملة في الحميات منقوع الفواكه مثل تمر الهندي والاجاص والتلك
والمشمش والخيارشنبر والعناب والسبستان ونقيع في ماء الورد وماء الرمان المز
المشوم ويستنبط مثل الشيرخشت او الترنجبين او السكر او شراب الورد او شراب البنفسج

بقدر الحاجة الى الحلاوة والمرارة والحموضة ومنها الطف النقوعات واطيبها وقد ينقع فلوس
الخيار شنبر في ماء الهندباء المعصور وماء ورق عنب الثعلب وماء الرازيانج لامراض الكبد وفي
ماء الشاهترج وماء الكشوث وماء اللبلاب وماء الهندباء المجرب في المواد الحارة ويلقى عليه
سقمونيا وبنفسج واهليلج اصفر حيث يراد تقويتها واما النقوعات المتخذة من
الادوية فهي والمطبوخات سواء في التركيب واذا اخذت نقعت في الماء بقدر ما يغمرها
الماء اصبعين ثلثة ويوضع في الشمس بالنهار في قنينة مشدودة الراس وفي التبن او اللبد
بالليل ويسقى بعد ثلثة ايام معصورة باليد مصفاة بخرقة متواة وغير متواة وقد ينقع
الصبر في العصارات والنقوعات لتنقية المعدة والدماغ والصبر على شرب نقيع الصبر
اشد على اكثر المرضى من احتمال المرض فان كان ولا بد فينبغي ان يحبب ويلبس كل حبة قميصا
من الناطف ويسقى قبل النقوع بساعة وقد ينقع التربد مجرشا ويوضع في الشمس اياما
حتى ياخذ الماء قوته ويخلط به ما انحل فيه من لبنه وصمغه وبعض اجزائه الصغار ثم يوخذ
ذلك الماء ويعقد في الشمس فيصير الطف ما يكون واخفه على الطبع وابعد من الغائلة و
كذلك يفعل بالهليلج الاصفر الباب الخامس في الحقن والشيافات والفرازج
واما تركيب الحقن المسهلة فقريب من تركيب المطبوخات لانها مركبة من ادوية مسهلة
وادوية ملطفة يلقى عليها السرداروج كما يلقى على المطبوخات لكن بعض المسهلات لا يدخل
لها في الحقن كالصبر والهليلجات كما لا يدخل بعض ادوية الحقن في المطبوخات من
الملينات والمزلقات وهي انما تستعمل في الحميات واورام الاحشاء ويبوسة

الثقل تتخذ من الاشياء التي تسهل بالتليين والازلاق واجداد بنفسج وخطمي وسمسم
والنخالة والعناب والسبستان والسلق وورق الهندباء وحب ... ونيلوفر
والخطمي وبزر الكتان واصل السوس والزبيب ونحوه وتحقن بالادهان الباردة
الرطبة كدهن البنفسج ودهن النيلوفر ودهن اللوز والبنفسج و... وخيار شنبر
والسكر ويزاد عليها في القولنج البارد الكرنب والاكليل والبابونج والبورق و...
تستعمل في القولنج البارد ونحوه من الامراض الباردة وتتخذ من الاشياء التي تسهل مع...
والتحليل ومن المحللات القوية مثل القنطوريون والسذاب والقيصوم والفوتنج والترمس
وشحم الحنظل والبسفايج والاكليل والبابونج والشبت والكرنب وورقه وحب حرمل
المدقوق والحلبة والتين وورقه والزبيب والصعتر والحسك والشهدانج والحرمل
وبزر الرازيانج والكرفس والكمون والانيسون والمرزنجوش والخروع المرضوض ونحوها
وتحقن بالادهان الحارة كدهن الزيت والزنبق والخيري واللوز المر ودهن البزر و
ماء العسل والفانيد والمري ويلقى عليها الزبد وشحم الحنظل والملح الهندي والجاوشير
والسكبينج والمقل والاشق والجندبيدستر تستعمل منها بقدر الحاجة وسهولة العلة
وصعوبتها ومراعاة قوانين التركيب ومحافظة النسب منها واذا اتخذت لاوجاع المفاصل
المزمنة زيدت الملطفات كالعاقرقرحا والزنجبيل والحاشا وحب الغار والمرماحوز
والابهل واصل الكبر والمسهلات المخصوصة بها مثل السورنجان والبوزيدان والماهيزهرج
وكذلك اذا زيدت للاخلاط السوداوية زيد فيها الافتيمون ونحوه وان حقنت للديدان

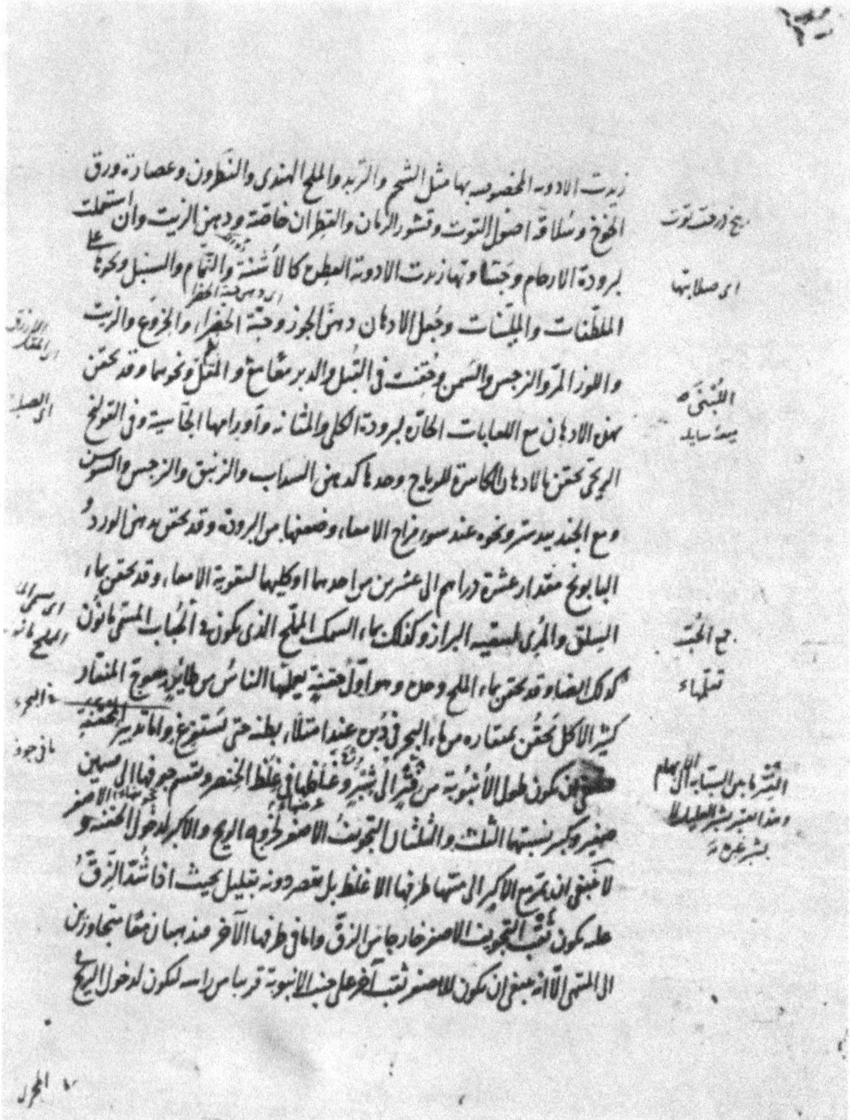

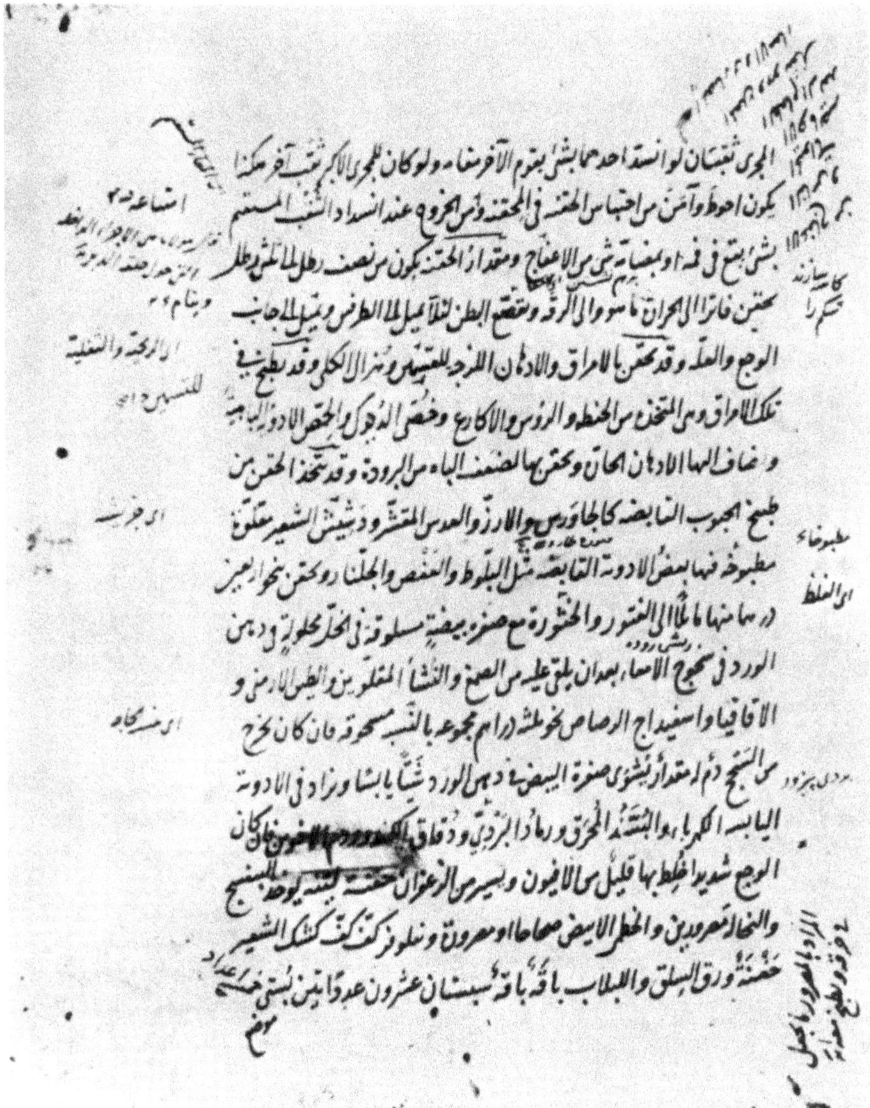

المجرى ثقبتان لو انسد احدهما بشيء يقوم الآخر مقامه ولو كان للمجرى الاكبر ثقب آخر لكان هذا
يكون احوط وآمن من احتباس الحقنة في المحقنة ومن الخروج عند انسداد الثقب المستقيم
بشيء يقع في فمه او بغضاضة شيء من الاعفاج ومقدار الحقنة يكون من نصف رطل الى ثلثي رطل
تحقن فاترا الى الحرارة ما هو والى الرقة وتقعقع البطن لئلا يميل الى الطرفين ويميل الى جانب
الوجع والعلة وقد تحقن بالامراق والادهان اللزجة للعتيقين ومن زال الكلى وقد يطبخ في
تلك الامراق وهي المتخذة من الحنطة والرؤوس والاكارع وخصى الديوك والحقن الادوية الباهية
ويضاف اليها الادهان الحارة وتحقن بها لضعف الباه من البرودة وقد تتخذ الحقن من
طبيخ الحبوب القابضة كالجاورس والارز والعدس المقشر وسويق الشعير مقلوة
مطبوخة فيها بعض الادوية القابضة مثل البلوط والعفص والجلنار وتحقن بنحو اربعة
دراهم منها ما يمال الى الفتور والخثورة مع صفرة بيضة مسلوقة في الخل محلولة ودهن
الورد في تجوج(?) الامعاء بعد ان يلقى عليه من الصمغ والنشا المقلوين والطين الارمني و
الاقاقيا واسفيذاج الرصاص نحو ثلثة دراهم مجموعة بالتبن(?) محروقة فان كان يخرج
من السحج دم لمقدار يشوى صفرة البيض في دهن الورد شيئا يابسا ويزاد في الادوية
اليابسة الكهربا والبسذ المحرق ورماد البردي ودقاق الكندر ودم الاخوين فان كان
الوجع شديدا خلط بها قليل من الافيون ويسير من الزعفران حقنة ليست يوخذ البنج
والنخالة مصروفين والخطمي الابيض صحاحا او مصروفة ونيلوفر كف كف كشك الشعير
حفنة وورق السلق والبلاب باقة باقة سبستان عشرون عددا تين بستي خمسة عدد
مويز(?)

غافث عشرة اعواد يطبخ برطلين ماء حتى يبقى ثلث رطل ويصفى ويخلط بلعاب بزر قطونا و
دهن الخل والسكر الاحمر والمري من كل واحد اوقية حقنة حادة قنطوريون ثلثة دراهم
حلبة ولب القرطم المرضوض وبزر الكتان [illegible] اكليل الملك وبابونج اوقية اوقية
شبث وسذاب وورق الكرنب وورق السلق والنونخواه الجبلي حزمة حزمة سبستان
مرضوض نصف اوقية كمون وبزر الانجدان كف كف تين عشرة اعداد يطبخ الجميع بخمسة
ارطال ماء حتى يرجع الى رطلين ثم يصفى ويحقن بثلثي رطل مع دهن الشونيز شحم الحنظل
وانطاكي والملح الهندي من كل واحد دانق ونصف بورق وتربد ابيض من كل واحد [illegible]
درهم سكبينج وجاوشير وسنبل من كل واحد ثلثة دراهم فانيذ ودهن الياسمين ومري
من كل واحد اوقية واما الشيافات المسهلة المستعملة في تليين البطن في القولنج وبقية
الامعاء وما يليها فحالها حال الحقن في اللين والخشونة ونسبتها الى الحقن المسهلة نسبة
الحبوب المسهلة الى المطبوخات المسهلة وهي طوال في طول الاصبع وازيد لتصل الى
المعاء المستقيم ويصل اثرها الى القولون اذا اريدت لعلاج القولنج واما اذا اتخذت
لوجع الورك والنسا فتجعل فرازج مدحرجة لتطول بقاؤها في موضع قريب من المقعدة
واما اللينة المستعملة منها في الحيات فالسهلة [illegible] وابسطها الرخبين الذي
هو باقية اللبن المنعقد ثم الناطف المتخذ من السكر الاحمر فانه يقتر عليه عند العقد قليل
ملح مسحوق ثم فرزجة الفار يعجن بالناطف وقد يجمع منهما جميعا وتتوى بالبورق الارمني
المسحوق وقد يزاد عليها الحنظل والبنفسج سمر قيس وقد يحمل عند يبوسة الامعاء و

قنطوريون

سبستان

سنبل الورق والحاجب [illegible]

البرزجة هي قطعة [illegible] الشيافات

صنعة الناطف ان يعقد السكر المحلول او العسل على نار هادئة وبساط [illegible] بحيث اذا اخذ منه وبرد يكسر [illegible]

جفاف النيل شيافة تتخذ من الزبد شديدة الانجاد بالثلج واقوى من الجميع شياف
السكبينج وصنعته سكبينج وسكر احمر ورخبين من كل واحد خمسة دراهم سقمونيا وتربد
وبورق من كل واحد ثلثة دراهم وهذه الثلثة الاخرى اقوى فعلا واشد كيفية
بالقياس الى الثلثة الاولى فيقلل مقدارها ويكثر مقدار تلك ملح هندي درهمان
ويقلل مقدار الملح جدا لاجتماع سببي التحليل وهما شدة التوق ووجود ادوية
المركب بفعل فعله ويشاركه في المنفعة واختص بالتحليل دونها وان كانت الاربعة
جميعا شديدة التوق مشتركة النفع لتلك منفعتها بالقياس اليها وهي التوق الاسهالية
مذاب السكر والرخبين ويذر عليها الادوية ويشيف واما الحادة المحتاج
اليها في القولنج البارد وتسخين الظهر واسهال البلغم من نواحيه فاحدها واسرعها
اسهالا الصابون وخصوصا الرقي اذا خرطت منه شيافة واحتملت او
جمع مع الفانيذ والعسل على النار ويذر عليها الملح المسحوق والبورق والتربد
والزنجبيل وشحم الحنظل وسقمونيا ونحوها من الادوية المسهلة والمحللة للرياح مثل
الشونيز والكمون والجندبيدستر ونحوها او يجمع هذه مع الصموغ الحادة كالجاوشير
والسكبينج والاشق والمقل بحسب الحاجة اليها على نسبة موافقة لتوافق المركب
اسم دواء مركب شيافة حادة تحل القولنج سكبينج جاوشير مقل اشق ملح هندي شحم الحنظل
بورق سقمونيا حب النيل يجمع متساوية لمساواة بعضها بعضا في التوق والمنفعة
وتحل الصموغ بماء السذاب ويجمع بها الباقي مدقوقة منخولة وتشيف وكذ

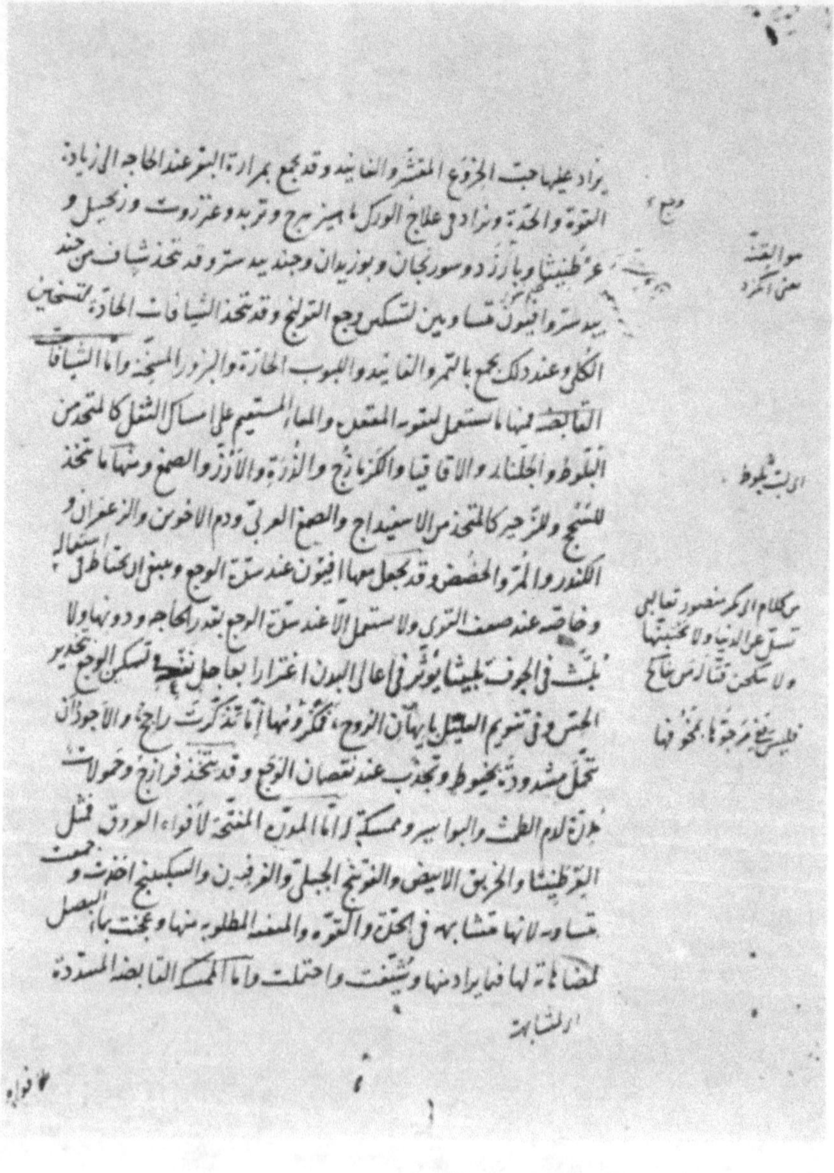

يراد عليها حب الخروع المقشر والعابد وقد يجمع بمرارة البقر عند الحاجة الى زيادة
القوة والحدة ويزاد في علاج الورك ماميزهرج وتربد وعنزروت وزنجبيل و
عرطنيثا وبارزد وسورنجان وبوزيدان وجندبيدستر وقد يتخذ شياف من جند
بيدستر وافيون متساوين لتسكين وجع القولنج وقد تتخذ الشيافات الحادة لتسخين
الكلى وعند ذلك يجمع بالتمر والعابد واللبوب الحارة والبزور المسخنة واما الشيافات
القابضة فمنها ما يستعمل لنتوء المقعد والمعا المستقيم على مساك الثقل كما يتخذ من
البلوط والجلنار والاقاقيا والكزمازج والذرة والارز والصمغ ومنها ما يتخذ
للسحج والزحير كالمتخذ من الاسفيداج والصمغ العربي ودم الاخوين والزعفران و
الكندر والمر والحضض وقد يجعل معها افيون عند شدة الوجع وينبغي ان يحتاط في استعمال
وخاصة عند ضعف القوى ولا يستعمل الا عند شدة الوجع بقدر الحاجة ودونها ولا
يلبث في الجوف طويلا ليؤثر في اعالي البدن اعتزازا بعاجل نفعه في تسكين الوجع بتخدير
الحس وفي تنويم العليل لا ليهابان الروح فكثر منها اما اتخذت راتجة والاجود ان
تحمل مشدودة بخيوط وتجذب عند نقصان الوجع وقد يتخذ فرازج وحمولات
لدرور الطمث والبواسير ومسكة واما الدرور المنتجة لافواه العروق فمثل
الفرطنيثا والخربق الابيض والشونيز الجبلي والفربيون والسكبينج اخذت وجمعت و
متساوية لانها متشابهة في الحق والقوة والمنفعة المطلوبة منها وعجنت بماء البصل
لمضادة لها فيما يراد منها ويشفت واحتملت واما المسكة القابضة المسددة
المشابهة

لا فواه تلك العروق مثل الكحل والعفص والشب والقاقيا والشكاعى والكندر
والجلنار ومن الادوية قريبة ايضا بعضها من بعض متساوية اوزانها الا الكندر
تقلل الحرارة وتجمع الجميع بالصمغ العربي وتتخذ منه شيافات صغار مثل نوى
الغبيراء وكذلك كل ما حمل في النبل من الزرازيج المعينة على الحبل تتخذ من الاقاقيا
والطيوب والصموغ وغير ذلك وقد تتخذ شيافات لديدان البطن من شحم الحنظل
والقنبيل وحب النيل والشيح والافسنتين ونوى المشمش المر وماء ورق الخوخ
محلولا فيه الصبر الباب السادس في ادوية التي المغذيات في اجناس جنس
تنقي الصفراء وجنس تنقي السوداء اما التي تنقي الصفراء اما من قبيل الاغذية
فماء الشعير والخيار والبطيخ النضيجان بشحمها واوراق البقول اللينة كالرجلة
والاسفاناخ والملوخية واليمانية وورق السلق واوراق الزرايج واطراف
الخرفان والسمك الطري والاحساء الدسمة بدهن الحل والترنجبين واما من قبيل
الادوية فالسكنجبين مع ماء الشعير الذي طبخ فيه اللوبيا الاحمر وقشور البطيخ و
اصول الملوخية المقطوعة وكذلك لحم البطيخ المقدد والفقاع المتخذ بدقيق الشعير
وبزر الرمق وبزر البطيخ واما التي تنقي البلغم اما من قبيل الاغذية فمرق الكشكية
كشك الحنطة بالشبث واللفتية والجزرية والنخلية وطبيخ الحلبة ودبس الرطب
والطبيخ والكوامخ مثل المري وكامخ الكبر وصباغ الخردل وزيتون الماء والعسل
واما من قبيل الادوية فالسكنجبين العسلي والعنصلي بماء النخل وماء الشبث والبورق

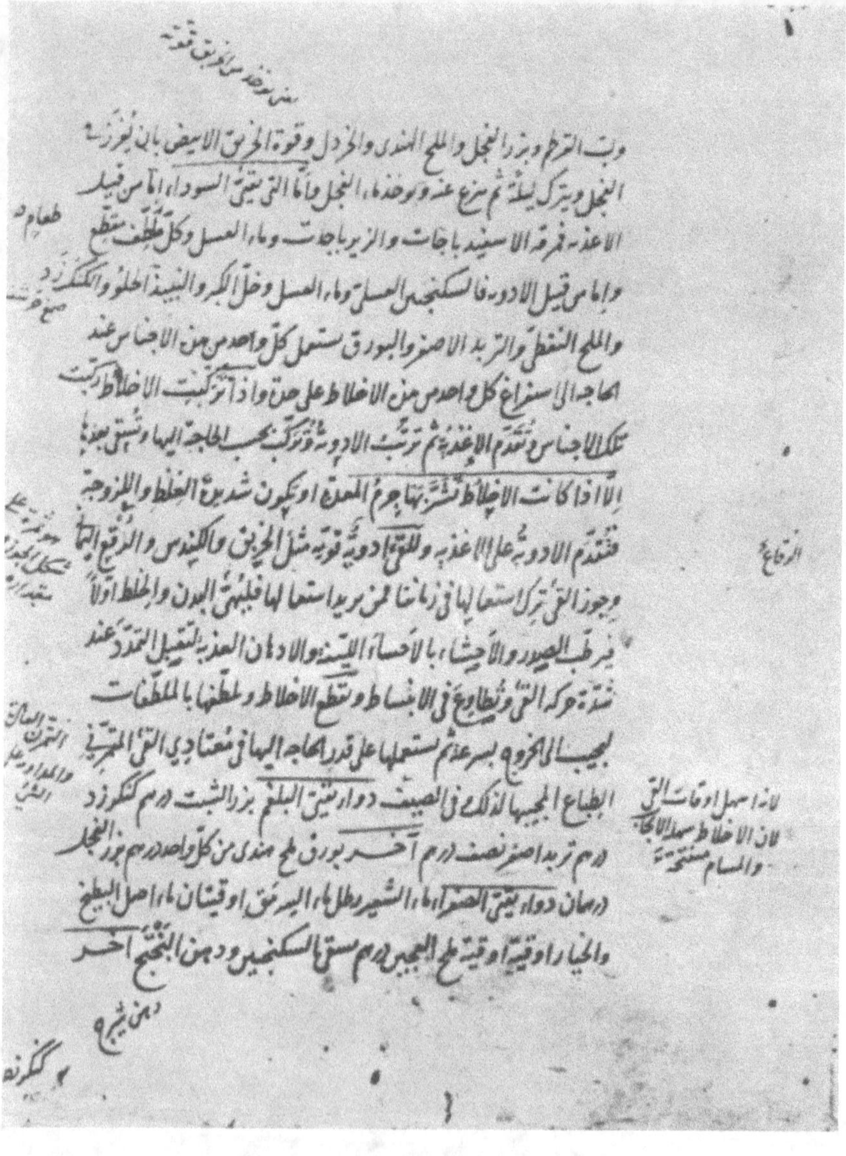
وب الترمس وبزر النجل والملح الهندي والخردل وقوة الخربق الابيض بان يغرز في
النجل ويترك ليلة ثم ينزع عنه ويوخذ ماء النجل واما التي تنقي السوداء اما من قبيل
الاغذية فمرقة الاسفيدباجات والزيرباجات وماء العسل وكل لطيف مقطع
واما من قبيل الادوية فالسكنجبين العسلي وماء العسل وخل الكرم والنبيذ الحلو والكنكرزد
والملح النفطي والزبد الاصغر والبورق يستعمل كل واحد من الاجناس عند
الحاجة الى استفراغ كل واحد من الاخلاط على حدة واذا تركبت الاخلاط تركبت
تلك الاجناس وتقدم الاغذية ثم ترتب الادوية وتركب بحسب الحاجة اليها وتسقى بعدها
الا اذا كانت الاخلاط تشربها جرم المعدة او يكون شديد الغلظ واللزوجة
فتقدم الادوية على الاغذية وللقي ادوية قوية مثل الخربق والكندس و[illegible]
وجوز القي ترك استعمالها في زماننا لمن يريد استعمالها فلينقي البدن والخلط اولا
بترطيب الصدور والاحشاء بالاحساء اللينة والادهان العذبة لتقبل التمدد عند
شدة حركة القي وتطاوع في الانبساط وتقطع الاخلاط ولطفها بالملطفات
ليجيب الى الخروج بيسر عنده ثم تستعملها على قدر الحاجة اليها في معتادي القي المتمرنين
الطباع المجيبها الذكرة في الصيف دواء تنقي البلغم بزر الشبث درهم كنكرزد
درهم تربد اصفر نصف درهم آخر بورق ملح هندي من كل واحد درهم بزر النجل
درهمان دواء تنقي الصفراء ماء الشعير رطل ماء [illegible] او قيشان ماء اصل البطيخ
والخيار اوقية او قية ملح العجين درهم يسقى بالسكنجبين ودهن البنفسج آخر

كنكرزد درهم تربجبين عشرة دراهم مع وحب مقيئ يخرج السودا ملح هندي تربد اسفر
وبورق درهم درهم خرفق درهم الباب السابع في اللعوقات واما اللعوقات
فهي اشيا رطبة ذات قوام كالناطف واللوذجات الرقيقة تلعق بالملعقة وتمسك في الفم و
يبلع ما يتحلل منها قليلا قليلا ليطول مدة عبورها في جوار القصبة فتنفذ اليها والى الرية
بالرشح والسيلان اللطيف من الرطوبات وتعديلها وازالة الخشونة عن آلات الصوت
والنفس وما يليها فمنها باردة تستعمل لتليين خشونتها عند السعال اليابس وعند النزلات
الرقيقة الحادة لتمتزج بها وتكسر حدتها وتغريها قواما صالحا لكي ينفذ عنها وانفاثها
ومن اللعابات الباردة والاشياء اللعابية والدهنية مثل بزرقطونا وحب السفرجل وبزر
الخطمي والبنفسج وبزر الخرفع والخيارين والخس والخشخاش والجبازي والقرع واللوز و
السمسم المقشرين ودهنهما والعناب والسبستان والنشا والصمغ والكثيرا ورب
السوس ولب الخيارشنبر والترنجبين ونحوها ومنها حارة تستعمل لانضاج الرطوبات
وتلطيفها وتقطيعها وجلائها كالزوفا والايرسا وحب الصنوبر واللوز المر والكرسنة
وبرسياوشان والصعتر والفلفل والدار فلفل واصل السوس والزعفران وبزر
الكتان والحلبة ولب حب القطن والعنصل والتمر والتين والزبيب والعسل و
الفانيذ ونحوها تركب منها بحسب الحاجة اليها في نوع نوع من السعال وفي مزاج مزاج لعوقات
مختلفة التراكيب محفوظة الاصول والقوانين ان لم تف المفردات بدفع الخطوب
على انفرادها لعوق بارد للسعال اليابس والحرارة والنزلة الحادة الى الصدر والرية

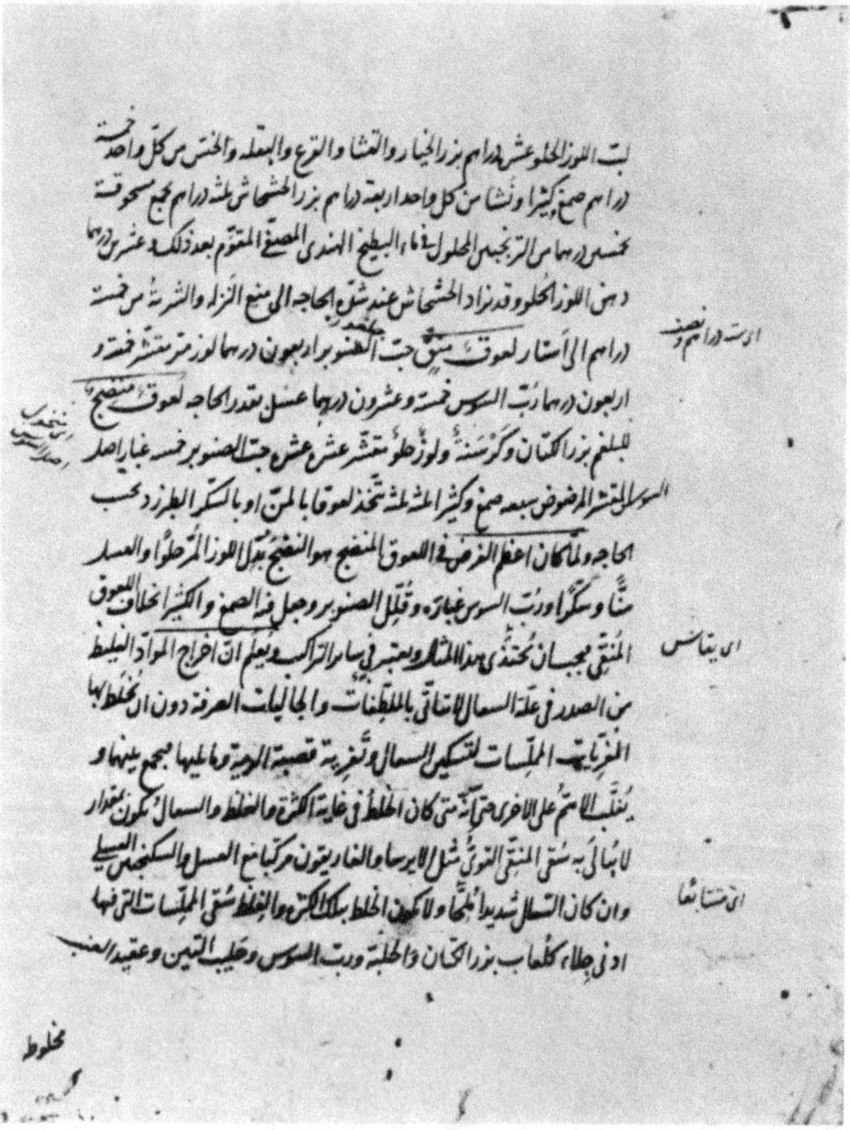

لب اللوز الحلو عشرة دراهم بزر الخيار والقثاء والقرع والبقلة والخس من كل واحد خمسة
دراهم صمغ وكثيرا ونشا من كل واحد اربعة دراهم بزر الخشخاش ثلثة دراهم يجمع مسحوقة
تخلط بماء الترنجبين المحلول في ماء البطيخ الهندي المصفى المقوم بعد ذلك بعشرين درهما
دهن اللوز الحلو وقد يزاد الخشخاش عند شدة الحاجة الى منع النزلة والشربة من خمسة
دراهم الى اسثار لعوق مشمش حب الصنوبر اربعون درهما لوز مقشر خمسة و
اربعون درهما رب السوس خمسة وعشرون درهما عسل بقدر الحاجة لعوق منضج
للبلغم بزر الكتان وكرسنة ولوز حلو مقشر عشرة عشرة حب الصنوبر خمسة غبار اصل
السوس المقشر المرضوض سبعة صمغ وكثيرا ثلثة ثلثة تتخذ لعوقا بالمن او بالسكر الطبرزد بحسب
الحاجة ولما كان اعظم الغرض في العوق المنضج هو النضج بدل اللوز المر حلوا والعسل
فانيذا وسكرا ورب السوس غبارة وقلل الصنوبر وجعل فيه الصمغ والكثيرا بخلاف العوق
المنقي فيجب ان تحتذي بهذا المثال وتعتبر في سائر التراكيب ويعلم ان اخراج المواد الغليظة
من الصدر في علة السعال لا تتاتى بالملطفات والجاليات المعروفة دون ان تخلط بها
الغروبات الملينات لتسكين السعال وتعرية قصبة الرئة وما يليها فيجمع بينهما و
يغلب احدهما على الاخرى حتى انه متى كان الخلط في غاية الكثرة والغلظ والسعال يكون بمقدار
لا يبالي به سقي المنقي القوي مثل الايرساء والغاريقون مركبا مع العسل والسكنجبين العسلي
وان كان السعال شديدا ملحا ولا يكون الخلط بتلك الكثرة والغلظ سقي الملينات التي فيها
ادنى جلاء كلعاب بزر الكتان والحلبة ورب السوس وحليب التين وعقيد العنب

مخلوطة بصمغ الاجاص والكثيرا ونحوها واذا تساوى الغرضان يستوي بينهما والله اعلم بالصواب

الباب الثامن في الاقراص من المركبات التي تركب لاغراض شتى

ولا يراد ادخارها زمانا طويلا كادخار المعجونات كما ان السفوفات مركبات يراد
استعمالها في الحال ولا تدخر كثيرا للاستبار لسرعة بطلان قواها ووشك انفعالها من
كيفيات الهواء المداخلة بها فمنها باردة تركب لحرارة المزاج والحميات الحادة تتخذ
من بزر الهندبا والخس والقرع والخيارين والورد والنيلوفر والبنفسج والانبرباريس
والصندل والطباشير والكافور ونحوها ومنها حارة تركب لتفتيح سدد الاحشاء و
صلابتها واورامها تتخذ من الانيسون والرازيانج والسنبل والمصطكي والاذخر والغافت
والافسنتين والكشوث والريوند واللك ونحوها ومنها مركبة من الحارة والباردة
تستعمل في الحميات المزمنة والحميات المركبة ومنها اقراص حابسة للدم وممسكة للبطن
ومدملة لقروح الجوف ونكتب من كل صنف من الاقراص على طريق المثال قرص الكافور
للحميات الحادة والخفقان مع الحرارة طباشير ورد صندل ابيض بزر الخيارين
والهندبا والخس والبقلة اجزاء سواء تجمع مسحوقة وتخلط بكل مثقال من الجميع نصف
طسوج كافور الطسوج وزن شعيرة الى نصف قيراط بمقدار الحاجة ويعجن بماء التفاح
ويقرص اقراصا رقاقا وتجفف في الظل وتحفظ من النكرج والشربة مثقال وانما جعل
الصندل والورد والطباشير مع البزور الخمسة متساوية لان كل واحد من الصنفين يوجب
التكثير ذاك لكثرة المانع وذا لضعف القوة فاستوت اوزانها وجعل الكافور قليلا
المانع

اللك

من كافوره

قيراط الاطباء
اربع شعيرات

اي البزور وغير
ذلك ... الصندل
والورد والكافور

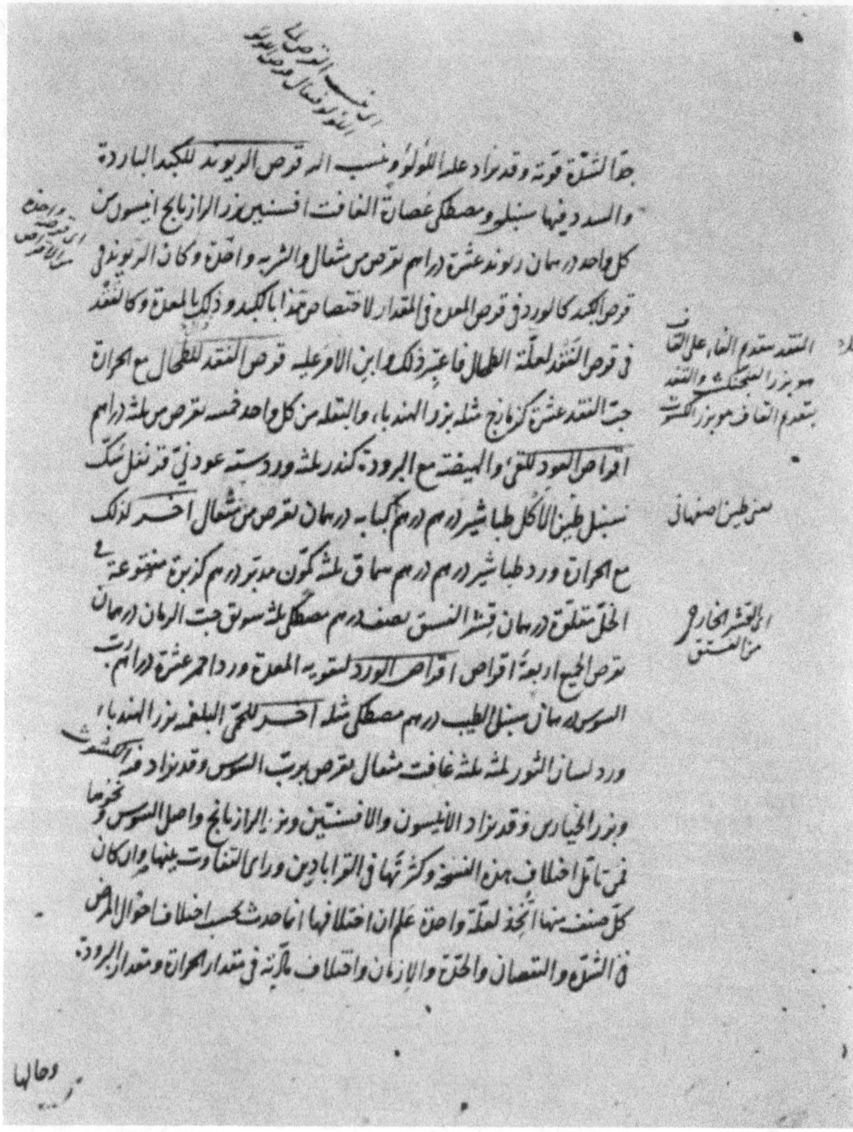

جدا السنق قوية وقد يزاد عليه اللؤلؤ وينسب اليه قرص الريوند للكبد الباردة
والسدد فيها سنبل ومصطكى عصارة الغافت افسنتين بزر الرازيانج انيسون من
كل واحد درهمان ريوند عشرة دراهم يقرص من مثقال والشربة واحد وكان الريوند في
قرص الكبد كالورد في قرص المعدة في المقدار لاختصاص هذا بالكبد وذلك بالمعدة وكان النقد
في قرص النقد لعلة الاطفال فاعتبر ذلك وابن الامر عليه قرص النقد للاطفال مع الحرارة
حب النقد عشرة كزمازج ثلثة بزر الهندبا والبقلة من كل واحد خمسة يقرص من ثلثة دراهم
اقراص العود للقي والمعدة مع البرودة كندر ثلثة ورد ستة عود ني قرنفل سك
سنبل طين الاكل طباشير درهم درهم كبابه درهمان يقرص من مثقال اخر لذلك
مع الحرارة ورد طباشير درهم درهم سماق ثلثة كمون مدبر درهم كزبرة منقوعة في
الخل مقلو درهمان قشر الفستق نصف درهم مصطكى ثلثة سويق حب الرمان درهمان
يقرص الجميع اربعة اقراص اقراص الورد لتقوية المعدة ورد احمر عشرة دراهم رب
السوس درهمان سنبل الطيب درهم مصطكى ثلثة اخرى للحمى البلغمية بزر الهندبا
ورد لسان الثور ثلثة ثلثة غافت مثقال يقرص برب السوس وقد يزاد فيه الكشوث
وبزر الخيارين وقد يزاد الانيسون والافسنتين وبزر الرازيانج واصل السوس ونحوها
فمن تامل اختلاف هذه النسخ وكثرتها في القراباذين ورأى التفاوت بينها وان كان
كل صنف منها لعلة واحدة علم ان اختلافها انما حدث بحسب اختلاف احوال المرض
في الشدة والنقصان والحدة والازمان واختلاف ما في مقدار الحرارة ومقدار البرودة

وحالها في الغلظ واللطافة والتركيب والبساطة والقلة والكثرة وبحسب اختلاف احوال
المريض في القوة والضعف واوقات مرضه في التزيد والابتداء والانحطاط والانتهاء
وعوارض تعرض له في مرضه فان القدماء انما اضطروا الى ان ركبوا لمريض واحد في مرض
واحد تركيبات مختلفة في كل حين بل في كل يوم بل في كل ساعة بحسب حدوث حال
وزوال حال فتقوى قلة عند ذلك ويزيد في النسخ وينقص منها بحسب ما يراه مصلحة
ويركب ما اراد تركيبه منشرح الصدر متسع المجال متمسكا بالاصول والقوانين و
قرص الورد دواء شريف نافع لامراض المعدة خاصة عند ضعفها في الحميات
المزمنة والمركبة لاضعافها المعدة ولا نزول من الا بتقويتها واصلاح حالها ونسبة
الورد الى المعدة عند الحاجة الى تقويتها في الحميات لشدة موافقته لها في تلك الحال
نسبة الهليلجات اليها في غير الحميات وكما ان الهليلجات هي الجبيرة والاصل
للاطريفلات كذلك الورد لاقراص الورد وتكثر منه فيها حتى يقع في شربة منها
درهم من الورد واول ما يضاف الى الورد ويجمع معه اصل السوس والسنبل على
نسبة النصف الى الربع ثم بعد ذلك تختلف نسخه باختلاف الحميات فتارة يقع فيها
الادوية الباردة المبردة اكثر وتارة يقع فيها الحارة اكثر بحسب الحاجة اليها واما
الاقراص القابضة فهي المتخذة من الادوية الممسكة لاسهال الصفراء والمانعة لاسهال
البلغم النافعة من الاسترخاء الحادث في الات الغذاء والحابسة للدم النافعة من
النسيج المفرية لها والمدملة للقروح اما التي تصلح لاسهال الصفراء فكاقابض

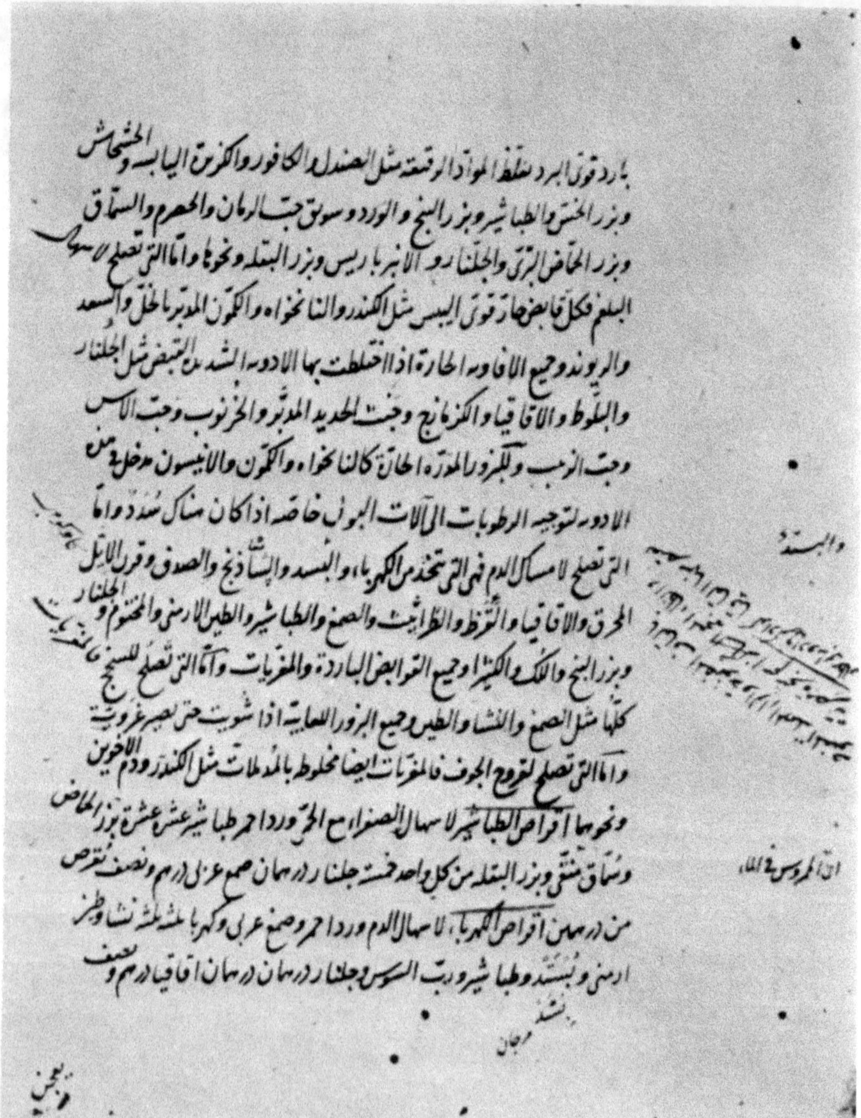

بارد قوي البرد يغلظ المواد الرقيقة مثل الصندل والكافور والكزبرة اليابسة والخشخاش
وبزر الخس والطباشير وبزر البنج والورد وسويق حب الرمان والحصرم والسماق
وبزر الحماض البري والجلنار و[illegible] الانبرباريس وبزر البقلة ونحوها واما التي تصلح لاسهال
البلغم فكل قابض حار قوي اليبس مثل الكندر والنانخواه والكمون المدبر بالخل والسعد
والراوند وجميع الافاويه الحارة اذا اختلطت بها الادوية الشديدة القبض مثل الجلنار
والبلوط والاقاقيا والكزمازج وخبث الحديد المدبر والخرنوب وحب الآس
وحب الزبيب والكندر والبزور الحارة كالنانخواه والكمون والانيسون مدخلة في
الادوية لتوجيه الرطوبات الى آلات البول خاصة اذا كان هناك سدد واما
التي تصلح لاسهال الدم فهي التي تتخذ من الكهرباء والبسد والشاذنج والصدف وقرن الايل
المحرق والاقاقيا والقرظ والطراثيث والصمغ والطباشير والطين الارمني والمختوم والجلنار
وبزر البنج والكك والكثيرا وجميع القوابض الباردة والمغريات واما التي تصلح للسحج
فكلها مثل الصمغ والنشا والطين وجميع البزور اللعابية اذا شويت حتى تصير غروية
واما التي تصلح لقروح الجوف فالمغريات ايضا مخلوطة بالمدملات مثل الكندر ودم الاخوين
ونحوها اقراص الطباشير لاسهال الصفراء مع الحمى ورد احمر طباشير عشرة عشرة بزر الحماض
وسماق منقى وبزر البقلة من كل واحد خمسة جلنار درهمان صمغ عربي درهم ونصف تقرص
من درهمين اقراص الكهرباء لاسهال الدم ورد احمر وصمغ عربي وكهربا ثلثة ثلثة نشا وطين
ارمني وبسد وطباشير ورب السوس وجلنار درهمان درهمان اقاقيا درهم ونصف

يعجن برب الآس الشربة مثقال اقراص البسد لنفث الدم صمغ عربي وطين ارمني
خمسة خمسة بسد كهربا ماذبح من كل واحد درهم ونصف رب السوس ونشا ودم
الاخوين درهمان درهمان بزر البنج ودارصيني درهم درهم تقرص من عشرة دراهم ولما كان
مسلك الدواء بعيدا جعل فيه بزر البنج ودارصيني حتى تحفظ احدهما قوة الدواء مع تخديره
لتسكين السعال الذي هو سبب زيادة نفث الدم والآخر ينفذه ويبدرقه الى اقصى مقصده
اقراص الكاكنج بليغة في قروح الكلى والمثانة منها تجربة ولبن والحام للقرحة وتسكين
لشدة الوجع والحرقة عند البول بزر الخيار وحب الكاكنج ولوز حلو مقشر ورب السوس
ونشا وكثيرا وطين ارمني وصمغ عربي ودم الاخوين وكندر درهم عشرة عشرة بزر الكرفس
درهمان افيون درهم تقرص من ثلثة دراهم ويسقى واحد بشراب البنفسج بزر الكرفس و
الافيون في هذه النسخة كالدارصيني مع بزر البنج في اقراص البسد والسلك المصلحة بينهما
اقراص السبح ورد احمر بزر الحماض المقلو ثلثة ثلثة صمغ مقلو ونشا وكثيرا من كل واحد درهم
ونصف تقرص بلعاب بزر قطونا من شعاليس ويسقى برب الآس الباب
التاسع في السفوفات والقمايح فاما السفوفات فهي المركبات التي تركيبها
بحسب اجرام مفرداتها فقط لا بحسب قواها وانفعال بعضها عن بعض حتى يحصل بينها
مزاج اخر فلذلك استعملت في الوقت ولما ذكر من فسادها سريعا بسبب تشتتها
وتخلخلها واكثر ما يستعمل من الادوية سفوفا هي الادوية اليابسة القابضة تستف
وتبلع لتنشيف رطوبات المعدة والامعاء واسهال البطن والبول وقد تتخذ غير ما كن

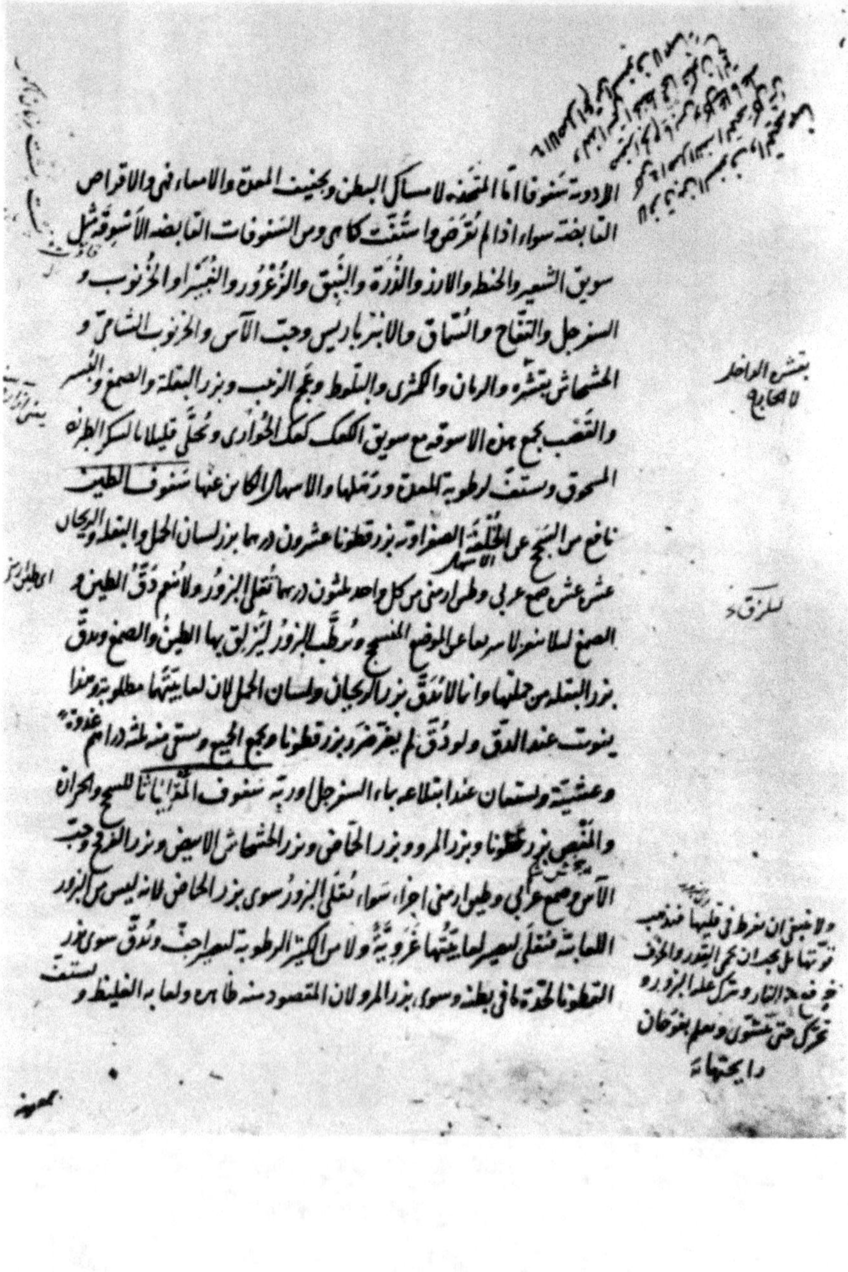

ومعه رب السفرجل او رب الآس اذا كان هناك سعال سفوف البزور لحرقة البول
بزر البطيخ المقشر مثقالين درهما بزر الخيار المقشر والقرع وبزر البقلة والخشخاش من كل واحد
عشرة دراهم نشا وكثيرا ورب السوس من كل واحد ثلثة بزر السبح درهمان سكر مثل الجميع والشربة
منه ثلثة دراهم غدوة وعشية بشراب البنفسج او الجلاب سفوف يمسك البول ويمنع
بلا حرقة والعطش غالب بلوط خمسون درهما كندر ثلثون درهما كزبرة يابسة وطين ارمني وصمغ عربي
عشرة عشرة ستة الشربة منه ثلثة دراهم غدوة وعشية اخرى لاكل كمون كندر حب الآس بلوط
اجزاء متساوية الشربة ثلثة دراهم سفوف السورنجان سورنجان درهم بنفسج درهمان
دانق ونصف ماميزهرج دانق ونصف انطاكي دانق ونصف انيسون دانق ورد
احمر دانق سكر ضعف الجميع وهي شربة والله اعلم الباب العاشر في الاضمدة والاطلية
والكمادات فاما الاضمدة فهي المركبات التي قوامها قوام المعاجين توضع على الاعضاء الظاهرة
وتشد عليها والاطلية ما كان منها ارق قواما بحيث اذا مسحت بها الاعضاء لصقت بها
وانفرشت على سطوحها ولم يحتج الى الشد والعصب عليها والاطلية الطف واسرع نفوذا
وتحليلا والاضمدة اغلظ واكثر ملازمة للعضو وحصرا للحرارة فلذلك اكثر ما تستعمل للتحليل و
الانضاج والكمادات اما رطبة واما يابسة فالرطبة كالمثانات المملوءة مياها حارة والخرق
المشربة مياها حارة توضع على الاعضاء لتسخينها مع الترطيب وقد تغلى في تلك المياه ادوية
ملينة مرخية محللة مثل الخطمي والشبت والخبازي والاكليل والبابونج والبنفسج والمرزنجوش
ونحوها وقد تكمد بتلك الادوية نفسها مطبوخة واما الكمادات اليابسة فهي مثل الملح المسخن

اي شد العصابة عليها

اي اكثر ما استعمل للتحليل والانضاج

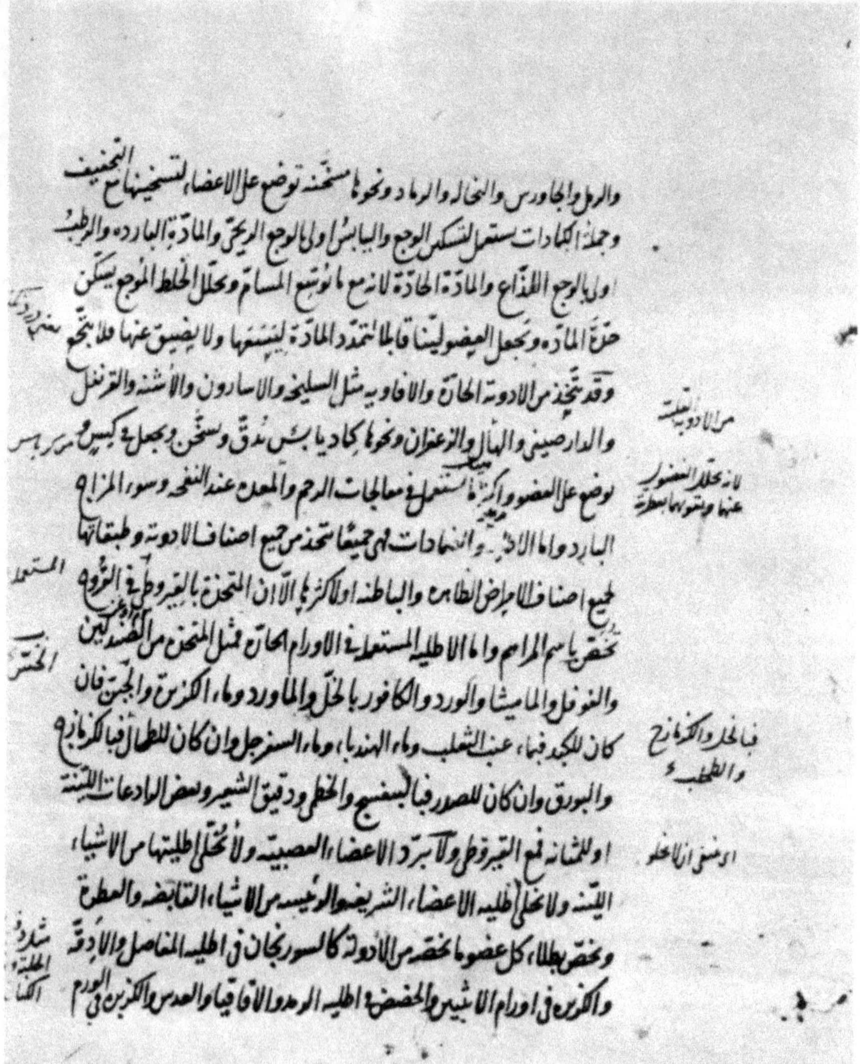

والرمل والجاورس والنخالة والرماد ونحوها مسخنة توضع على الاعضاء لتسخينها مع التجفيف
وجملة الكمادات تستعمل لتسكين الوجع واليابس اولى بالوجع الريحي والمادة الباردة والرطب
اولى بالوجع اللذاع والمادة الحادة لانه مع ما توسع المسام وتحلل الخلط الموجع يسكن
حدة المادة وتجعل العضو لينا قابلا لتمدد المادة لينبسط بها ولا يضيق عنها فلا يتوجع
وقد تتخذ من الادوية الحارة والافاويه مثل السليخة والاسارون والاشنة والقرنفل
والدارصيني والهال والزعفران ونحوها كادية يابسة تدق وتسخن وتجعل في كيس ثم
توضع على العضو واكثر ما تستعمل في معالجات الرحم والمعدة عند النفخة وسوء المزاج
البارد واما الاضمدة والنطولات فهي جميعا تتخذ من جميع اصناف الادوية وطبقاتها
لجميع اصناف الامراض الظاهرة والباطنة الا ان اكثرها التي تتخذ بالقيروطي في القروح
تخص باسم المراهم واما الاطلية المستعملة في الاورام الحارة فمثل المتخذ من الصندلين
والفوفل والماميثا والورد والكافور بالخل والماورد وماء الكزبرة والجبن فان
كان للكبد فبماء عنب الثعلب وماء الهندباء وماء السفرجل وان كان للطحال فبالكزمازج
والبورق وان كان للصدر فبالبنفسج والخطمي ودقيق الشعير وبعض الادهان اللينة
او للمثانة فمع القيروطي ولا تبرد الاعضاء العصبية ولا تخلى طليتها من الاشياء
اللينة ولا تخلى اطلية الاعضاء الشريفة الرئيسة من الاشياء القابضة والعطرة
ويخص ايضا كل عضو ما يختص من الادوية كالسورنجان في اطلية المفاصل والادقة
والكزبرة في اورام الانثيين والحضض في اطلية الرمد والاقاقيا والعدس والكزبرة في الورم

الوسمه وجرادة القرع والخس ولسان الحمل في الورم الصفراوي واما الادوية المستعملة
في ضمادات الاورام البارده فمثل الاكليل والبابونج والمرزنجوش والقيصوم و
الخطمي والشبت ثم ان كانت في الكبد يضاف اليها السنبل والريوند والزعفران
والمر ونحوهما او في الطحال يضاف السداب والبورق والاشق والغوتنج واصل الكبر — اليهاء
او في المعدة يضاف اليها المصطكى والسليخة والقسط والافسنتين والاذخر او
في الخصية والثديين يضاف اليها الكمون ولحم الزبيب ودقيق الحلبة وبزر الكتان — اليهاء
او في المفاصل يضاف اليها المقل وسنام الجمل والامخاخ والشحوم والادهان لما علم
من ضمادات اورام الاعضاء العصبية او في العنق ومن جنس الخنازير يضاف اليها
الايرسا والزفت وكذلك يخص بطلاء كل ورم ما يخصه مثل الملح والرماد والبورق
والخل والسعد في الورم الرخو والسداب والابهل والسرو في الورم الريحي واسفيداج — اى ورق السرو
الاسرب والتوتيا المغسول وعصارات البقول البارده واللعابات في السرطان
واما انضاج الخراجات فيكون باضمدة لزجة غروية مثل بزر الكتان والحلبة والتين
والخير ونحوهما واما الاضمدة القابضة المستعملة عند الاسهال فمثل ورق الاس و
قشر الرمان والجلنار والاقاقيا والمر والرامك والكندر والكعك والسعد وماء
السفرجل العفص وماء لب الكروم ولا ينبغي ان يستعمل هذا الضماد في الحمى لانه يسد — اطراف رطب من الكروم
المسام ويحبس الحرارة فتزيد الحمى حدة واما المسهلة للبطن والقاتلة للديدان فهي
مثل حب النيل وحب الملوك والبورق والشونيز والتربد والترمس وشحم الحنظل

باقلى

والمازريون والشيح والسقمونيا والصبر اذا اتخذت ضمادا بماء ورق الخوخ و
الافسنتين والحنظل ومرارة البقر ومن اكثر ما يؤثر في الصبيان ونحوهم للين مزاجهم
ووصول قوى الادوية الى امعائهم ويجب ان تطلى بطونهم بها وراء كاغدة رقيقة
لئلا تخرق جلودهم وتقرحها واما الاضمدة التي تنشف المائية من المستسقين واصحاب
الترهل المائي فهي مثل بعر الغنم واخثاء البقر والسعد والبورق ودقيق الشعير ورماد
الطرفاء ورماد الودع بالخل واما ضماد الكسر والخلع والوثي فيتخذ من مثل المغاث
والسرو والآس ودقيق الماش والعدس والطين الارمني والاقاقيا والصندلين
والنوفل والماميثا والبوش والخطمي وتطلى في الصداع الحار والبارد باطلية الاورام
الحارة والباردة ويزاد في الحار الاشياء المخدرة مثل ورق الخشخاش والخس واللفاح
والبنج والافيون ان كان الوجع شديدا وفي البارد الجندبيدستر والمسك والصبر و
الفربيون عند الحاجة اليها واما الاطلية التي لامراض الجلد واضمدتها ما يتعلق بالزينة
فهي جلاءة مثل البورق والخردل والكندس والفربيون وزبد البحر وقشور شجر التين
محرقين والشونيز والقنبيل والشيطرج والخل والزرنيخ والنفط والعنابرتي و
نحوها واما اطلية الجرب والسعفة فهي مركبة من الحارة الجلاءة والباردة القابضة والرطبة
اللينة للجذب والتنقية والردع والمنع وكسر الحدة وتليين الجلد وترطيب الخلط فلذلك
كثرت هذه المركبات وتنوعت بحسب هذه الاغراض وتفاوتت هذه الحاجة اليها بحسب
المواد وانواعها حتى فاتت الحصر والعد والكل موافق للكلام اذا وضعت مواضعها

طلا للثوباء صبر مر حضض درهم درهم زعفران دانقان طلا للرعاف عدس مقشر
خطمي صندل شياف ماميثا طين حر شيء من الكافور يطلى على الجبهة بماء الآس ضماد
للسكتة خردل جندبيدستر سعتان بالخل ويضمد به طلا للنعش مصطكي قشار الكندر ضماد
جوز السرو وورقه وبزر وابهل وعنزروت وانزراش وغرا السمك اجزاء سواء
يذاب الغرا بالخل ويجمع به طلا يجلب النوم بزر البنج وبزر الخشخاش وافيون ولفاح
يطلى على الجبهة بطبيخ الخشخاش والله اعلم الباب الحادي عشر في الادهان
واما الادهان فتركب بعضها مع بعض كسائر الادوية اما لتقوية قواها وكيفياتها واما
لحدوث مزاج مطلوب يحدث من اجتماعها وقد تركب الادهان مع قوى الادوية بواسطة
الماء والنار اما بان يطبخ الادوية في الماء حتى ياخذ الماء قوتها ثم يمزج ذلك الماء بالدهن
ويغلى حتى يذهب الماء ويبقى القوة في الدهن واما بان تلقى وهي غضة طرية في الدهن و
تشمس حتى تتوسط ما بينها ما بين قواها والدهن في الاخذ والاعطاء قبل الفناء وقد تركب
الادهان مع قوى الادوية بوساطة الهواء بان يجمع الرياحين الرطبة واللبوب الدهنية بواسطة
في خرائط صفيقة وتستوثق من رؤوسها حتى تذبل ثم تبدل ويجدد عليها غضة طرية ويكرر
ذلك حتى ياخذ من قواها وروائحها شيئا صالحا فتعصر اللبوب عند الحاجة ويوخذ ادهانها
وهذا ضعيف جدا بالقياس الى الصنفين المتقدمين وقد استاثروا هذا الطريق في اي اختاروا
الادهان الباردة الرطبة مثل دهن السمسم المقشر واللوز الحلو المقشر وحب القرع
المقشر ونحو ذلك والرياحين الباردة الرطبة مثل البنفسج والنيلوفر ونحوهما احترازا

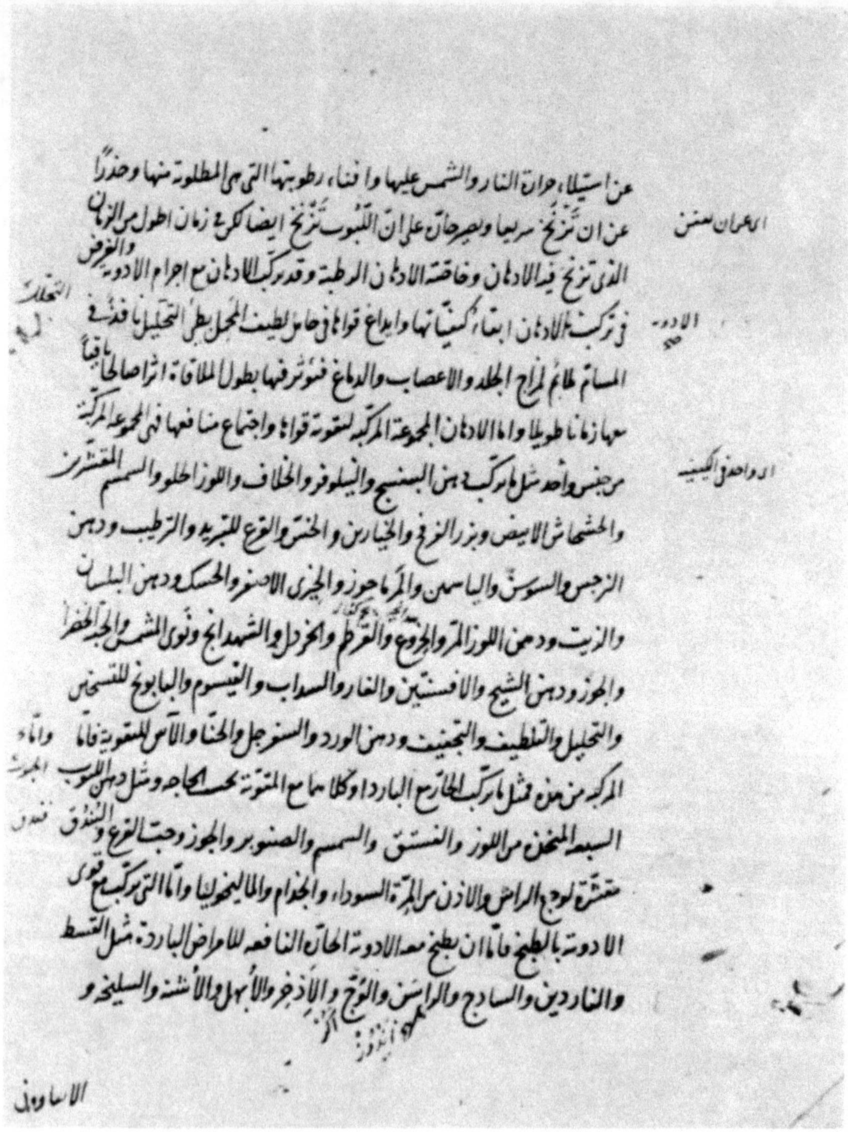

عن استيلاء حرارة النار والشمس عليها وافناء رطوبتها التي هي المطلوبة منها وحذرا
عن ان تزنخ سريعا وبرهان على ان اللبوب تزنخ ايضا لكن في زمان اطول من الزمان
الذي تزنخ فيه الادهان وخاصة الادهان الرطبة وقد تركب الادهان مع اجرام الادوية والغرض
في تركيب الادهان ابقاء كيفياتها وايداع قواها في حامل لطيف المحل بطيء التحليل نافذ في
المسام ملائم لمزاج الجلد والاعصاب والدماغ فيؤثر فيها بطول الملاقاة اثرا صالحا باقيا
معها زمانا طويلا واما الادهان المجموعة المركبة لتقوية قواها واجتماع منافعها في المجموع المركب
من جنس واحد مثل ما تركب من دهن البنفسج والنيلوفر والخلاف واللوز الحلو والسمسم المقشر
والخشخاش الابيض وبزر القرع والخيارين والخس والقرع للتبريد والترطيب ودهن
النرجس والسوسن والياسمين والمرزنجوش والخيري الاصفر والحسك ودهن البلسان
والزيت ودهن اللوز المر والخروع والقرطم والخردل والشهدانج ونوى المشمش والحبة الخضراء
والجوز ودهن الشبث والافسنتين والغار والسذاب والقيصوم والبابونج للتسخين
والتحليل والتلطيف والتجفيف ودهن الورد والسفرجل والحنا والآس للتقوية فاما
المركب من نوعين فمثل ما تركب من الحار والبارد وكلاهما مع المتنوعة بحسب الحاجة ومثل دهن اللبوب
السبعة المتخذ من اللوز والفستق والسمسم والصنوبر والجوز وحب القرع والبندق
[illegible] لوجع الراس والاذن من المرة السوداء والجذام والماليخوليا واما التي تركب مع قوى
الادوية بالطبخ فاما ان يطبخ معه الادوية الحارة النافعة للامراض الباردة مثل القسط
والناردين والساذج والراسن والوج والاذخر والابهل والاشنة والسليخة و

الاسارون والزنجبيل والعاقرقرحا والمرماحوز والسعد والبرداما والمرزنجوش
والسنبل والمر والقرنفل والجوزبوا والبيعة والزعفران ونحوها وقد تكرر الادوية على
مقدار من الدهن لاجتماع قواها فيه واشتدادها وقد تكرر الدهن على مقدار من الادوية
ويعاد طبخها ثانيا للاستقصاء في استخراج قواها واما ان نطبخ مع الادوية القابضة لما
من العرق مثل الآس والورد والسفرجل والجلنار ونحوها واما ان نطبخ مع الادوية المقوية
للشعر الحارة والباردة مثل ورق الآس والاملج وورد الشقائق والبرسياوشان وسنبل
الطيب وسعد وبزر السلق والعفص والهليلج الكابلي وورق السدر ونحوها واما التي
تتخذ وتركب بالتشميس اما الباردة فدهن البنفسج والنيلوفر والخلاف والورد والآس و
اللفاح وقد تتخذ من الخضر والرياحين الباردة واما الحارة فدهن النرجس والسوسن والياسمين
والشاهسفرم والمرزنجوش والنمام والخيري الاصفر والنسرين والاقحوان والشيح والزعفران
واما الادهان المركبة مع اجرام الادوية فمثل الجندبيدستر والفرفيون والزعفران والمر
والزنجبيل والعاقرقرحا والفلفل تنقع في الادهان الحارة وتمرخ بها للفالج والاسترخاء — اي تحجر
والشخوص والاعلال الباردة مثل العنبر والمسك والزعفران والعود الهندي والدارصيني — المبهور العين
والمصطكي والقرنفل والافاويه الطيبة تنقع في الادهان الطيبة وتمرخ بها للعلل الباردة — العلل
في الاعضاء الرئيسة والرحم واعضاء التناسل دهن القسط ينفع من الفالج قسط اوقية
فلفل عاقرقرحا فرفيون من كل واحد ثلث اوقية جندبيدستر نصف اوقية تنقع
الجميع في نصف رطل دهن الخيري او دهن الزنبق ويمرخ به الاعضاء المسترخية دهن [illegible]

يستعمل في جميع الاعلال البارده. فنؤثر باعتدال ولا يحدث في العضو يبسا دهن الخيري
ودهن الياسمين ودهن البطم ودهن السوسن ودهن الخروع ودهن نوى المشمش
ودهن الغار اجزاء سواء يطرح عليها يسير من جندبيدستر ويسير من المسك ونغلي عليه
غلية خفيفة ويستعمل دهن بارد رطب للصداع الحار والبرسام واليبس بزر القرع وبزر
الخس ولب حب الخيار والقثاء ولب لوز الحلو وبزر الخشخاش الابيض وسمسم مقشر
اجزاء سواء يستخرج دهنها ويستعمل سعوطا ومروخا والسعوط منه نصف درهم في
غاية النفع الباب الثاني عشر في ادوية العين منها الاكحال وشيافات ومنها برودات
وذرورات وقطورات ومنها ضمادات واطلية اما الضمادات والاطلية فيستعمل عند
ابتداء اورام العين وانصباب المواد اليها وهي الاطلية الرادعة المتخذة من مثل
اطراف عنب الثعلب وعصا الراعي وبقلة الرجلة والكزبرة الرطبة والخس وزهر القرع
والخشخاش والبنفسج والورد المنقى او شل الحضض والصندل والاقاقيا والماميثا
والنوفل والطين الارمني والصمغ والافيون ونحوها عند شدة الوجع اذا بولغ في
التسكين وامالة المادة عنها وقد يجمع بعضها الزعفران والصبر عند الحاجة الى تحليل
يسير ويضاف اليها الكزبرة اليابسة والاكليل وبزر الكتان والكعك عند الحاجة الى تحليل
اكثر حيث يكون المادة اغلظ والادوية الرادعة لا تسكن الوجع الحادث من مادة غليظة
وعند ذلك يجمع الادوية بالشراب ويكبت على بخاره وبخار طبيخ المرزنجوش والبابونج
والشبث وتبن الحنطة خاصة عند برد الهواء وتكاثف الجلد وقد يكمد بالاسفنج ابتدريا

والماء الحار او بياض البيض وماء الورد عند الابتداء ونضمد عند ضربه تصيبها بصفرة
البيض وماء الكزبرة ودهن الورد ونضمد في الورد ينفع فيه المخلوط بقشور الفستق وبحب
الرمان والعدس والحمص والهندباء واما القطورات فهي الين ادوية العين
واولى ان تستعمل في اوائلها عند الابتداء ومع ذلك حيث لا تحتمل شي صلابة الميل
وثقله والين القطورات المستعملة في اوائل الرمد وانفعها بياض البيض الرقيق
لتعديله مزاج العين وغسله لها وتسكين الوجع ثم لعاب بزر القطونا ولعاب حب
السفرجل مع لبن الجارية ثم الذي فيه ادنى تحليل كالماء الذي طبخ فيه الشعير المقشور وحب
السفرجل والطلوغ المقشر والخشخاش المخرش ويسير من العنزروت في اناء مضاعف
طبخا جيدا ثم القطورات التي قد خلطت فيها الشيافات اللينة واما القطورات
التي تستعمل لنضج البثور فمثل لعاب بزر المرو وبزر الكتان والحلبة باللبن
ويتلو القطورات في خفة الاستعمال وقلة ايلام العين الذرورات وتستعمل
عند كثرة الرمص ليبوستها ونشفها وهي تتخذ من الانزروت الابيض الجلال
المربى بلبن الجواري في الظل وقليل من النشا وتتخذ ايضا من الانزروت وزبد
البحر والسكر او من الانزروت وشياف ماميثا والحضض والزعفران والصبر
والمر وزبد البحر بحسب شدة الحرارة ونقصانها وكثرة الحاجة الى الجلاء وقلتها وكيف
ما كان في الاصل فيها هو الانزروت ونسبة كل واحد ما يضاف اليه نسبة العشر و
الخمس والثلث بحسب قواها ومنافعها والحاجة اليها وقد يزاد عليها الافيون او الكافور

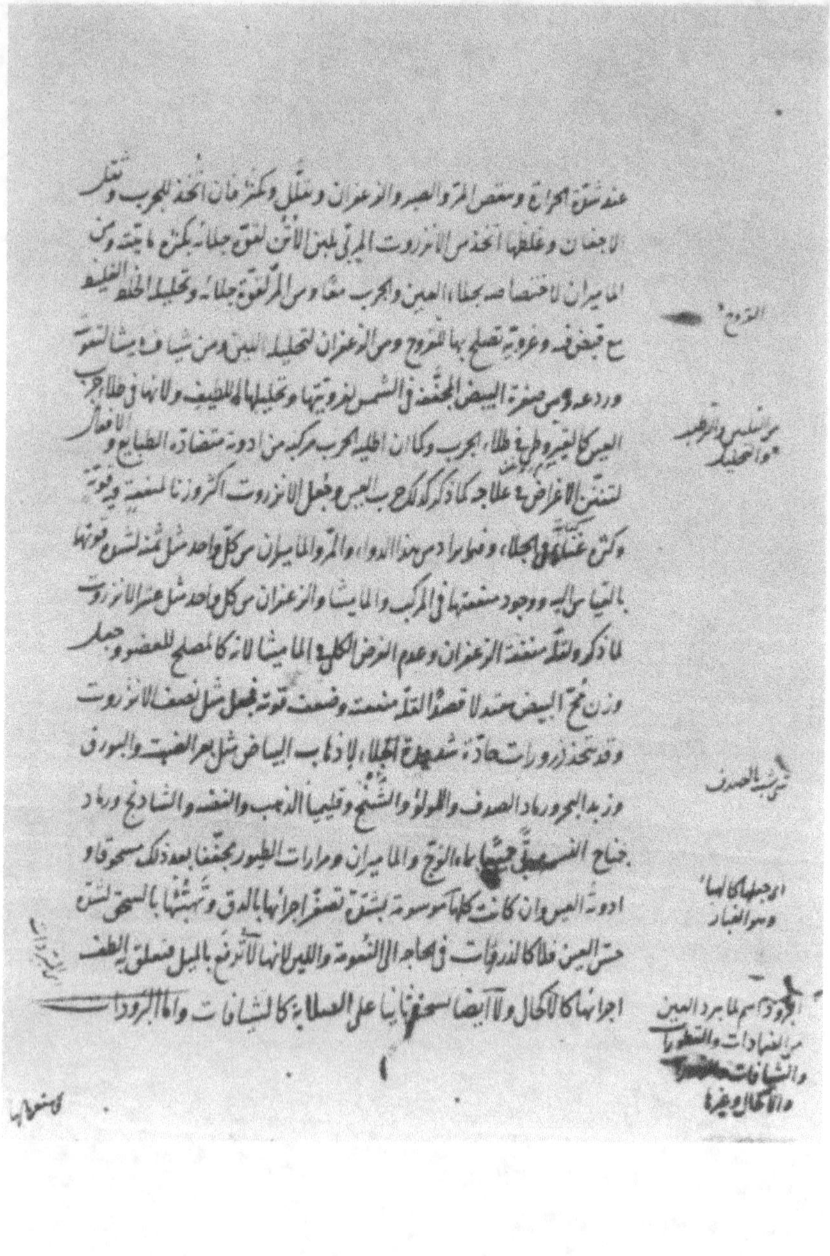

فاستعمالها مثل استعمال الاكحال الابرود الرمان فانه يستعمل مفردا واكثر ما يستعمل في
تسكين العين عند هيجانها ونحوها من الادوية الحارة مثل المتخذ من ورد البنفسج و
الكزبرة المحرقة والنشا والصمغ والكثيرا مربى جميعا بالخل وعن اقليميا والانزروت
المربى والرصاص المحرق وزبد البحر والافيون ومثل برود الرمان وبرود الزعفران
وهي وان اتخذت من ادوية حادة جلاءة مضافة للعين مثل علاج السلاق والطفرة
ونحوها فلا تخلو من الكافور والافيون ونحو ذلك برودات وكانها برودات بالقياس الى
غيرها من الاكحال الحارة واما الاكحال فلما كانت اكثر ما تستعمل في تقوية العين وجلائها و
تصقيلها والعين عضو رطب اكثر ضررها من الرطوبة وجب ان تكون ادويتها
الجالية لها الحافظة لصحتها يابسة الكحال واما الشيافات فلما كانت مستعملة
في امراض العين وادويتها غير مقصورة على الجلاء والتقوية بل مركبة من اصناف مختلفة
لاغراض شتى وجب ان تكون استعمالها كاستعمال الاطلية والضمادات مستغنية
لاستبقاء قوتها معه للكحل والطلى بالميل والعين وان كانت ذكية الحس لا تحتمل
الادوية القوية الكيفية لكنها عصبية غشائية لا تؤثر فيها الادوية الضعيفة عند استعمالها
في تلطيف المواد الغليظة وتحليل فضلاتها الراسخة فيها خصوصا والادوية لا يمكن
توضع عليها وضعها على الاعضاء الاخرى كما توضع الاطلية والضمادات لعلة احتمالها
بالنسبة اليها ولدوام حركتها فجعلت الاكحال والشيافات حادة واستعملت في اوقات
متباعدة ليحصل الغرض منها ولصلابة اغشية العين ومناسبتها الادوية الحجرية جعل

اكثر ادويتها منها المراد من بقائها فيها واما الادوية التي تصلح للاكحال القوية الجالية
فمثل التوتيا والاثمد المصوّلين بماء المطر المربّيين بماء الرازيانج وماء المرزنجوش و
الاقليميا والمارقشيثا واللولؤ والبسد والشادنج والروسختج والسرطان البحري
مشويّة مصولة والسادج الهندي والزعفران والزنجبيل والفلفل والدار فلفل
والماميران والفلفل الابيض وزبد البحر والحضض والماميثا والكافور والهليلج
الاصفر والمسك والملح الاندراني والسنبل والاشنة والعروق ونحوها والتي تصلح
لانبات الاشفار فمثل نوى التمر المحرق ودخان الكندر والسنبل الهندي وحب البلسان اى الاهداب
وحجر اللازورد والشنج المحرق والصنوبر المحرق والاقاقيا والمداد اليابس وعصير البصل
والكواث والتي تصلح لقطع الدمعة فالتوتيا وحكاك الهليلج الاصفر والصبر والفلفل و
الدار فلفل والزنجبيل والملح الهندي وزبد البحر والماميران والزعفران والكحل والمارقشيثا
والعاقرقرحا والاصداف المكلّسة والنوشادر وماء الحصرم واما الشيافات فالّتي
منها تتخذ من اسفيداج الرصاص والصمغ العربي والكثيرا والنشا والعنزروت المربّى و
زبد البحر وبزر الخس والماميثا والزعفران والكافور والورد والافيون والقليميا
واما الشيافات الحادة تتخذ من مثل الزاج والفلفل والزنجار والدهنج والشادنج و
الزرنيخ والنوشادر وزبد البحر والبورق والاشق والزنجفر والسكبينج والفرفيون
وشحم الحنظل والدار فلفل والزنجبيل والسادج والاقليميا والملح الهندي والشنج
المحرق وبعر الضب وخرء الخطاطيف وقشور البيض المدبّر والمرارات ولا تبلغ

خشاش

اى من الادوية اللينة

ان تحل الادوية الحادة من اللينة المسكنة للحدة مثل النشا والكثيرا والصمغ واسفيداج

الرصاص بمقدار الحاجة الى تسكين حدتها وحفظ العين من حرارتها ونكايتها فلان تتبلد

فعلها وبطوا اثرها ويطول زمان استعمالها اولى واذن لما السلامة من تهيج العين

وايجاعها شديدا بعير بذلك غرضا لانصباب المواد اليها واما الشيافات

فى قروح العين هى المتخذة من الادوية التى تجلو وتجفف من غير لذع لحاجة القروح الى ذلك

ولذكاء حاسة العين ولما كانت قروحها لا تخلو من ورم وشق ووجع فتحتاج مع ذلك

الى المسكنات والمغريات اما الاولى اعنى التى تجلو وتجفف من غير لذع فمثل التوتيا

والرصاص المحرق والاثمد المحرق والقليميا والشبح والشادنج واللؤلؤ مغسولة

والكحل والكندر المصلى وصمغ المصطكى والانزروت المربى ودم الاخوين واما الاخر اى

المسكنات المغريات فمثل الماميثا والنشا والكثيرا والصمغ وبزر الورد والزعفران

والافيون والبنج واليبروح وعلى الطبيب ان يركب بحسب حالات القروح وادواتها على

التدريج والترتيب والجمع بين الشيافات اللينة والحادة على المساواة او على

التغليب وتداف الشياف فى اوائل الرمد والبثور فى اللبن للتسكين وتعديل ما عسى

تنح فيها من الافيون والكافور وفى اواخره فى الماء لئلا تنكسر وتتبلد قوا[ه]ا فى التلطيف

والتحليل لبقايا الرمد ضماد للحكة بزر الهندبا النعنع تهيأ منه رفادتان ويضمد

بها مسوحة بدهن الورد اخضر عدس مقشر سماق ورد احمر شحم الرمان تخبص

ويضمد طلا للتهيج وورم الاجفان ورد شياف ماميثا اقاقيا حضض عروق صفر

ای النحاس

ای نصف فعلها

ای يدق ويجعل منه رفادتان

ای يدق ناعما ويطبخ حتى يصير خبيصا

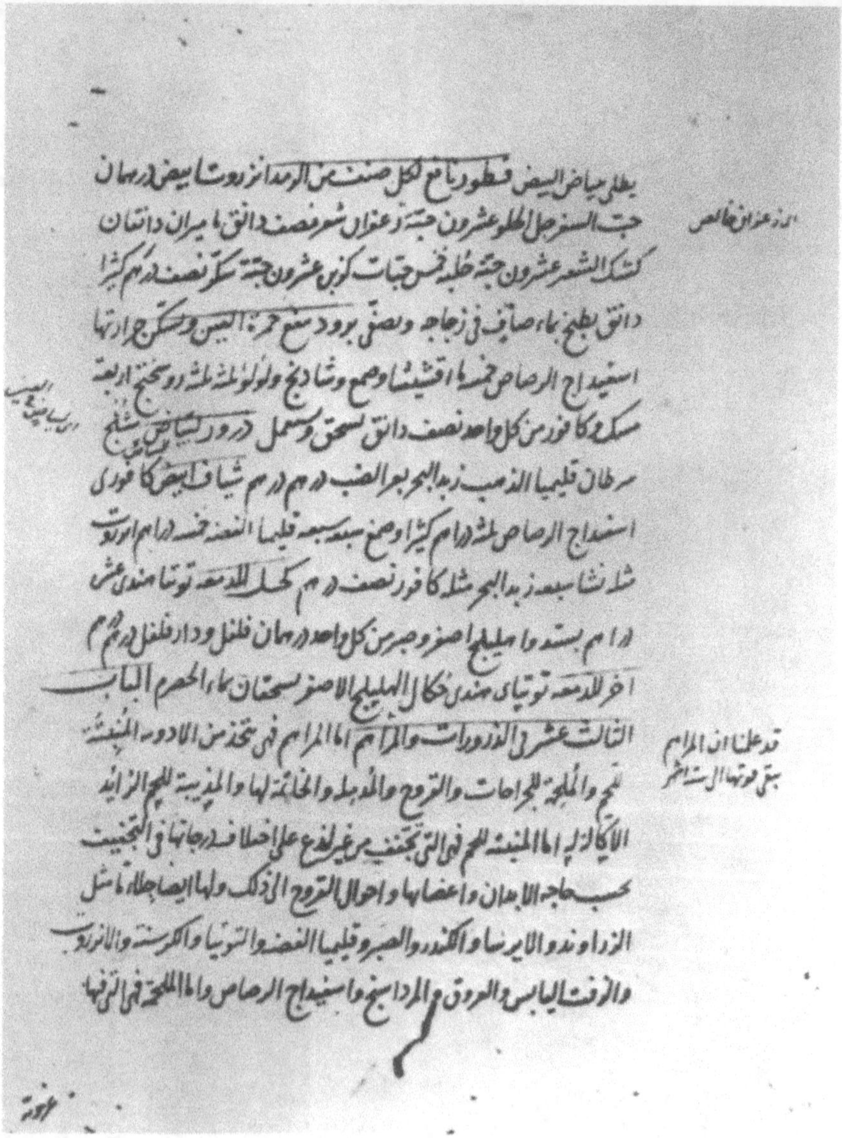

يطلى بياض البيض قطوريا مع لكل صنف من الرمد انزروت ابيض درهمان
حب السفرجل الحلو عشرون حبة زعفران شعر نصف دانق ماميران دانقان
كشك الشعير عشرون حبة حلبة خمس حبات كزبرة عشرون حبة سكر نصف درهم كثيرا
دانق يطبخ بماء صاف في زجاجة ويصفى برود سنج حمرة العين وسكن حرارتها
اسفيداج الرصاص خمسة اقليميا وصمغ وشادنج ولؤلؤ ثلثة ثلثة روسختج اربعة
مسك وكافور من كل واحد نصف دانق يسحق ويستعمل درور للبياض شيلنج
سرطان قليميا الذهب زبد البحر بعر الضب درهم درهم شياف ابيض كافوري
اسفيداج الرصاص ثلثة دراهم كثيرا وصمغ سبعة سبعة قليميا الفضة خمسة دراهم انزروت
ثلثة نشا سبعة زبد البحر ثلثة كافور نصف درهم كحل للدمعة توتيا هندي عشرة
دراهم بسفايج هليلج اصفر وصبر من كل واحد درهمان فلفل ودار فلفل درهم درهم
آخر للدمعة توتياى هندي كحل الهليلج الاصفر يسحقان بماء الحصرم الباب
الثالث عشر في الذرورات والمراهم اما المراهم فهي تتخذ من الادوية المنبتة
للحم والملحمة للجراحات والقروح والمدملة والخاتمة لها والمذيبة للحم الزائد
الاكال لها اما المنبتة للحم فهي التي تجفف من غير لذع على اختلاف درجاتها في التجفيف
بحسب حاجة الابدان واعضائها واحوال القروح الى ذلك ولها ايضا جلاء ما مثل
الزراوند والايرسا والكندر والصبر وقليميا الفضة والتوتيا والكرسنة والانزروت
والزفت اليابس والعروق والمرداسنج واسفيداج الرصاص واما الملحمة فهي التي فيها

انزروت خالص

قد علمنا ان المراهم يبقى قوتها الى ستة اشهر

عروية ولصوق يسد الدم الوارد قواما والنزف فمثل دم الاخوين والراتينج و
البنج والمقل والمصطكي والاشق وعلك البطم والجاوشير والصبر والكندر و
المر واما المدملة فهي التي تصلب لحم القرحة وهي المجففة باعتدال والخاتمة هي المجففة
القوية بجفف سطحها الذي قد ساوى سطح الجلد وبجعله كالجلد في اليبوسة ولذلك
سميت خاتمة والادوية التي تفعل هذين الفعلين كل دواء قابض قليل القبض
او كثيره مثل الجلنار والورد وبزره وقشر الرمان وورق السوس والعفص
الشب والقلقطار المحرق والكحل والزنجار والنحاس المحرق المغسول والصبر
والروسختج واما الاكالة للحم الزائد المجففة للقروح العتيقة فهي مثل الزنجار والنوشادر
والزرنيخ والنورة الحية اذا اتخذت مرهما ومثل الادوية المجففة من غير قبض
كالمرداسنج والصدف المحرق اذا استعملت ذرورا وقد تصير الادوية الاكالة
المذيبة للحم مدملة بطريق العرض وتجفف باعتدال اذا استعمل منها المقدار
اليسير مع الزيت والشمع مرهما فمن هذه الادوية تتخذ المراهم على انحاء التراكيب
بانواع انواع القروح ولما كانت القروح يحتاج في الاكثر الى جميع هذه الاغراض من
انبات اللحم والالحام والادمال والختم والجلاء والتذويب جعلت المراهم مركبة
منها اي من تلك الاصناف والطبقات على اختلاف الحاجة اليها وربما اجتمع في دواء
واحد مفرد منها غرضان او اكثر من تلك الاغراض فينفع في اكثر المراهم بسبب ذلك
واذا كانت الادوية اليابسة لا تلتصق اكثر القروح ولا تثبت عليها ذرورا ومنثورا

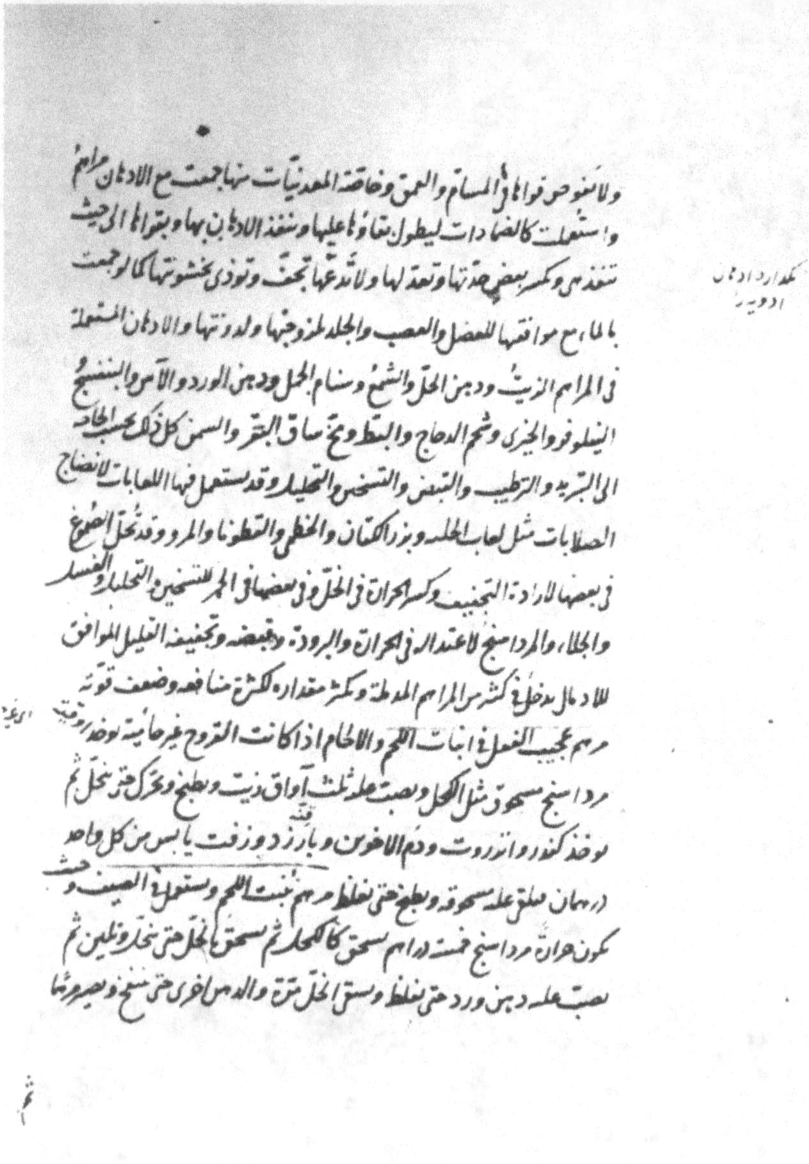

ولا ينوص قواما في المسام والعمق وخاصة المعدنيات منها جمعت مع الادهان مراهم
واستعملت كالضمادات ليطول بقاؤها عليها وتنفذ الادهان بها وبقوامها الى حيث
تنفذ هي وتكسر بعض حدتها وتعدلها ولا تدعها تجف وتؤذي بخشونتها كما لو جمعت
بالماء مع موافقتها للعضل والعصب والجلد لمزوجتها ولدونتها والادهان المستعملة
في المراهم الزيت ودهن الحل والشمع وسنام الجمل ودهن الورد والآس والبنفسج و
النيلوفر والخيري وشحم الدجاج والبط ومخ ساق البقر والسمن كل ذلك بحسب الحاجة
الى التبريد والترطيب والتيبيس والتسخين والتحليل وقد تستعمل فيها اللعابات لانضاج
الصلابات مثل لعاب الحلبة وبزر الكتان والخطمي والقطونا والمر وقد تحل الصموغ
في بعضها لارادة التجفيف وكسر الحرارة في الخل وفي بعضها في الخمر للتسخين والتحليل والغسل
والجلاء والمرداسنج لاعتداله في الحرارة والبرودة وقبضه وتجفيفه القليل الموافق
للادمال يدخل في كثير من المراهم المدملة ويكثر مقداره لكثرة منافعه وضعف قوته
مرهم عجيب الفعل في انبات اللحم والالحام اذا كانت القروح غير جاسية يؤخذ اوقية
مرداسنج مسحوق مثل الكحل ويصب عليه ثلث اواق زيت ويطبخ ويحرك حتى ينحل ثم
يؤخذ كندر وانزروت ودم الاخوين وبارزد وزفت يابس من كل واحد
درهمان ويلقى عليه مسحوقة ويطبخ حتى يغلظ مرهم ينبت اللحم ويستعمل في الصيف و
يكون حرارة مرداسنج خمسة دراهم يسحق كالكحل ثم يسحق بالخل حتى ينحل ويلين ثم
يصب عليه دهن ورد حتى يغلظ ويسقى الخل مرة والدهن اخرى حتى ينعقد ويصير مرهما

ثم يلقى عليه قسط دراهم اسفيداج الرصاص وقليل كافور مرهم يصلح النواصير وينفع
كل قرحة وضربة وسحجة ويأكل اللحم الميت زنجار اوقية انزروت واشق من كل
واحد نصف اوقية يسحق الجميع بخل ثم يعجن بعسل ويستعمل مرهم آخر يسحق انزروت
مسحوق ومثله عسل واما الذرورات فينثر على المراهم لاحد ثلث اما الالحام
جراحات طرية مستوية لا تحتاج الى غير الالحام والالزاق وتتخذ من مثل الصبر و
دم الاخوين والاقاقيا وقشار الكندر والسندروس والكهربا والجوز خوارزمي
والانزروت والمر وجرادة الاديم ولحا الصنوبر محرقين وصمغ البلوط ونحوها
واما لتجفيف قروح رطبة كثيرة الوضر والصديد وتتخذ من مثل تراب الكندر
والجلنار والمرداسنج والقرطاس المحرق والحناء والكرسنة اليابسة وقشور شجر
البق وقشور القرع اليابس محرقة وقشور البلوط وورق السوسن واصل السوسن
والزراوند وزبد البحر وقشر الرمان والشب والعفص ودقيق الشعير وسويقه و
شقائق النعمان ونحوها واما لاحراق اللحم الردي العفن وكيه واستيصاله و
تتخذ من الادوية الحادة الكاوية مثل الزاج والزنجار والنوشادر والزرنيخ و
النورة والقلي والاشنان والزيبق المقتول المصعد والشب ومن القابضة
القوية التجفيف مثل توبال الحديد والروسختج وقشور النحاس والعفص والقيسور
المحرق والاقاقيا ونحوها وينبغي ان يحتاط في استعمالها وتوقى اللحم الصحيح منها ولابد
بعد استعمالها من استعمال السمن لاسقاط الخشكريشة وتسكين اللذع والوجع اللذين بهما

وهو جوهر حكة الرجل

ان يحذر ان يوضع على اللحم الصحيح

دليلان على فناء اللحم الردي ووصول الدواء الى اللحم الصحيح ذرور آخر كندر انزروت
ومر مكي ودم الاخوين اجزاء سواء وهو المعروف باربعة الادوية ذرور آخر جفت
مرداسنج وورق السوس قشور الهليلج عفص من كل جزء جزء قشور الرمان وعروق نصف
جزء نصف جزء ذرور الاكال قلقطار محرق عفص زنجار انزروت اجزاء سواء

الباب الرابع عشر في السنونات ولما كانت الاسنان عظمية يابسة المزاج
فصحتها ان تكون على مزاجها اليابس وهي مع ذلك موضوعة بين رطوبات الفم وعلى
ممر الطعام والشراب متعرضة لملاقاة الابخرة الدخانية الخارجة بالتنفس ابدا وبخار
الاخلاط الغليظة والاطعمة الصاعدة من المعدة اليها وجب ان يكون حفظ صحتها
بالسنونات وهي ادوية يابسة تسحق وتنثر عليها لتجلو ما يتراكم عليها من الرطوبات
وتلزج وتلتصق بها من خارج وتجففها مع ذلك اما الجالية منها التي يدلك بها الاسنان
لتنقيتها من الحفر والقلح فهي التي تتخذ من اللؤلؤ والبسد والزجاج الشامي وزبد البحر
وسنجشونيا والملح المحرق بالعسل وخزف الجرار الخضر والقلي والفنيكي والزراوند
ورماد الصدف والشعر المحرق والبورق والعود المحرق ونحوها واما اليابسة
القابضة التي تنثر عليها وعلى اصولها لتحركها واسترخاء ما يحيط بها من اللثات
والتمور اما عند البرودة وعدم الحمرة والحرارة في اللثة فقرن الايل المحرق والسعد
والكزمازج والساذج الهندي وجفت البلوط والاثل والجلنار والسنبل و
الشب والاذخر والعفص والسليخة والورد والعود والاقاقيا والايرسا و

يعني إذا سُرّحت

هو الرطوبة المتحجرة بين الاسنان

القاقوله

العاقرقرحا والسك والمصطكى والقرنفل وإن عند استرخاء اللثات من حرارة و
حمرتها واورامها وتبيغ الدم منها فمثل الطباشير وبزر الورد والسماق والعفص
والقرظ والصندل وقماع الكرم والنوفل والكافور والكزبرة اليابسة والعدس
المقشر وقشور الرمان الحامض والكزبرة والهليلج والبليلج والاملج والاقاقيا
والجلنار والطين المختوم ودقيق الكرسنة ونحوها تركب من كل طبقة مركبات بحسب
الحاجة الى الاجلى والاقبض والاحر والابرد ويركب من جميعها سنونات مركبة من
الافعال عند اجتماع تلك الاغراض وبحسب الاستمام والغنا بكل واحد منها سنون
يجلو الاسنان ويذهب بالحفر زجاج شامي وفينك سوسة سحم يسحق ويدلك
به الاسنان ويقوى اللثة آخر زبد البحر ملح دراني محرق حرف رماد الصدف
شعير محرق رماد اصل القصب زراوند مدحرج اجزاء سواء سنون يشد اللثة
والاسنان قرن ايل محرق ملح دراني هليلج اصفر ورد جلنار عفص
والله اعلم بالصواب الباب الخامس عشر في الغراغر واما الغرغرات
فاما ان تستعمل لتلطيف الاخلاط الغليظة التي تكون في الراس واحدارها من طريق
الحنك واما لمنع الرقيقة من النزول بتغليظها وتضييق مسالكها واما لتحليل اورام
الحلق وانضاجها اما التي تستعمل لتلطيف الاخلاط الغليظة وانزالها من الدماغ فهي
حارة حادة تتخذ من مثل العاقرقرحا والزنجبيل والصعتر والمويزج والوج والخردل
والشونيز وقشور اصل الكبر والايرسا والبورق والفلافل والمرزنجوش والثمام و

الاجاص وماء العسل والمري او السكنجبين السكري او العسلي او العنصلي واما التي تستعمل
لنفع النزلات فكل بارد قابض طبخ في الماء ويتغرغر به مثل الورد والجلنار والخرنوب
الشامي والعدس وحب الآس والخشخاش ونحوها واما التي تستعمل في اورام الحلق
اما عند ابتداء الاورام الحارة فعصارات البقول الباردة الرادعة كعنب الثعلب
والخس والكزبرة الرطبة والهندبا ونحوها او مياه الفواكه الباردة كالتوت الشامي
والرمان الحامض والسماق ونحوها واللعابات الباردة كلعابات بزر القطونا و
لسان الحمل والشاهسفرم وحب السفرجل ونحوها وسلاقات الادوية الباردة
القابضة كالجلنار والورد والاقاقيا والكزمازج والكزبرة اليابسة ونحوها واما بعد
الابتداء وعند الحاجة الى التحليل فسلاقات البقول الحارة كالكرفس والكرنب و
الرازيانج والكشوث ونحوها وسلاقات الفواكه الحارة كالتين والزبيب والخيارشنبر
والعناب ونحوها واللعابات الحارة كلعاب الحلبة وبزر الكتان والمرو وحب
الرشاد ونحوها وسلاقات الادوية الحارة كاصل السوس والسوسن والخطمي واصول
الرازيانج والقسط ونحوها ومن منضجات اورام الحلق الخبز المنقوع في اللبن او في
التين والبنفسج وماء الكرنب وماء الشعير المركب وغيره المركب مع ... الخيارشنبر
الباب السادس عشر في المربيات معنى التربية ههنا ادخار بعض الثمار مثل
الهليلج والاملج والاترج والتفاح والسفرجل ونحوها وبعض الانوار مثل الورد و البنفسج
والنيلوفر وازهار كثيرة من الاشجار كورد السفرجل ونحوها وبعض اصول النبات كالزنجبيل

اي المدبر مع العناب والبستان

و

والشقاقل والجزر والقنبيط ونحوها على طراوتها محفوظة رطوباتها عليها وذلك اما
تهيئتها بوضعها في العسل وايداعها اياه لانه اجود ما تحفظ به الاشياء الرطبة عن التغير
والفساد مع ما يزيدها لطافة ونفوذا وتحببها الى الطبع وقوانين تربيتها اما في الثمار
بان يسلب عنها المرارة وكل كيفية قوية فيها بالانقاع والسلق ثم توضع في مقدار
من العسل لا يغمرها كثيرا وتوضع في الشمس مستوثقا عنها واما الازهار والانوار فان
تؤخذ بعد التفتح التام اوراقا منتقاة عن اكمامها وتوضع كل رطل منها في اربعة ارطال
من العسل وتشمس كذلك وقد يجعل بدل العسل عسل القصب او عسل المن او الغايد
المذاب على حسب مقتضى ما يراد منها وقد تتخذ بالسكر الطبرزد بان يدق معها وتشمس
عندما يراد استعمالها في الامراض والامزجة الحارة واما اصول النبات فان يفعل بها
ما يفعل بالثمار ويبالغ في تعذيبها مبالغة اشد ولو بسلقها في الماء الملح وغسلها
مرارا وتقطيعها وتشقيقها ثم توضع في العسل على مثال ما توضع الثمار وقد يخلط بها
بالثمار ايضا عند التربية بعض الافاويه كالزعفران والقرنفل والفوذنج والبهار
ونحوها مسحوقة الباب السابع عشر في السعوطات والقطورات والبخورات
والشمومات الادوية التي يستعمل من طريق مجرى الانف اما سعوطات وتستعمل
قطورا او مما حارة يابسة ينفط بها لتنفض بقايا الفضول البلغمية من الدماغ وتفتح
سدد الراس وتسخين مزاجه في اواخر العلل الباردة مثل الصرع والفالج واللقوة و
الصداع البارد ونحوها وتتخذ من مثل جندبيدستر والنوشادر والترمد والشونيز

والحرمل والصبر والمر والجاوشير والبورق والسعتر والفلافل والحلتيت والاشق
والافربيون والمسك والعاقرقرحا والملح الهندي والعدس المر والساقيثا و
مرارات الطيور وغيرها وابوال الجمال وماء البصل والمرزنجوش والسداب والسقو و
الخل ودهن اللوز المر والنرجس والسوسن ونحوها واما باردة رطبة تستعمل لترطيب
الدماغ وترطيبه في العلل الحارة اليابسة مثل الصداع الحار والبرسام والسهر ونحوها
وتتخذ من مثل عصارات الخس والهندبا وعنب الثعلب وماء الخيار والقرع ودهن البنفسج
والنيلوفر ودهن حب القرع ودهن الورد والافيون والكافور والطباشير ونحوها
واما عطوسات وتستعمل لتفتيح مجاري الاشتمام ونفض الفضول الباردة منها — اى يعطس بها
وهي الادوية الحارة مثل الكندس والعرطنيثا والحبة السوداء والبورق والجندبيدستر
والفربيون والزراوند وحب البلسان والعاقرقرحا والمسك وابوال الابل مجففة
والفلافل والسداب والسعتر والموبزج والخربق والخردل والصبر والمرزنجوش
والنوشادر والزنجبيل والمرارات ومنها بخورات البخورات اما رطبة واما
يابسة والبخورات الرطبة اما حارة تستعمل لتفتيح الخياشيم وتلطيف المواد وهي
المتخذة من مثل المرزنجوش والنمام والشيح والقيصوم والاكليل والبابونج والافسنتين
والرازيانج والنعناع والزوفا والشبث والسداب والسعتر والكرنب ونحوه
وتستعمل هي ايضا لتفتيح الصماخ وتسييل المواد والاوساخ وتحليل الرياح ويطبخ في القمقم
وتحاذى بمبزالها الانف والاذن او ينكب عليها متزملا وقد يجعل معها الملح والخل — اى متدثرا بالكساء

يحب

بحسب الحاجة وقد يستعمل التبخير بالشراب وبالمرى بان يرش على حجارة الرحى المحماة واما
باردة رطبة تستعمل لتبريد الدماغ وترطيبه عند السهر وحرارة الدماغ ويبوسته تتخذ من
البنفسج والنيلوفر والكزبرة الرطبة والخس والخبازى والبقلة والخلاف والخيار و
ورق القرع وجرادته والخشخاش وقشوره والورد وتفاح شاهسفرغم وحى العالم
ولسان الحمل والخطمى والشعير المرضوض ونحوها تطبخ ويصب فيها اللبن ودهن البنفسج
ونحوه من الادهان ويلقى فيها الحجارة المحماة ويتلقى بخارها من بعد بحيث لا يسخن الراس
ويصل البخارات اليه فاترة وقد يستعمل التبخير بالخل بان يرش على حجارة محماة ويكب عليه
واما البخورات اليابسة فهي الدخن التي يتدخن بها اما لتقوية الراس والدماغ مثل
المسك والكافور والعود والصندل والقسط والعنبر والسك واما للزكام ومنع النزلة
الحارة مثل نخالة الحوارى تنقع في الخل ويجفف بعد ذلك ومثل دقيق الشعير ودقيق
الباقلى والصندل الابيض والورد والبنفسج وثمرة الطرفاء والكافور والسكر الطبرزد
واما للزكام البارد ومنع النزلة الباردة مثل الكندر والميعة اليابسة والقسط و
السعد والسندروس والكاغد والعود والعنبر ونحوها وقد يبخر للسعال الكثير
الرطوبة بالكبريت والقسط والقنة والمر والسليخة والزعفران والكبابة والزراوند
والكندر والزرنيخ الاحمر في قمع من طريق الفم وقد يبخر لعسر الولادة واخراج المشيمة
بالجاوشير والكبريت والمر والقنة ومرارة الثور تجمع في الفتيل واما المشمومات
فمنها حارة وتستعمل لتعديل مزاج الدماغ البارد وهي اما رياحين كالياسمين والنرجس و

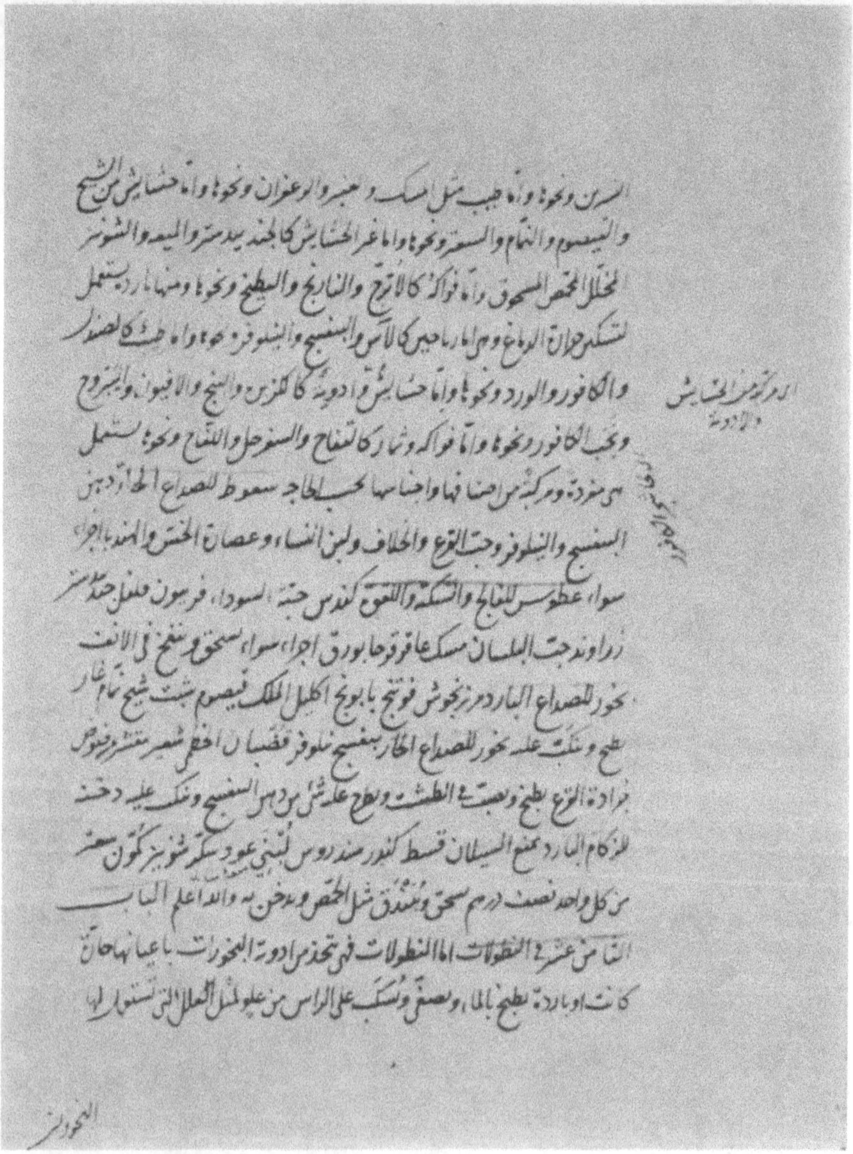

السرين ونحوها واما طيب مثل المسك والعنبر والزعفران ونحوها واما حشايش من الشيح
والقيصوم والنمام والسعتر ونحوها واما غير الحشايش كالجندبيدستر والميعة والشونيز
المحلل المحمص المسحوق واما فواكه كالاترج والنارنج والبطيخ ونحوها ومنها بارد يستعمل
لتسكين حرارة الدماغ وهي اما رياحين كالآس والبنفسج والنيلوفر ونحوها واما طيب كالصندل
والكافور والورد ونحوها واما حشايش وادوية كالكزبرة والبنج والافيون واليبروح
وحب الكافور ونحوها واما فواكه وثمار كالتفاح والسفرجل واللفاح ونحوها تستعمل
هي مفردة ومركبة من اجناسها واجناسها بحسب الحاجة سعوط للصداع الحار دهن
البنفسج والنيلوفر وحب القرع والخلاف ولبن النساء وعصارة الخس والهندبا اجزاء
سواء عطوس للفالج والسكتة واللقوة كندس حبة السوداء فربيون فلفل جندبيدستر
زراوند حب البلسان مسك عاقرقرحا بورق اجزاء سواء يسحق وينفخ في الانف
بخور للصداع البارد مرزنجوش فوتنج بابونج اكليل الملك قيصوم شبت شيح نمام غار
يطبخ وينكب عليه بخور للصداع الحار بنفسج نيلوفر قضبان الخس شعير مقشر خشخاش
برادة القرع يطبخ ويصب في الطشت ويطرح عليه شيء من دهن البنفسج وينكب عليه دخنة
للزكام البارد يمنع السيلان قسط كندر سندروس لبني عود سكر شونيز كمون من
من كل واحد نصف درهم يسحق ويندق مثل الحمص ويدخن به والله اعلم الباب
الثامن عشر في النطولات اما النطولات فهي تتخذ من ادوية البخورات باعيانها حارة
كانت او باردة تطبخ بالماء ويصفى ويسكب على الراس من علو مثل العلل التي تستعمل لها

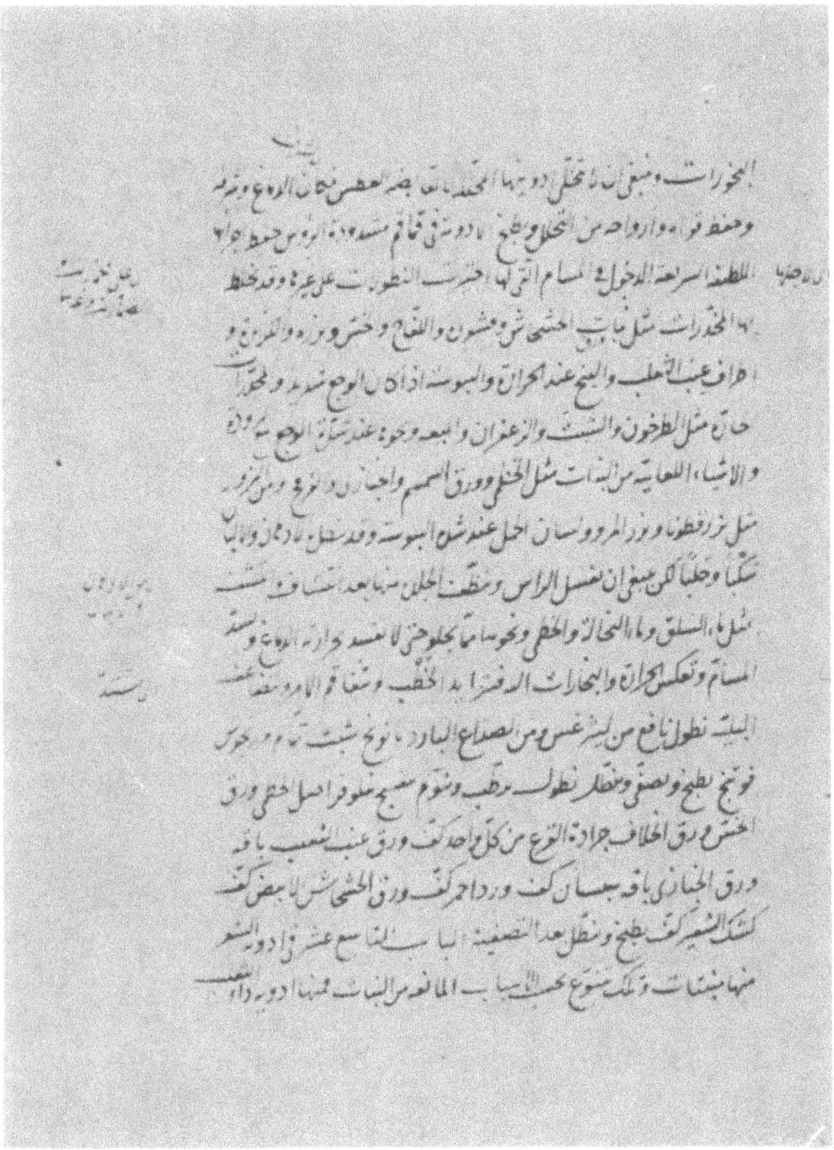

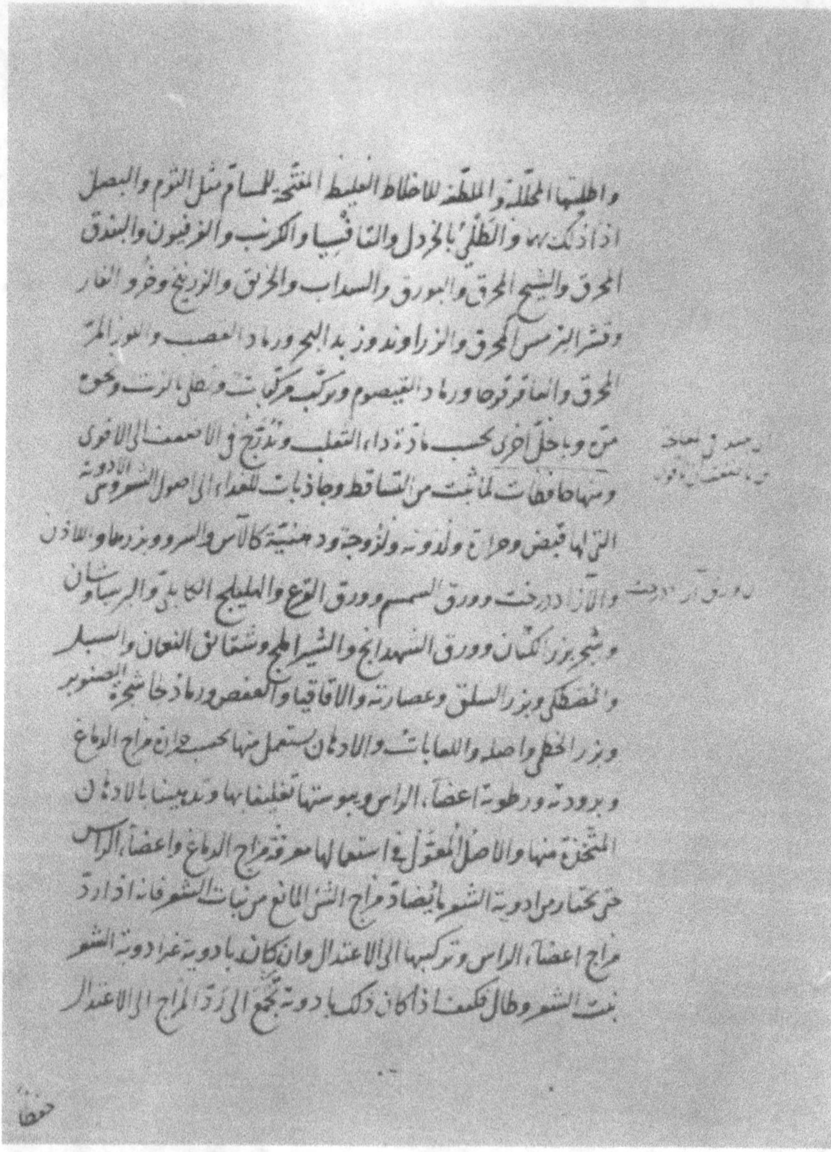

والطلبها المحللة والملطفة للاخلاط الغليظة المفتحة للمسام مثل الثوم والبصل
اذا دلك بها والطلي بالخردل والثافسيا والكرنب والفرفيون والبندق
المحرق والشيح المحرق والبورق والسداب والحرمل والزرنيخ وخرء الفار
وقشر النرجس المحرق والزراوند وزبد البحر ورماد القصب والعود المر
المحرق والماء قرحا ورماد القيصوم ويركب مركبات ويطلى بالزيت وحده
مرة وبالخل اخرى بحسب مادة داء الثعلب وتدرج في الاضعف الى الاقوى
ومنها حافظات لما ثبت من التساقط وجاذبات للغذاء الى اصول الشعر والادوية هي
التي لها قبض وحرارة ولدونة ولزوجة ودهنية كالآس والسرو وبزرهما واللاذن
والآزاددرخت وورق السمسم وورق القرع والهليلج الكابلي والبرسياوشان
وشحم بزر الكتان وورق الشهدانج والشيرالج وشقائق النعمان والسنبل
والمصطكي وبزر السلق وعصارته والاقاقيا والعفص ورماد خشب الصنوبر
وبزر الخطمي واصله واللعابات والادهان يستعمل منها بحسب حرارة مزاج الدماغ
وبرودته ورطوبة اعضاء الراس ويبوستها تغليظا بها وتدهينا بالادهان
المتخذة منها والاصل المعول في استعمالها معرفة مزاج الدماغ واعضاء الراس
حتى يختار من ادوية الشعر ما يضاد مزاج الشيء المانع من نبات الشعر فانه اذا رد
مزاج اعضاء الراس وتركيبها الى الاعتدال وان كان بادوية غير ادوية الشعر
نبت الشعر وطال فكيف اذا كان ذلك بادوية تجمع الى رد المزاج الى الاعتدال

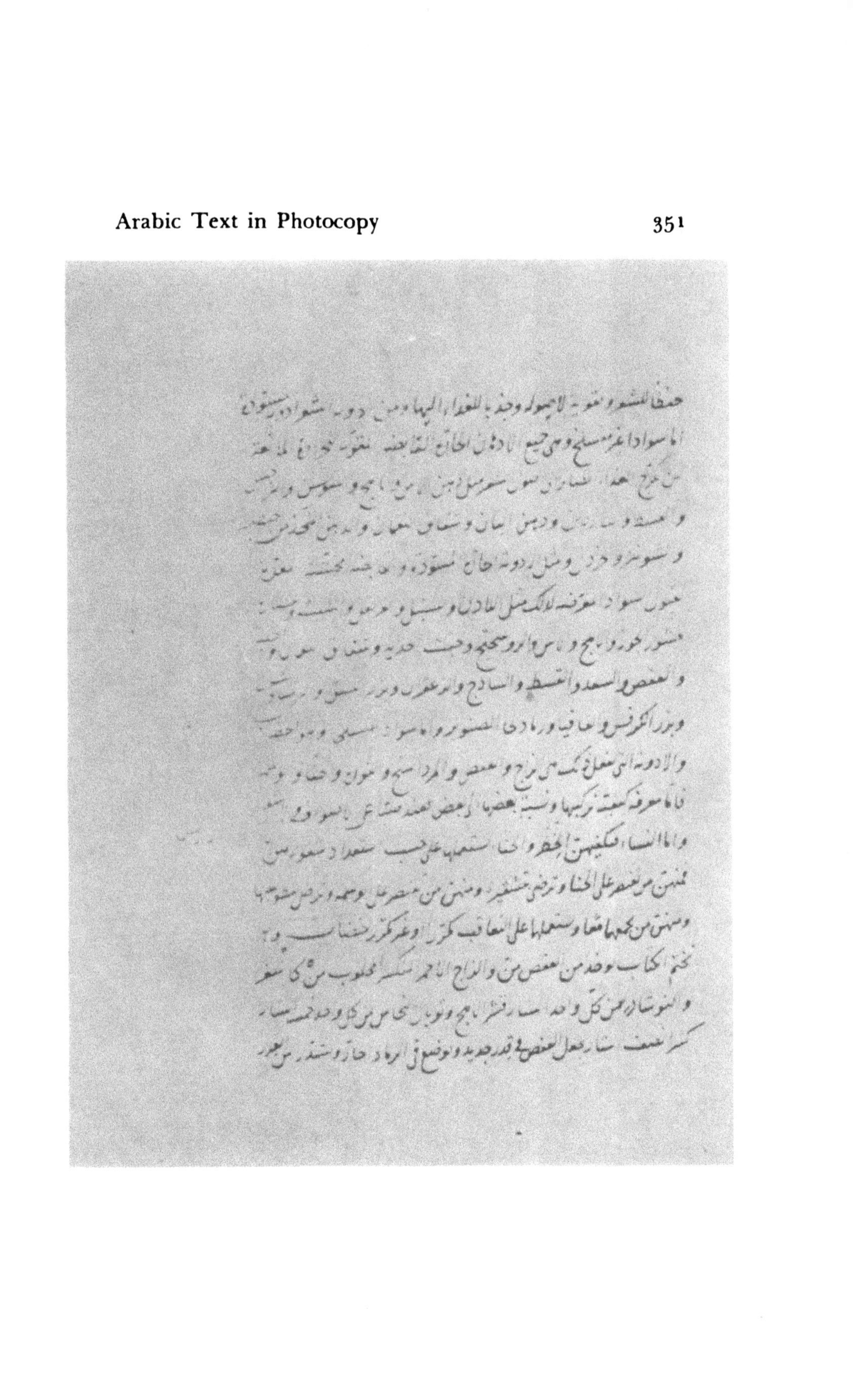

[illegible]

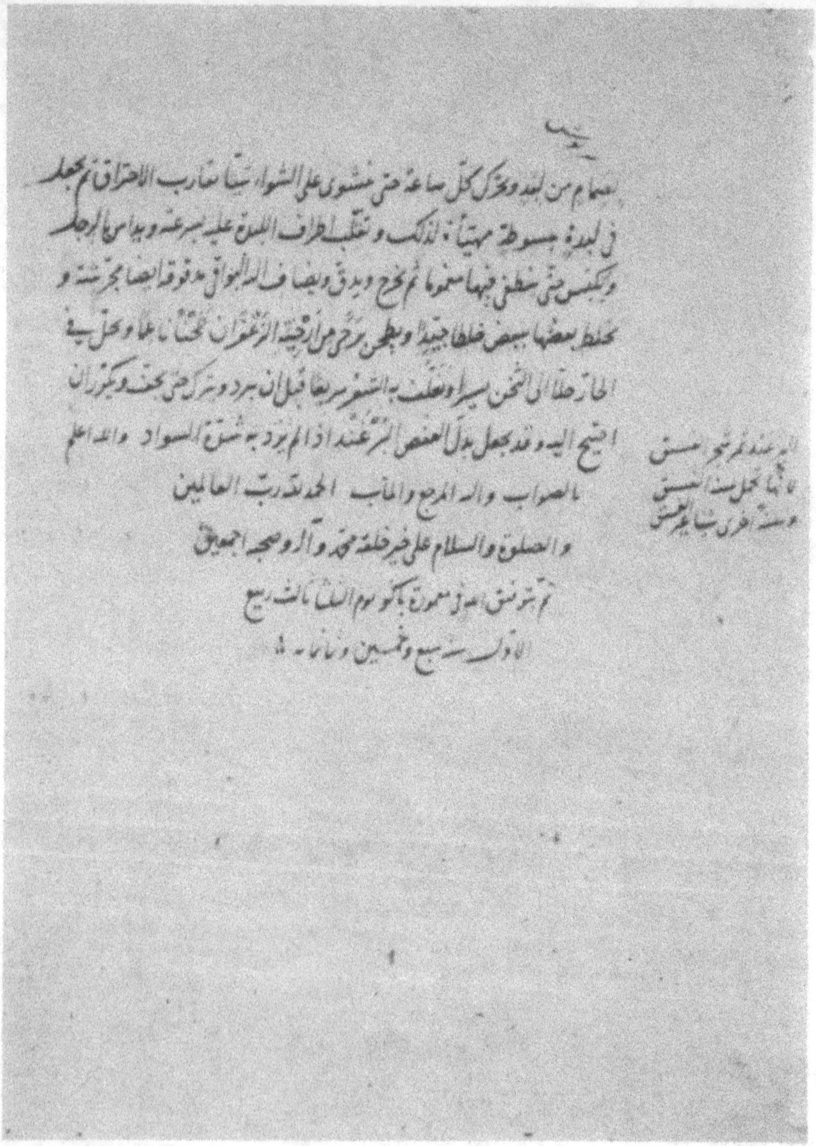

بعمام من لبده ويحرك كل ساعة حتى يشوى على الشواء شيا يقارب الاحتراق ثم يجعل
في لبدة مبسوطة مهيأة لذلك و تقلب اطراف اللبد عليه ثم يعصر ويداس بالرجل
ويكبس حتى ينطفى فيها سموما ثم يخرج ويدق ويضاف اليه الحوائج المذكورة ايضا مجرشة و
يخلط بعضها ببعض خلطا جيدا ويطحن برحى من [illegible] الزعفران طحنا ناعما ويحل في
الماء حلا الى الثخن يسيرا ويغلف به الشعر سريعا قبل ان يبرد ويترك حتى يجف ويكرر ان
احتيج اليه وقد يجعل بدل العفص [illegible] اذا لم يرد به شدة السواد والله اعلم
بالصواب واليه المرجع والمآب الحمد لله رب العالمين
والصلوة والسلام على خير خلقه محمد وآله وصحبه اجمعين
تم [illegible] يوم الثلثاء ثالث ربيع
الاول سنة سبع وخمسين وثمانمائة

Greek Index

Foreign Words (Except Greek)

General Index

Botanical Index

www.ingramcontent.com/pod-product-compliance
Lightning Source LLC
LaVergne TN
LVHW011821200926
848484LV00005B/1272
9781512803914